Leukocyte and Stromal Cell Molecules

The CD Markers

D1611215

Leukocyte and Stromal Cell Molecules

The CD Markers

Heddy Zola

Child Health Research Institute
North Adelaide, Australia

University of Adelaide
Adelaide, Australia

Cooperative Research Center for Diagnostics
Adelaide, Australia

Bernadette Swart

Child Health Research Institute
North Adelaide, Australia

Ian Nicholson

Child Health Research Institute
North Adelaide, Australia

University of Adelaide
Adelaide, Australia

Cooperative Research Center for Diagnostics
Adelaide, Australia

Elena Voss

Child Health Research Institute
North Adelaide, Australia

WILEY-LISS

A John Wiley & Sons, Inc., Publication

Library of Congress Cataloging-in-Publication Data

Leukocyte and stromal cell molecules : the CD markers / Heddy Zola . . . [et al.].
    p. ; cm.
   Includes bibliographical references.
   ISBN-13: 978-0-471-70132-3 (pbk.)
   ISBN-10: 0-471-70132-7 (pbk.)
   1. CD antigens. I. Zola, Heddy.
  [DNLM: 1. Antigens, CD–classification. 2. HLA Antigens–classification. QW 573.5.H7 L652 2006]
  QR186.6.C42L485 2006
  571.9′6–dc22

                                      2006036649

Printed in the United States of America

10 9 8 7 6 5 4 3 2 1

Contents

PREFACE   vii

ABBREVIATIONS   ix

ACKNOWLEDGMENTS   xi

PART 1:   INTRODUCTION AND BACKGROUND MATERIAL   1

Chapter 1: Leukocyte Membrane Molecules—An Introduction   3

Chapter 2: Web Resources for CD Molecules   17

PART 2:   MOLECULE PROFILES CD1–CD350   37

         How to Use the Molecule Profiles   39
         Symbols Used to Denote Domains, Motifs, and Repeats   41
         Molecule Profiles CD1–CD350   42

INDEX   549

Preface

The CD markers are molecules, studied primarily on human blood cells that are targets for research, diagnostic, and therapeutic applications. CD markers are used ubiquitously in medical research, diagnosis, and treatment; examples include CD3, which is used to count circulating T cells and make treatment choices in patients with HIV AIDS, and CD20, the target for an antibody that generates over $1 billion in sales annually and has made a significant impact on the blood cancer lymphoma.

The CD markers derive from a series of workshops, the HLDA (Human Leukocyte Differentiation Antigen) Workshops. The first seven HLDA Workshops each produced a book (Leukocyte Typing I–VII). The books have served as core reference works containing the data on which the individual CD markers are based. Each book has also contained a user-friendly summary of the major properties of each CD molecule. The 8th Workshop, HLDA8, published the scientific papers in the peer-reviewed scientific press. Papers with a methodological emphasis were collected in a special issue of the *Journal of Immunological Methods* (Zola and Dandie, 2005a), whereas most of the other papers were grouped in a special issue of *Cellular Immunology* (Zola and Dandie, 2005b). Additional papers were published in *Cell Research*, and a summary of the conclusions was published in *Blood* (Zola et al., 2005).

Leukocyte and Stromal Cell Molecules: The CD Markers presents a profile of each CD molecule. The CD profiles are presented in a compact and easy-to-use format, with a set of common subheadings, and a schematic diagram indicating the major structural features, including protein domains, motifs, and post-translational modification. The molecular profiles are intended to be used by biologists, pathologists, and clinicians generally; they do not require special immunologic knowledge. The book has an index and two introductory chapters that allow the reader to navigate through the molecule profiles, explaining the use of technical terms and providing important links to the websites that provide more detailed information.

A few words about some choices we had to make. By and large, each molecule profile represents a gene. The gene may have multiple protein products through alternative splicing and post-translational modifications, and these differences may be important in applications of the antibody—CD45 RA and RO represent an example. Two isoforms of CD45 provide the biologically important distinction between naïve and memory (antigen-experienced) T lymphocytes. We felt that it would be easier to assimilate the information if it was in a single entry, rather than flicking from one to another.

In some instances, a CD number with a number of members (for example, CD156a, b, and c) represents three distinct but related gene products. Generally, we have given each a separate profile. There are instances, however, where two gene products are so similar that when we wrote two profiles, we found most of the information was repetitive. We merged them into one profile (CD167a and b, for example).

The book, and the nomenclature system it represents, have inconsistencies of this sort and more serious ones. For example, although the KIR (Killer Inhibitory Receptors) family is grouped together under one CD number, which allows for the addition of additional family members not yet characterized, there are other close-knit families whose members are scattered. The TNF receptor superfamily members, for example, include CD27, CD30, CD95, CD120a, CD120b, CD134, and CDw137. The issue here is a historical one. Had HLDA waited until the entire proteome was catalogued before assigning CD numbers, we could have had a satisfyingly logical and systematic nomenclature. But without the CD system, the field was at risk of being swallowed by a quicksand, and the CD system brought sufficient order and systematization to allow the field to progress.

REFERENCES

Zola H, Dandie G editors. The 8th International Workshop on Human Leukocyte Differentiation Antigens. Adelaide, Australia. 12–16. December 2004, Journal Immunological Methods: Special issue, Volume 305, Issue 1, Pages 1–106 (20 October 2005b).

Zola H, Dandie G editors. The 8th International Workshop on Human Leukocyte Differentiation Antigens, Adelaide, Australia. 12–16 December 2004, Cellular Immunology Volume 236, Issues 1–2, Pages 1–190 (July–August 2005a).

Zola H, Swart B, Nicholson I, Aasted B, Bensussan A, Boumsell L, et al. CD molecules 2005: Human cell differentiation molecules. Blood 2005 1;106(9):3123–3126.

Abbreviations

ADAM	A disintegrin and metalloproteinase
AIDS	Acquired immune deficiency syndrome
ALL	Acute lymphoblastic leukemia
AML	Acute myeloblastic leukemia
ATP	Adenosine triphosphate
BCR	B-cell receptor
CD	Original abbreviation for cluster of differentiation. Now best regarded as part of the nomenclature system for leukocyte and related molecules, for example CD20, in which the letters CD are not expanded to words
cDNA	Complementary DNA (complementary to a messenger RNA)
CLL	Chronic lymphocytic leukemia
DNA	Deoxyribonucleic acid
EGF	Epithelial growth factor
ELISA	Enzyme-linked immunoassay
FDC	Follicular dendritic cells
GAG	Glycosylamino glycan
gal	Galactose
Glc	Glucose
Gp	Glycoprotein—often used in naming glycoproteins—e.g., gp130 is a 130-kDa glycoprotein of MWt 130 kDa
GPI	Glycosyl-phosphatidylinositol
GPCR	G-protein-coupled receptor
HCDM	Human cell differentiation molecules
HIV	Human immunodeficiency virus
HLDA	Human leukocyte differentiation antigens
ICAM	Intracellular adhesion molecule
Ig	Immunoglobulin
IgSF	Ig superfamily

ITAM	Immunotyrosine-linked activation motif
ITIM	Immunotyrosine-linked inhibition motif
kD, kDa	kilo Daltons (1 Dalton is the atomic weight of hydrogen)
KIR	Killer inhibitory receptors
LDLR	Low density lipoprotein receptor
LFA	Leukocyte function-associated antigen (name used for a particular family of molecules)
LILR	Leukocyte Immunoglobulin-like Receptors
LRR	Leucine-rich repeat
MHC	Major histocompatibility complex (the major polymorphic molecules involved in antigen presentation and in transplant rejection. MHC class I (MHC I) molecules present antigen peptides to CD8 cells, whereas MHC II molecules present peptides to CD4 cells
MWt, Mol.Wt	Molecular weight (strictly, relative molecular mass)
MS4A	Membrane-spanning 4, subfamily A (the name of a family of proteins that spans the membrane 4 times)
NCBI	National Center for Biotechnology Information
NK	Natural killer
PCR	Polymerase chain reaction
RNA	Ribonucleic acid
SCR	Short consensus repeat
SEMA	Semaphorin
SF	Superfamily (applied to genes or proteins)
SIGLEC	Sialic acid binding Ig-like lectin
SNP	Single nucleotide polymorphism
TCR	T-cell receptor
TGF	Transforming growth factor
TH1	T-helper type 1 cell
TH2	T-helper type 2 cell
TNF	Tumor necrosis factor
TNFR	TNF receptor
TNFRSF	TNF receptor superfamily
WWW	World Wide Web

Acknowledgments

The authors' work in the field of human leukocyte molecules has been supported over many years by a number of funding bodies, in particular the Australian National Health and Medical Research Council and the South Australian Cancer Foundation. Recently, work that led directly to this book was carried out in part under the auspices of the Co-operative Research Centre for Diagnostics (supported by the Australian Commonwealth Government), and in large part through the 8th Human Leukocyte Differentiation Antigens (HLDA) Workshop. The 8th HLDA Workshop, which was chaired by one of us (HZ) and managed by one of us (BS), was supported financially by the South Australian Cancer Foundation, the Australian Government through the International Science Linkages Program, and a number of companies in the field of monoclonal antibodies against CD molecules. These companies were BD Biosciences, DakoCytomation, R&D Systems, Beckman Coulter, Miltenyi Biotec, Serotec, Caltag, and Diaclone.

Although the book represents the hard labors of the authors, it owes a debt of gratitude to the pioneers of the HLDA concept, Laurence Boumsell and Alain Bernard, and the other stalwarts of the early HLDA Workshops, including Stuart Schlossman, Andrew McMichael, and the late Walter Knapp. The book covers the CD molecules characterized in Workshops HLDA I through HLDA VIII and HCDM1, and we are particularly indebted to the Section Chairs and Council members for HLDA8: Bent Aasted, Armand Bensussan, Chris Buckley, Georgina Clark, Pablo Engel, Derek Hart, Václav Horejsí Clare Isacke, Peter Macardle, Fabio Malavasi, Armin Saalmueller, Reinhard Schwartz-Albiez, Paul Simmons, Mariagrazia Uguccioni, and Hilary Warren.

The book, and the field as a whole, also owes a debt of gratitude to the late Alan Williams, Neil Barclay, and co-authors, for their *Leukocyte Antigens Facts Book* (Academic Press). This has been an extraordinarily useful book, and we would probably not have embarked on our book had it not been for our understanding that there was no third edition of the "Facts Book" in the foreseeable future.

The production of this book has been facilitated greatly by Thom Moore and Kris Parrish at Wiley. It has been a pleasure dealing with our publisher.

Finally, it is a pleasure to acknowledge a number of colleagues who provided us with a great deal of help in preparing the book. Debbrah Millard and Christos Mavrangelos provided invaluable help with the figures and the collection of information for the book and for the "Web Resources" link in the www.hcdm.org website. The following scientists were kind enough to look through the chapters and a selection of molecule profiles and provide us with suggestions as to how to make them as useful and accessible as possible: Drs. Peter Macardle, Allison Cowin, Greg Hodge, Michael Abdo, Mary-Louise Rogers, and Alice Beare. We thank these people for their help, but we retain responsibility for any flaws or omissions.

Part 1

Introduction and Background Material

1

Leukocyte Membrane Molecules—An Introduction

1.1 HISTORY

In the late 1970s and early 1980s, as immunologists came to appreciate the power of monoclonal antibodies as reagents, large numbers of new antibodies were made, analyzed, and published. It was difficult to know whether two different antibodies were directed against the same antigen. The antigen that was later named CD9 is a good example. Five antibodies were described independently; they shared some features: precipitation of a protein band of 24–26 kD, reactivity with platelets, and non-T-non-B acute lymphoblastic leukemia. There were some apparently important differences: one antibody was described as reacting with 26% of normal blood lymphocytes, whereas the other four were reported to react with less than 2%; only one of the five was reported to react with monocytes and polymorphs; there were differences in reported reactivity with chronic lymphocytic leukemia. Later analysis, under

"Workshop conditions" (multiple laboratories examining coded panels of antibodies), demonstrated that the antibodies all reacted with the same antigen. The differences in the individual descriptions reflected differences in technique, antibody affinity, and interpretation.

A small group of immunologists recognized the problem and devised a solution: multi-laboratory blind analysis and statistical evaluation of the results. This solution led to the First International Workshop on Human Leukocyte Differentiation Antigens (HLDA), organized in Paris by Laurence Boumsell and Alain Bernard in 1984 (Bernard et al., 1984). The purpose of this and subsequent workshops was to standardize reagents and, through the use of standardized reagents, to develop an understanding of the structure and function of leukocyte cell surface molecules and their utility as diagnostic and therapeutic targets.

Important tools in this process were a nomenclature (the CD nomenclature) and

Leukocyte and Stromal Cell Molecules: The CD Markers, by Heddy Zola, Bernadette Swart, Ian Nicholson, and Elena Voss

the publication of books (Leukocyte Typing I-VII), which contained the conclusions of the workshops and the data on which these conclusions were based.

1.1.1 The Significance of the CD Nomenclature and HLDA Workshops

The CD nomenclature, supported by the HLDA workshops and the Leukocyte Typing volumes, has become accepted universally. All immunology journals and journals in other fields that deal with these molecules use the CD nomenclature. The U.S. Food and Drug Administration (FDA) has mandated the workshops in the sense that antibodies that seek approval as diagnostic reagents against CD molecules must have been validated through the HLDA workshops. The World Health Organization (WHO) and the International Union of Immunological Societies have mandated the CD nomenclature.

Nevertheless, there have been major changes in the nature and importance of the contribution made by HLDA workshops in the years since the first one was conducted. The main business of the early HLDA workshops was to identify new human leukocyte cell surface molecules, using antibodies that had been made by immunizing mice with whole cells or cell membranes. The major tools were analysis of reactivity of antibodies with a variety of cell types and statistical analysis of the resulting expression data. The statistical procedure used to identify antibodies with a high probability of reacting with the same molecule was cluster analysis, hence, the name "Cluster of Differentiation." Information of a confirmatory nature was often contributed by protein analysis—Western blotting or immunoprecipitation followed by gel electrophoresis. By the third HLDA workshop, antibodies were also being used to identify antigen expressed in cDNA libraries, allowing the cloning of the cDNA and molecular characterization of the antigen. However, antibody was still the primary tool for antigen discovery and characterization.

As molecular technologies improved, new human proteins were increasingly identified by first cloning the gene, either through sequence homology with a gene of animal origin or by searching for genes with sequence similarity to known molecules. With increasing frequency, the antibody was made after the protein had been identified, expressed, and characterized.

The quality and reliability of good molecular data has changed the methodologic focus of the HLDA workshops. The primary focus of HLDA has moved to the functional molecules (the "antigens"); the antibodies are tools used in their study. In the late 1970s and early 1980s, the question behind many studies was "What does my antibody react with?" Today we can focus on much more fundamental questions about intercellular interactions and cell–molecule interactions. The ligands and receptors involved in these interactions still need to be described, detected, and measured, and monoclonal antibodies are still the most powerful tools for achieving an understanding of these interactions.

1.1.2 Why Does HLDA Focus on Surface Membrane Molecules?

The early studies (1970s–1980s) focused on the cell surface simply because that was the major focus of immunology at the time—immunologists wanted to know how cells interacted with other lymphocytes, with endothelium, and with antigen. Without the tools to identify, visualize in tissue, and isolate individual cell types, many of the questions that have engaged immunologists for the last generation could not even be formulated, let alone addressed. Diagnostic distinctions, for example, between different types of leukemia, seemed at the time to be capable of being addressed with cell surface markers. From the start of the monoclonal antibody era (and indeed earlier, using polyclonal antisera), therapy using antibodies to knock out cancer cells or immune cells (to prevent organ graft rejection) was a major driver of research, and here the targets were clearly cell surface molecules.

Once we had an extensive catalog of cell surface molecules, and the tools with which to study their function, cell signaling became a new front in the development of understanding of the immune system. The myriad intracellular molecules—syk, zap, cbl, and their ilk—cry out for a nomenclature accessible to scientists from other fields. The HLDA considered on several occasions whether to extend the CD system to cover these molecules and decided on several occasions not to. The reasons included an anxiety that if the CD nomenclature covered these many hundreds of additional molecules it would lose its focus and ability to help scientists classify and remember them, and the concern that many reagents were polyclonal and so of uncertain specificity.

Recognition of the significant capacity of intracellular molecules to serve as markers of differentiation stage [see, for example, Marafioti et al., (2003)] and that the workshops could perform a useful task without necessarily allocating CD names, finally led the HLDA Council to include intracellular markers of differentiation (Zola et al., 2005), in a set of major changes.

1.1.3 Are We Nearly There?

Any parent will recognize this question—asked by children at any stage in a journey, including the very early stages. The child has no concept of the length of the journey, so it's a reasonable question. If the journey of the HLDA is from the early chaos described earlier in this chapter to the goal of having a complete catalog of the leukocyte cell surface molecules, how far do we have still to travel?

We cannot be sure, but the evidence suggests that we are less than halfway there. Estimates of the numbers of surface molecules expressed by one functional category of leukocyte, the T lymphocytes, arrive at a number around 1000 (Zola and Swart, 2003). The number of T cell markers currently known to be on T cell surfaces is 100–200. The T cells are the best characterized leucocytes, so the journey is unlikely to be more advanced in the other leukocyte families.

The estimate of the total number of molecules is based on counting of proteins or messenger RNA species expressed by cells and multiplying by the estimated proportion of expressed proteins that are membrane proteins. Some known proteins that have not been identified on T cells may nevertheless be expressed on T cells. In arriving at the estimated number of molecules, we have not taken into account post-translational modifications. Clearly, there is room for error in either direction. But the conclusion that we are nowhere nearly "there" receives some support from two other lines of evidence.

First, for the recent Eighth HLDA Workshop, we identified 180 known molecules that could qualify for CD status, and half of them were given CD status at the end of the workshop (Zola et al., 2005). This yield is better than any previous HLDA workshop (Fig. 1.1). If we were nearly at the end of the list, we would expect to be seeing diminishing returns.

Second, several proteomics-based discovery projects have found more new molecules than known ones, (Peirce et al., 2004; Nicholson et al., 2005; Loyet et al., 2005; Watarai et al., 2005). Again, there is no evidence of the diminishing returns we would expect to see if we had a near-complete catalog of leukocyte molecules.

The availability of genomic sequence, coupled with recent developments in proteomics technology, indicates that there is a window of opportunity over the next 5–10

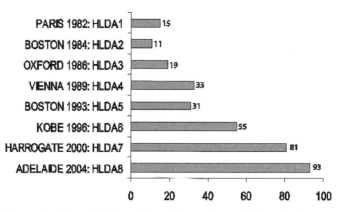

Figure 1.1. *New CDs assigned per HLDA workshop. The numbers of CD molecules assigned have continued to increase, suggesting that we have not yet characterized the majority of leukocyte membrane molecules.*

years to complete the discovery process. Based on the number of CD molecules known currently that serve as targets for diagnosis and therapy, we can reasonably expect to find many new diagnostic and therapeutic targets among the molecules to be discovered.

1.2 STRUCTURE AND FUNCTION

Most molecules that serve as useful markers of differentiation on leukocyte membranes are glycoproteins. There is enormous variation of structure, but there are also recognizable themes and motifs. Structural features of proteins are summarized in Boxes 1.1 to 1.4. Function depends on structure, so structure can predict function to a significant degree. Determination of the three-dimensional structure of a molecule depends on X-ray diffraction analysis or nuclear magnetic resonance studies, which are complex and require time and resources. Only a few leukocyte membrane molecules have their structure analyzed at this level, but as the number of "solved" structures increases, our ability to predict the tertiary structure of proteins from amino acid sequence improves.

Thus, given an amino acid sequence, usually translated from a DNA sequence, we can predict the structure, and at least some likely functions, for any protein. Structural prediction is most effectively done with Web-based resources, which will be described in Chapter 2. It is important to remember that such structures, and derived functions, are predictions and will almost certainly be wrong in some aspect.

The functional requirements of immune cells are diverse, and the molecules that mediate surface interactions are correspondingly diverse in structure. Nevertheless, several molecular themes recur, and classifying the molecules according to their molecular structure is helpful in understanding both structure and function.

1.2.1 Protein Domains

Protein domains (see Box 1.1) are distinct subunits of proteins that are associated with a particular molecular function, such as protein–protein interactions or kinase activity. One characteristic of domains, which is used in identifying them, is that interactions between residues within a domain are generally stronger than interactions between residues in different domains. Domains usually occur as individ-

---

Box 1.1. TERMS USED IN DESCRIBING STRUCTURAL FEATURES OF PROTEINS

Domain: A protein domain is a distinct subunit of a protein. Many proteins are composed of several domains, separated by short or long sequences that may act as "hinge" regions or "spacers." Domains have characteristic structural features, and about 20 domains have been described (Table 1.1). Domain structure dictates domain function. It is believed that there are domain structures still to be discovered.

Module: The term "module" can be used interchangeably with domain. It tends to be used when describing a domain in a protein that has several different domains—a modular protein.

Motif: Motif is used to describe a shorter sequence than a domain or module, but a sequence associated with a particular structural or functional feature.

Family: Proteins are grouped together in families based on structural similarities. Because the structural features that allow the family relationship to be discerned are largely located in the domains, and many proteins have multiple different domains, a protein may be assigned to several families. The term "family" is applied to the gene as well as the protein.

Superfamily: Superfamilies are broader groupings that include several families that show similarity.

---

ual regions of a protein sequence that have a defined three-dimensional structure. Domains may be present in both the extracellular and the intracellular regions of a protein. Extracellular domains are likely to be involved in interactions with other cells, extracellular matrix or extracellular signals, whereas intracellular domains are likely to be involved in signaling to trigger the cellular response to the extracellular interactions. The association of a domain with a particular function is useful in assigning probable cellular functions to otherwise poorly characterized proteins.

At least 20 functional domain types have been identified within the CD molecules (Table 1.1). Individual proteins may have multiple copies of a single domain, for example, CD22, which has five adjacent Ig-like domains, and CD30 (TNFRSF8), which has three consecutive TNFR domains, or they may contain a mixture of different domains, for example, CD62L, which contains c-type lectin, EGF, and sushi (short complement-like repeat) domains.

Differences in the intracellular domains can result in proteins with identical or similar extracellular domains having opposite functions. For example, the four TRAIL receptors (CD261, CD262, CD263, and CD264) that are encoded by separate genes all have a single extracellular TNFR domain, but they differ by the presence, absence, or truncation of an intracellular Death domain.

The sequencing of the human genome has lead to the development of programs that can annotate conserved protein domains automatically. These annotations can be used to assign some function to proteins that have not been identified using antibodies. The InterPro database (www.ebi.ac.uk/interpro) (Mulder et al., 2005) provides a single access resource for the major protein domain signature databases.

1.2.2 Protein Families

The classification of proteins into families originally relied on the presence of a shared protein domain and could therefore

TABLE 1.1. Protein domains found commonly in leukocyte surface molecules

Domain	Structure	Functions	Example CD Molecules
ABC Transporter	Multiple transmembrane domains coupled to nucleotide binding domain	ATP-dependent transport of substances across membranes	CD243, CD338
Cadherin	A beta-sandwich formed of seven strands in two sheets. Ca++ ions bind residues from neighboring domains.	Adhesion	CD144, CD324, CD325
C-type Lectin	Open structure consisting of five beta strands and two alpha helices, with four loops of relatively unstructured sequence.	Calcium-dependent sugar binding	CD62L, CD72, CD141 CD205, CD303
CUB	Ig-like beta barrel with four conserved cysteines that probably form two disulphide bridges (C1–C2, C3–C4).	Complement components	CD304
DEATH	A homotypic protein interaction module composed of a bundle of six alpha-helices.	Regulation of apoptosis and inflammation through the activation of caspases and NF-kappaB	CD95, CD261, CD271
EGF	A two-stranded beta-sheet followed by a loop to a C-terminal short two-stranded sheet. The domain includes six cysteine residues that have been shown to be involved in disulphide bonds.	Unknown	CD62L, CD97, CD141, CD339
Fibronectin 2	The domain contains four conserved cysteines involved in disulphide bonds and is part of the collagen-binding region of fibronectin.	Protein binding	CD205, CD206, CD222
Fibronectin 3	Seven beta-strands modeled to fold into antiparallel beta-sandwiches with a topology that is similar to immunoglobulin constant domains.	Protein binding	CD122, CD130, CD171
GPCR	Seven-transmembrane helices, G-protein binding loop.	Receptors	CD97, CD195, CD294
Ig-like	The fold consists of a beta-sandwich formed of seven strands in two sheets, usually stabilized by intradomain disulfide bonds.	Protein–protein and protein–ligand interactions	CD3, CD19, CD50, CD80, CD171, CD226, CD300a

LDLR	Complement-like cysteine-rich repeats	CD91
Link	Two alpha helices and two antiparallel beta sheets arranged around a large hydrophobic core similar to that of C-type lectin.	CD44
LRR	2–45 motifs of 20–30 amino acids in length that generally folds into an arc or horseshoe shape.	CD180, CD281
Protein tyrosine kinase	Cytoplasmic protein kinases.	CD117, CD136, CD167a, CD331
SCR	Domain contains four repeats of a well-conserved region, which spans 115 amino acids, and contains six conserved cysteines	CD5, CD6, CD163
Semaphorin	A variation of the beta propeller topology, with seven blades radially arranged around a central axis. Each blade contains a four-stranded (strands A to D) antiparallel beta sheet.	CD100, CD108, CD136
Sushi	The structure is based on a beta-sandwich arrangement; one face made up of three beta-strands hydrogen-bonded to form a triple-stranded region at its center and the other face formed from two separate beta-strands.	CD21, CD25, CD35, CD62L
TNF	Central beta sheet.	CD153, CD154, CD178
TNFR	Repeats containing six conserved cysteines, all of which are involved in intrachain disulphide bonds.	CD30, CD40, CD95
Phosphotyrosine phosphatase	Cytoplasmic tyrosine-specific protein phosphatases.	CD45, CD148

Bind multiple ligands
Hyaluronan(HA)-binding region

Protein–protein interactions

Catalyses the addition of a phosphate group to a tyrosine residue
Protein binding

Detect and respond to chemical signals

Protein binding

Trimeric cytokines
Binding of TNF ligand domains

Catalyzes the removal of a phosphate group attached to a tyrosine residue

Box 1.2. CARBOHYDRATE STRUCTURES

Carbohydrates may be attached to protein (glycoprotein) or lipid (glycolipid).

The monosaccharides that occur most often in leukocyte antigens are as follows:

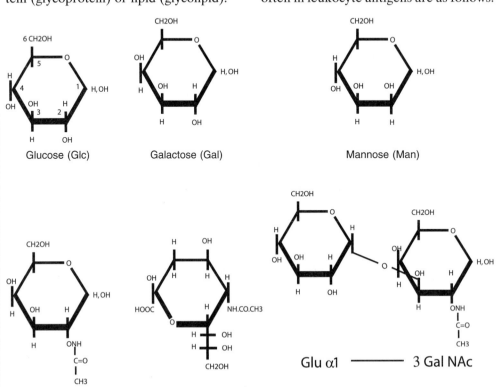

Glucose (Glc)   Galactose (Gal)   Mannose (Man)

N-acetyl galactosamine (GalNac)   Sialic acid (N-acetyl neuraminic acid)

Glu α1 ————— 3 Gal NAc

Monosaccharides are linked together to form oligosaccharides or polysaccharides.

Each linkage is described as follows: Glc-alpha1-3GalNac means glucose is linked from its number 1 carbon to carbon 3 of N-acetyl galactosamine. The formation of the link changes the #1 carbon of the glucose from a state that allows free rotation to a state in which it is fixed in one of two mirror-image orientations alpha or beta. In the example given, it is the alpha orientation.

Glycosamino glycans (GAGs) are polysaccharides that are chains of disaccharides or longer oligosaccharides that include an amino sugar. The amino sugar is generally glucosamine or galactosamine, and it is often acetylated or sulfated. The major GAGs found in leukocyte membrane molecules are chondroitin sulfate and heparin or heparan sulfate.

Box 1.3. MEMBRANE ATTACHMENT AND ORIENTATION OF PROTEINS

Integral membrane proteins cross the lipid bilayer. In the simplest form, an integral membrane protein consists of an extracellular region, a membrane spanning region, and a cytoplasmic region. The membrane spanning region is generally an alpha helix consisting largely of hydrophobic amino acids, allowing it to be stable in the hydrophobic lipid environment. Some proteins include a charged residue in the membrane-spanning region, which interacts with charged residues on other proteins.

Type I integral membrane proteins have the N-terminus outside the cell and the C terminus in the cytoplasm. A signal sequence is cleaved from the N terminus before export to the cell surface.

Type II integral membrane proteins have their C terminus outside the cell and the N-terminus in the (generally short) cytoplasmic sequence. The membrane-spanning sequence is uncleaved but resembles a signal sequence for protein secretion.

Type III integral membrane proteins pass the membrane several times. Examples are found ranging from two to seven passes through the membrane.

Type IV integral membrane proteins are multipass proteins, like type III proteins. However, in type IV proteins, the proteins form a hydrophilic pore through the membrane.

Type V refers to proteins that do not pass through the membrane but are attached to it by their C-terminus via glycosyl-phosphatidylinositol (a GPI link). In more detail, the C-terminal amino acid is linked to ethanolamine, which is in turn linked through a phosphodiester link to a short string of sugars that link via myoinostol through a phosphodiester to glycerol and thence to the membrane fatty acids.

In addition, proteins may be linked to the membrane through other proteins, via salt bridges, disulphide bonds, or non-covalent interactions.

Proteins that do not pass through the membrane, or have a short cytoplasmic sequence devoid of signal-initiating motifs, may nevertheless transducer signals to cells through interaction with other proteins that do have signaling capacity. Receptors often consist of two or more protein chains, where one binds the ligand and the other transmits the signal.

---

group proteins that appear very distinct. The largest family that includes CD molecules is the immunoglobulin superfamily, which includes proteins such as CD3, CD19, CD80, CD90, and CD200. Other large families that include multiple leukocyte cell surface antigens are the TNF and TNFR superfamilies, the C-type lectin superfamily, and the tetraspanins (Table 1.2). Even though many leukocyte cell surface proteins contain different domains,

the assignment to a family is usually based on a single domain that can be associated with a common protein function. There have been recent efforts to formalize the assignment of protein to families, based on aspects of the evolutionary relationship between proteins (Wu et al., 2004).

The members of those families that are more closely related tend to occur in clusters in the genome, such as the KIR family of immunoreceptors, which are located on

TABLE 1.2. Some protein families that have CD molecules as members

Family	Domain	Functions	Example CD Molecules
ADAMs	Metallopeptidase	Matrix degradation	CD158a, CD158c
Cadherins	Cadherin	Adhesion	CD144, CD324, CD325
IgSF	Ig-like, ICAM	Protein–protein and protein–ligand interactions	CD3, CD19, CD80, CD171, CD226, CD300a, CD50, CD242
Integrins	Heterodimer of alpha and beta chains	Adhesion	CD18, CD41, CD61, CD49a, CD103
LILR	Ig-like	Immunoreceptors	CD85-family, CD335
MS4A	4-transmembrane domain	Various	CD20
Rhodopsin GPCR	7-transmembrane domain	Receptors	CD191, CD193, CD294
Secretin GPCR	7-transmembrane domain	Receptors	CD97
Selectins	Lectin, EGF, sushi	Adhesion	CD62I, CD62E, CD62P
SEMA	Semaphorin, plexin	Cell migration	CD100, CD108,
SIGLECs	Sialic acid-recognizing Ig-superfamily lectins	Adhesion	CD22, CD33, CD170
Tetraspanins	Four transmembrane domain	Various	CD9, CD37, CD81, CD151
TNFRSF	TNFR	Binding of TNF ligand domains	CD27, CD30, CD40, CD95, CD271
TNFSF	TNF	Trimeric cytokines	CD70, CD153, CD154, CD178, CD252

Note: The domains listed are characteristic domains of the families. The functions are indicative of a function for the family.

Box 1.4. POST-TRANSLATIONAL PROTEIN MODIFICATION

Carbohydrate attachment to protein is either through asparagine (N-linked glycosylation) or through the OH of serine or threonine (O-linked glycosylation).

Asparagine is glycosylated only if the sequence is Asn-X-Ser or Asn-X-Thr, but not if X is Pro. Even with the right neighboring amino acids, gycosylation is not automatic and may vary for the same protein depending on the tissue and other conditions, so that these sequences are referred to as *potential* N-glycosylation sites.

O-glycosylation can occur at any Ser or Thr, but it is more likely in regions rich in Ser, Thr, and Pro.

Proteoglycans are proteins linked to glyosylaminoglycans (GAGs) (see Box 1.2). The GAGs are generally linked to protein through serine or threonine.

Glycosylation varies from tissue to tissue and between stages of activation and differentiation.

Proteins can be phosphorylated either at tyrosine or at serine and threonine, which occurs generally in the cytoplasmic part of the molecule. Phosphorylation (by kinases) or dephosphorylation (by phosphatases) is often the first stage of a signaling cascade leading to activation of gene transcription.

Proteins may be sulfated, at tyrosine, serine, or threonine.

Covalent acylation affects protein compartmentalization and function. Proteins may be acylated as follows:

- Palmitoylation through thioester linkage to (usually) cysteine residues
- Myristoylation through amide linkage to the N terminal glycine
- Prenylation through thioether linkage to C terminal cysteine
- Glypiation through phophatidylinositol linked to the C-terminal amino acid after removal of the signal sequence

Palmitoylation and glypiation affect predominantly membrane proteins and direct them into lipid raft regions.

Proteins are frequently cleaved into two or more components by proteases after synthesis and before they can be expressed or function. A common example is the removal of a signal sequence in proteins expressed with the N terminus outside the cell. When proteins are cleaved, the fragments may stay together, held by disulphide bonds or by noncovalent interactions.

---

chromosome 19 in humans, or the MS4A family of which CD20 is a member, which is located on chromosome 11. Other families can be spread throughout the genome: There are members of the Ig-like superfamily on each chromosome.

1.3 UTILITY IN RESEARCH, DIAGNOSIS, AND THERAPY

The availability of the full human genome sequence (Venter et al., 2001; McPhersen et al., 2001) has changed the world irreversibly. As with all significant knowledge, once we have it, we cannot revert to not having it, and if we ignore it, we risk becoming irrelevant. However, the euphoria that accompanied the publication of the genome sequence was quickly followed by a reassessment of what we still need to know, to make use of the genomic information. Even before completion of the sequence, those involved were turning their attention back to function and hence to proteins (Broder and Venter, 2000), the rapidly developing field known as proteomics.

Knowing the DNA sequence is a starting point. From the genome we need to define the genes—the coding sequences. Every cell has the same genes (ignoring for the moment processes where parts of the genome are spliced out or mutated during the course of differentiation). What characterizes different cells with different functions is the set of genes that is expressed. So the emphasis shifts from gene sequencing to understanding the protein profile of cells and how it relates to function.

The sequence information is being converted rapidly into a catalog of genes, which can be searched for molecules of likely relevance to the immune system in a variety of ways. We can look for homologs to known human immunoreceptors or, more broadly, for members of molecular families that are known to be used by the immune system. From the sequence information, we can construct probes and use Northern blots, *in situ* hybridization, microarray technology, or polymerase chain reaction (PCR) to determine what is being expressed in cells of the immune system and what is differentially expressed in different cells or states of the immune system.

Antibodies remain uniquely useful tools in the analysis of expression and function of molecules, particularly surface membrane molecules. Although methods based on mRNA detection are improving in quantitative precision and accuracy, there is no direct and universal relationship between the amount of mRNA for a protein in the cell and the amount of protein actually present, and it is the protein that mediates the function. Flow cytometry has sophistication, precision, dynamic range, and ability to analyze on a single-cell basis that will be difficult to improve on, and it works particularly well with antibodies as probes. Immunohisto-

chemical methods, used together with video image analysis, allow studies of tissue sections, which approach flow cytometry in precision and sensitivity, and additionally provide information on spatial relationships. Several immunoassay formats provide sensitive and precise methods of measuring the concentration of molecules in solution, provided specific antibodies are available.

The ability of antibodies to act as agonists or antagonists facilitates the analysis of the functions of molecules, particularly those on the cell surface. Finally, antibodies can make therapeutic reagents, for example, in cancer (Grillo-Lopez et al., 1999) and in situations where we need to modulate immune reactivity (Nashan et al., 1997).

1.3.1 Major Applications of Antibodies

CD markers provide an outstanding example of the power of antibodies in identification, quantitation, and localization of cells in order to analyze function and disease state. (See Table 1.3 for major applications). Flow cytometry using multiple antibodies conjugated to different fluorescent dyes, beads, or nanoparticles allows the determination of cell lineage and sublineage using several different markers in widely available instruments. For example, T cells are identified by the expression of CD3, and the T cells of the "helper" subset (which interact with antigen-presenting cells using MHC Class II to present antigen) are identified by expression of CD4. Within the CD3/CD4 double-positive subpopulation, antigen-experienced (memory) cells are identified by the expression of CD45R0 and can be further subdivided into effector memory and central memory cells using one of several markers. This example of multiparameter analysis uses four antibodies and colors, in addition to two physical parame-

TABLE 1.3. Outline of applications of antibodies against leukocyte markers

Application	Feature	Example
Identification	Multiparameter, multiplex	Flow cytometric cell-by-cell analysis
		Antibody microarray
Localization	Multiparameter	Immunohistology
Quantitation	Multiplex	Cytometric bead array, ELISA
Isolation/purification	Multiparameter	Cell sorting, protein purification
Therapy	Specificity, potency	Transplantation and cancer therapy—e.g., CD3 and CD20 antibodies

ters, to identify lymphocytes if the analysis is done on whole blood (Rivino et al., 2004). The cells of a particular functional subset are not just identified by this procedure, but they are also counted. Furthermore, by performing the separation in a preparative fluorescence-activated cell sorter, the cells can be isolated for further analysis, for example, by extraction of mRNA for analysis of expression of other molecules (Seddiki et al., 2005).

The application of CD markers to cell localization has become routine in diagnostic immunopathology, as illustrated by the classification of lymphomas using the Revised European American Lymphoma (REAL) classification (www.pathnet.medsch.ucla.edu/educ/lecture/pathrev/lymphoma.htm).

Some of the same antibodies can be used therapeutically, generally by removing unwanted cells such as malignant B cells (CD20, (Hiddemann et al., 2005)) or T cells mediating organ transplant rejection (CD3, Shapiro et al., 2005).

The therapeutic applications of antibodies against CD molecules started early with the use of OKT3 to reverse rejection, but there was then a long period where additional successes were few. There has been a resurgence of the field recently, with several notable successes in the clinic that have profoundly changed the treatment of some cancers, and incidentally created billion-dollar markets (Weinberg et al., 2005).

REFERENCES

Bernard AR, Boumsell L, Dausset J, and Schlossman SF editors. Leukocyte Typing I. Berlin: Springer-Verlag; 1984.

Broder S, and Venter JC. Whole genomes: the foundation of new biology and medicine. Curr Opin Biotechnol 2000;11:581–585.

Grillo-Lopez AJ, White CA, Varns C, Shen D, Wei A, McClure A, and Dallaire BK. Overview of the clinical development of rituximab: first monoclonal antibody approved for the treatment of lymphoma. Semin Oncol 1999;26:66–73.

Hiddemann W, Buske C, Dreyling M, Weigert O, Lenz G, Forstpointner R, et al. Treatment strategies in follicular lymphomas: current status and future perspectives. J Clin Oncol. 2005;23(26):6394–6399. Review.

Loyet KM, Ouyang W, Eaton DL, and Stults JT. Proteomic profiling of surface proteins on Th1 and Th2 cells. J Proteome Res 2005;4:400–409.

Marafioti T, Jones M, Facchetti F, Diss TC, Du MQ, Isaacson PG, et al. Phenotype and genotype of interfollicular large B cells, a subpopulation of lymphocytes often with dendritic morphology. Blood 2003;102(8):2868–2876.

McPherson JD, Marra M, Hillier L, Waterston RH, Chinwalla A, Wallis J, et al. International Human Genome Mapping Consortium. A physical map of the human genome. Nature 2001;409:934–941.

Mulder NJ, Apweiler R, Attwood TK, Bairoch A, Bateman A, Binns D, et al. InterPro, progress and status in 2005. Nucleic Acids Res 2005;33(Database issue):D201–D205.

Nashan B, Moore R, Amlot P, Schmidt AG, Abeywickrama K, and Soulillou JP. Randomised trial of basiliximab versus placebo for control of acute cellular rejection in renal allograft recipients. CHIB 201 International Study Group [published erratum appears in Lancet 1997;350(9089):1484]. Lancet 1997; 350:1193–1198.

Nicholson IC, Mavrangelos C, Fung K, Ayhan M, Levichkin I, Johnston A, Zola H, Hoogenraad NJ, Characterisation of the protein composition of peripheral blood mononuclear cell microsomes by SDS-PAGE and mass spectrometry. J Imm Methods 2005;305(1): 84–93.

Peirce MJ, Wait R, Begum S, Saklatvala J, and Cope AP. Expression profiling of lymphocyte plasma membrane proteins. Molecular Cell Proteomics 2004;3:56–65.

Rivino L, Messi M, Jarrossay D, Lanzavecchia A, Sallusto F, and Geginat J. Chemokine receptor expression identifies Pre-T helper (Th)1, Pre-Th2, and nonpolarized cells among human CD4+ central memory T cells. J Exp Med 2004;200(6):725–735.

Seddiki N, Santner-Nanan B, Tangye SG, Alexander SI, Solomon M, Lee S, et al. Persistence of naive CD45RA+ regulatory T cells in adult life. Blood 2005; [Epub ahead of print].

Shapiro R, Young JB, Milford EL, Trotter JF, Bustami RT, and Leichtman AB. Immuno-suppression: evolution in practice and trends, 1993–2003. Am J Transplant 2005;5(4 Pt 2): 874–886.

Venter JC, Adams MD, Myers EW, Li PW, Mural RJ, Sutton GG, et al. The sequence of the human genome. Science 2001;291: 1304–1351.

Watarai H, Hinohara A, Nagafune J, Nakayama T, Taniguchi M, and Yamaguchi Y. Plasma membrane-focused proteomics: Dramatic changes in surface expression during the maturation of human dendritic cells. Proteomics 2005;5:4001–4011.

Weinberg WC, Frazier-Jessen MR, Wu WJ, Weir A, Hartsough M, Keegan P, and Fuchs C. Development and regulation of monoclonal antibody products: Challenges and opportunities. Cancer Metastasis Rev 2005;24(4): 569–584.

Wu CH, Nikolskaya A, Huang H, Yeh LS, Natale DA, Vinayaka CR, et al. PIRSF: family classification system at the Protein Information Resource. Nucleic Acids Res 2004;32(Database issue):D112–D114.

Zola H, and Swart BW. Human leucocyte differentiation antigens. Trends Immunol 2003; 24(7):353–354.

Zola H, Swart B, Nicholson I, Aasted B, Bensussan A, Boumsell L, et al. CD molecules 2005: human cell differentiation molecules. Blood 2005;106(9):3123–3126.

2

Web-Based Information Resources for Human Leukocyte Cell Surface Proteins

2.1 INTRODUCTION

The nature of the publication process places several limitations on the information that can be included in a book such as this one. It can only include information that is available up to a certain date and cannot pre-empt new information that may be published in the days, weeks, or years after that date. There are also limits on the type of information that can be included and how easy it is to make use of that information for other purposes.

This section introduces some of the many websites on the Internet through which information can be obtained that is up-to-date, or which can be used for additional analysis. The sites covered include information on the DNA and protein

sequences, the function of the protein, gene expression, the structure of the protein including the topology in the membrane, and some post-translational modifications. In most cases, multiple sites provide essentially the same information, although the overlap is not always complete. The CD-Hub website (www.hcdm.org/hub_index.htm) has been developed as a starting point to access different sources of information about the protein CD molecules.

2.2 NOMENCLATURE ISSUES

The first key to searching for information about a molecule is knowing how that molecule is referred to at a particular website. A name that can be used at one site may

1: CD40LG   CD40 ligand (TNF superfamily, member 5, hyper-IgM <u>E</u>
syndrome)   [*Homo sapiens*]
GeneID: 959   Locus tag: <u>HGNC:11935</u>; <u>MIM: 300386</u>   updated 18-Oct-2005

Summary   ⑦ ⬆

Official Symbol: CD40LG **and Name:** CD40 ligand (TNF superfamily, member 5, hyper-IgM syndrome) **provided by** <u>HUGO Gene Nomenclature Committee</u>
Gene type: protein coding
Gene name: CD40LG
Gene description: CD40 ligand (TNF superfamily, member 5, hyper-IgM syndrome)
RefSeq status: Reviewed
Organism: *Homo sapiens*
Lineage: *Eukaryota; Metazoa; Chordata; Craniata; Vertebrata; Euteleostomi; Mammalia; Eutheria; Euarchontoglires; Primates; Catarrhini; Hominidae; Homo*
Gene aliases: IGM; IMD3; TRAP; gp39; CD154; CD40L; HIGM1; T-BAM; TNFSF5; hCD40L
Summary: The protein encoded by this gene is expressed on the surface of T cells. It regulates B cell function by engaging CD40 on the B cell surface. A defect in this gene results in an inability to undergo immunoglobulin class switch and is associated with hyper-IgM syndrome.

Figure 2.1. Summary section of the NCBI EntrezGene page for CD40LG. The Official Symbol and Name are assigned by the Human Genome Nomenclature Committee. The gene aliases are other names that have been used to identify the molecule in the literature. There are links to the HGNC and OMIM pages.

not be useful at another, and it may not be obvious which name for the molecule should be used. Confusion over the naming of leukocyte cell surface molecules was a major factor in the initiation of the HLDA workshops. The different names arise for a variety of reasons, and in looking through past literature, one may not be aware that the protein referred to as "X" by one group is the same as protein "Y" studied elsewhere. Formal and informal names can indicate function (CD40-ligand), phenotype (HIGM; hyperIgM syndrome), membership of a gene family (TNFSF5), or they may be a reflection of the discovering laboratory. The examples that follow can illustrate some of the issues.

In the case of the gene known as CD40LG, or CD40 ligand (NCBI Entrez-Gene ID 959; HGNC entry 11935), the gene name indicates the function of the protein: it is the ligand for the CD40

protein. As shown in Figure 2.1, several aliases are listed at the EntrezGene site (IGM; IMD3; TRAP; gp39; CD154; CD40L; HIGM1; T-BAM; TNFSF5; hCD40L), which reflect the disease association of the protein (Hyper IgM syndrome), its physical characteristics (a 39 kDa glycoprotein), and its gene family (member 5 of the tumor necrosis factor (ligand) superfamily). A similar set of synonyms is listed in the UniProtKB-Swiss-Prot entry (Fig. 2.2). The receptor for this protein, which has the gene name CD40 (NCBI Entrez Gene ID 958; HGNC entry 11919), is member 5 of the tumor necrosis factor receptor superfamily (TNFRSF5). The same naming pattern has been used for another TNFSF ligand and receptor pair, which have the gene names FAS (NCBI Entrez Gene ID 355; HGNC entry 11920; also known as CD95 and TNFRSF6) and FASLG (NCBI Entrez Gene ID 356;

Entry name	**TNFL5_HUMAN**
Primary accession number	**P29965**
Secondary accession numbers	None
Entered in Swiss-Prot in	Release 25, April 1993
Sequence was last modified in	Release 25, April 1993
Annotations were last modified in	Release 48, September 2005
Name and origin of the protein	
Protein name	**Tumor necrosis factor ligand superfamily member 5**
Synonyms	**CD40 ligand**
	CD40-L
	TNF-related activation protein
	TRAP
	T cell antigen Gp39
	CD154 antigen
Contains	**Tumor necrosis factor ligand superfamily member 5, membrane form**
	Tumor necrosis factor ligand superfamily member 5, soluble form
Gene name	**Name: TNFSF5**
	Synonyms: CD40L, CD40LG, TRAP

Figure 2.2. *A section of the UniProtKB/Swiss-Prot entry for CD40LG, showing synonyms for the protein name and gene name. Note that the HGNC gene name shown in Figure 2.1 is listed as a synonym here.*

HGNC entry 11936; also known as CD178, CD95L and TNFSF6). In contrast, the gene superfamily name is used as the root for another pair of related genes: TNFRSF8 (NCBI Entrez Gene ID 943; HGNC entry 11923; also known as CD30) and its ligand TNFSF8 (NCBI Entrez Gene ID 944; HGNC entry 11938; also known as CD153 and CD30L). The linking of gene names for a ligand and its receptor will be useful to some researchers; the linking of different TNFRSF members will be useful for other researchers.

The use of single-letter suffixes in gene names can also be a source of confusion where the reasons for using a particular letter differ. Continuing the example above, the suffix "L" is used to indicate "ligand" in the unofficial but widely used CD40L (gene name CD40LG), "lympho-cyte" in CD62L (gene name SELL), and "like" in CD209L (gene name CLEC4M, and recently clustered at HLDA8 as CD299). It is also used in clusters of closely related genes such as CD85, where CD85L

has been used as the designation of the pseudogene ILTA9.

A single name for a protein may not be enough to locate the information about that protein at a particular website. The gene names being assigned by the HGNC are becoming widely used, but the incon-sistencies between the names given to members of the same gene family (as described above) may cause problems. The development of formal nomenclatures, such as the HLDA and the HGNC, means that fewer and fewer new protein names are derived from sources such as antibody or cDNA clone designations.

For the CD-Hub, the index page shows the CD number and the HGNC gene name. The alternative names listed by the NCBI and UniProtKB/Swiss-Prot are listed in a molecule's page. In other searches, one or more of the gene names, the NCBI RefSeq accession number, or the UniProtKB/Swiss-Prot accession number can usually be used to locate information about a molecule.

2.3   GENE INFORMATION

The completion of the human genome sequence has increased the amount of information that can be obtained about the gene encoding a protein. There are two major starting points for genetic information: the NCBI EntrezGene page (Maglott et al., 2005), and the EMBL Ensembl GeneView page (Hubbard et al., 2005). Similar information can be sourced through each page, although the Ensembl information seems to reflect its origins in the Human Genome sequencing effort, whereas the NCBI pages show more of the literature evidence.

The simplest facts about a gene are its chromosomal location and the structure of the coding sequence. The GeneView page reports the location by its position in the nucleotide sequence of a chromosome (Fig. 2.3), whereas EntrezGene includes more detail of the cytogenetic context (Fig. 2.4). Both link to source information such as contig sequences, which may be examined to confirm in-house sequencing of the genes.

The structure of the gene is usually shown as a map of the exons, indicating the orientation of the gene in the chromosome, the organization of the exons, and whether the linked mRNA transcripts include regions that are not translated. If the gene has multiple transcripts, then each of these are shown with an indication of which exons are not included in a variant.

The genomic context can be found using both sites, although it may not be immediately obvious where to look for the best information. From the EntrezGene page, the MapViewer link goes to a schematic of the chromosome, which can also display the equivalent regions in other species. Selecting the "show sequence" option from the menu on the image of the sequence then links to a graphical map of the chromosomal sequence of the region. This last page can be used to find the intron–exon bound-aries. The Ensembl representation of the genomic context can be found by following the link to the chromosomal location, which is indicated by the nucleotide range.

2.3.1   Splice Variants and Polymorphisms

Two sources of variation in the protein encoded by a gene arise from gene-level polymorphisms, such as single-nucleotide polymorphisms (SNPs) and from the generation of variant transcripts through differential mRNA splicing. Polymorphisms are alterations in the DNA sequence coding for the molecule, and they may or may not affect the amino acid sequence. These can be found on pages linked from the Ensembl GeneView page (under "Gene variation info") and from the NCBI EntrezGene page (under "SNP: GeneView"). The SNP are annotated according to their location and their effect on the amino acid sequence (Figs. 2.5 and 2.6). Each SNP has an accession number that is linked to a page showing complete details of the SNP. Differential splicing can lead to the production of soluble or membrane-bound isoforms of a protein, or proteins that are missing domains, or which have differential glycosylation. The splice variants are shown as part of the exon structure maps on the EntrezGene and GeneView pages, and indicate which exons are missing from each isoform (Figs. 2.1 and 2.2). There are also links to the nucleotide and amino acid sequences of each isoform, which will have unique accession numbers.

2.3.2   Orthologues

The interspecies differences in the amino acid and nucleotide sequences of proteins can be used to identify conserved regions and regions that may be immunogenic. Links to the identified homologues are present on the NCBI EntrezGene pages

Genomic Location	This gene can be found on Chromosome X at location: 135,455,889-135,468,069 This start of this gene is located in Contig AL135783.6.1.175706.
Description	Tumor necrosis factor ligand superfamily member 5 (CD40 ligand) (CD40- L) (TNF-related activation protein) (TRAP) (T cell antigen Gp39) (CD154 antigen). Source: Uniprot/SWISSPROT P29965
Prediction Method	Genes were annotated by the Ensembl automatic analysis pipeline using either a GeneWise model from a human/vertebrate protein, a set of aligned human cDNAs followed by GenomeWise for ORF prediction or from Genscan exons supported by protein, cDNA and EST evidence. GeneWise models are further combined with available aligned cDNAs to annotate UTRs.
Transcripts	ENST00000218368 ENSP00000218368 TNFL5_HUMAN [Transcript info] [Exon info] [Peptide info] 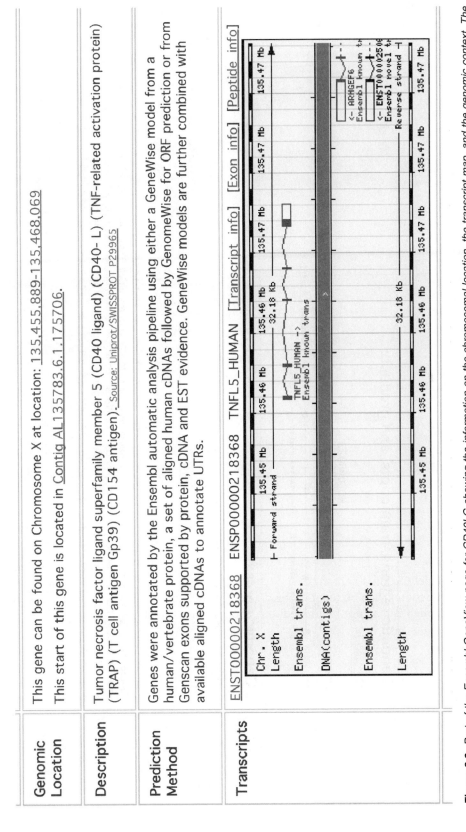

Figure 2.3. *Part of the Ensembl GeneView page for CD40LG showing the information on the chromosomal location, the transcript map, and the genomic context. The genomic location, "Transcript info," "Exon info," and "Peptide info" links can be used to obtain further information on the molecule.*

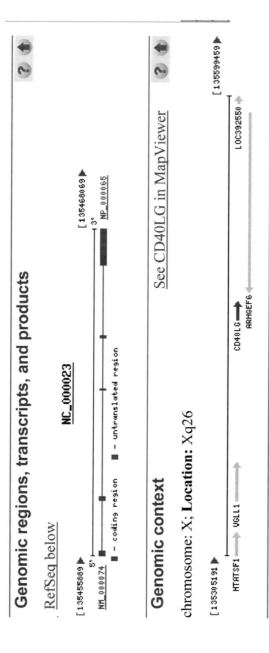

Figure 2.4. Exon structure and genomic context information for CD40LG from the NCBI EntrezGene page. The exon map shows that CD40 LG has five exons and has links to the mRNA and protein RefSeq entries for the single known CD40LG transcript. The genomic context indicates that CD40LG is located on the X chromosome and shows the neighboring genes. The MapViewer link can be used to obtain further genomic sequence information and to see the interspecies comparisons.

Variations in region of gene ENSG00000102245

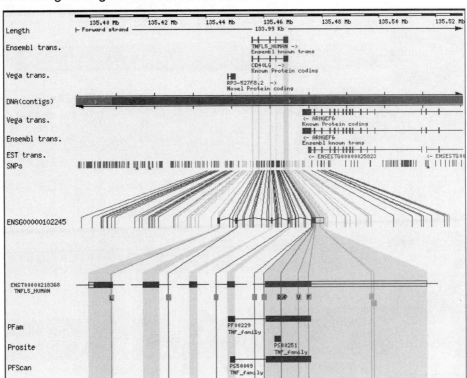

Figure 2.5. *Ensembl SNP map for CD40LG showing the location of single nucleotide polymorphisms in and around the coding sequence for CD40. The color of the listed SNPs indicates whether they are in a coding or noncoding region and whether they change the amino acid sequence.*

(Fig. 2.7) and the Ensembl GeneView pages (Fig. 2.8). Both sets of links can access alignments of the nucleotide and amino acid sequences (Fig. 2.9). The NCBI HomoloGene page [3] links to the Entrez-Gene page for the protein in each species and to other pages at the NCBI. The homologue of any one protein may not have been identified in a particular species, either because it may not be present or the region of the genome may not have been sequenced completely. It may also not be

possible to identify the homologues of particular isoforms of a protein.

2.4 PROTEIN INFORMATION

There are three major protein sequence databases: the NCBI RefSeq (Wheeler et al., 2005), ExPASy UniProtKB/Swiss-Prot, and the International Protein Index (IPI). These three are curated databases, meaning that they have been selected to

gene model (contig mRNA transcript):	Contig	mrna	protein	mrna orientation	transcript	sn
	NT_011786	NM_000074	NP_000065	forward	plus strand	3,

Contig position	dbSNP rs# cluster id	Hetero-zygosity	Validation	3D	OMIM	Function	dbSNP allele	Protein residue	Codon position	
19941903	rs1126535	0.258		H		synonymous	C	Leu [L]	1	
		0.258		H		contig reference	T	Leu [L]	1	
19941903	rs17424229	N.D.				synonymous	C	Leu [L]	1	
		N.D.				contig reference	T	Leu [L]	1	
19952904	rs3092922	0.049		Yes		synonymous	C	Phe [F]	3	
		0.049		Yes		contig reference	T	Phe [F]	3	

Variations in genomic region of CD40LG

Contig Accession	Contig position	dbSNP rs# cluster id	Hetero-zygosity	Validation	3D	OMIM	Function	dbSNP allele	Protein residue	Codor positic
NT_011786	19940951	rs3092946	0.082		H		locus			
NT_011786	19940957	rs3092945	0.182				locus			
NT_011786	19954104	rs6635311	N.D.				locus			
NT_011786	19954348	rs3092921	0.436		H		locus			

Figure 2.6. *Section of the NCBI SNP report for CD40LG. The SNPs listed at NCBI and Ensembl can be cross-referenced using the "rs" cluster id number.*

include high-quality sequences with minimal replication of sequences. The UniProtKB/Swiss-Prot entries are manually curated (Bairoch et al., 2005) and have the greatest detail for the annotation of protein features and modifications such as signal sequences, repeats, glycosylation sites, and disulfide bonds. The IPI database is a compilation of sequences from several sources, and it aims to minimize sequence duplication (Kersey et al., 2004). The Ensembl database also has peptide translations for each transcript that are annotated in its genome sequence, and that show the location of the intron–exon boundaries in the amino acid sequence. Many of these entries are cross-referenced to the other databases, although sometimes the cross-referenced entry is not the same isoform of the protein. Sequence data can be downloaded from all of these sites and can be copied for use in other Web-based analysis tools.

The amino acid sequence can be used to predict many chemical and physical properties, including the molecular weights and isoelectric points, which may be useful in identifying the protein in two-dimensional-electrophoresis, and to predict peptide fragments after enzymatic digestion, which

1: HomoloGene:56. Gene conserved in Amniota

Genes
Genes identified as putative homologs of one another during the construction of HomoloGene

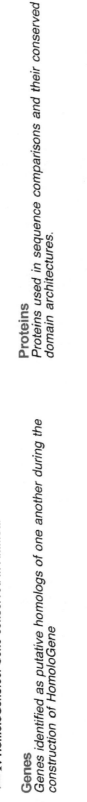
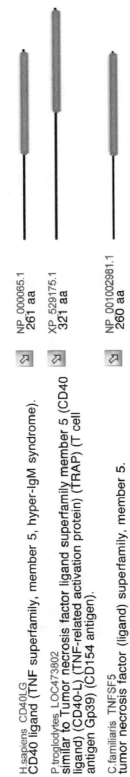
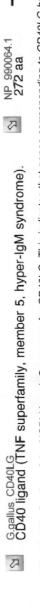

H.sapiens CD40LG
CD40 ligand (TNF superfamily, member 5, hyper-IgM syndrome).

P.troglodytes LOC473802
similar to Tumor necrosis factor ligand superfamily member 5 (CD40 ligand) (CD40-L) (TNF-related activation protein) (TRAP) (T cell antigen Gp39) (CD154 antigen).

C.familiaris TNFSF5
tumor necrosis factor (ligand) superfamily, member 5.

M.musculus Tnfsf5
tumor necrosis factor (ligand) superfamily, member 5.

R.norvegicus Tnfsf5
tumor necrosis factor (ligand) superfamily, member 5.

G.gallus CD40LG
CD40 ligand (TNF superfamily, member 5, hyper-IgM syndrome).

Proteins
Proteins used in sequence comparisons and their conserved domain architectures.

NP_000065.1
261 aa

XP_529175.1
321 aa

NP_001002981.1
260 aa

NP_035746.2
260 aa

NP_445805.1
260 aa

NP_990064.1
272 aa

Figure 2.7. *Section of the NCBI HomoloGene page for CD40LG. This indicates that genes corresponding to CD40LG have been identified in chimpanzees, dogs, mice, rats, and chickens. The illustration of the protein structure indicates that the chimpanzee protein is 60 amino acids longer than the protein in the other species listed. There are links to the EntrezGene and protein database pages for each of the homologues.*

Orthologue Prediction			

The following gene(s) have been identified as putative orthologues by reciprocal BLAST analysis:

Species	Type	dN/dS	Gene identifier
Pan troglodytes	DWGA		ENSPTRG00000022318 (TNFSF5) [MultiContigView] No description
Canis familiaris	UBRH	0.22220	ENSCAFG00000018945 (TNFL5_CANFA) [MultiContigView] [Align] Tumor necrosis factor ligand superfamily member 5 (CD40 ligand). [Source:Uniprot/SWISSPROT;Acc:O97626]
Gallus gallus	UBRH		ENSGALG00000006415 (TNFL5_CHICK) [MultiContigView] [Align] Tumor necrosis factor ligand superfamily member 5 (CD40 ligand) (CD40- L) (CD154 protein). [Source:Uniprot/SWISSPROT;Acc:Q918D8]
Xenopus tropicalis	UBRH		ENSXETG00000017494 (Novel Ensembl prediction) [MultiContigView] [Align] No description
Bos taurus	UBRH	0.16968	ENSBTAG00000017843 (TNFL5_BOVIN) [MultiContigView] [Align] Tumor necrosis factor ligand superfamily member 5 (CD40 ligand) (TNF- related activation protein) (TRAP) (T cell antigen GP39). [Source:Uniprot/SWISSPROT;Acc:P51749]
Rattus norvegicus	UBRH	0.33141	ENSRNOG00000000871 (TNFL5_RAT) [MultiContigView] [Align] Tumor necrosis factor ligand superfamily member 5 (CD40 ligand) (CD40- L). [Source:Uniprot/SWISSPROT;Acc:Q922V2]
Mus musculus	UBRH	0.27922	ENSMUSG00000031132 (Tnfsf5) [MultiContigView] [Align] tumor necrosis factor (ligand) superfamily, member 5 [Source:MarkerSymbol;Acc:MGI:88337]

View alignments of homologies.

UBRH = (U)nique (B)est (R)eciprocal (H)it
MBRH = one of (M)any (B)est (R)eciprocal (H)its
RHS = Reciprocal Hit based on Synteny around BRH
DWGA = Derived from Whole Genome Alignment

Figure 2.8. Section of the Ensembl GeneView page for CD40LG showing the homologues identified. In addition to those listed by the NCBI (Fig. 2.9), this page also lists homologues for cattle and xenopus. The links go to the GeneView page for the corresponding species and to an alignment of the human and homologue animo acid sequences.

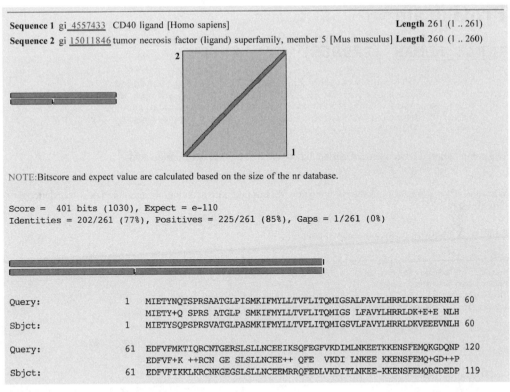

Sequence 1 gi 4557433 CD40 ligand [Homo sapiens]   **Length** 261 (1 .. 261)

Sequence 2 gi 15011846 tumor necrosis factor (ligand) superfamily, member 5 [Mus musculus] **Length** 260 (1 .. 260)

NOTE:Bitscore and expect value are calculated based on the size of the nr database.

```
Score =  401 bits (1030), Expect = e-110
Identities = 202/261 (77%), Positives = 225/261 (85%), Gaps = 1/261 (0%)
```

```
Query:      1   MIETYNQTSPRSAATGLPISMKIFMYLLTVFLITQMIGSALFAVYLHRRLDKIEDERNLH 60
                MIETY+Q SPRS ATGLP SMKIFMYLLTVFLITQMIGS LFAVYLHRRLDK+E+E NLH
Sbjct:      1   MIETYSQPSPRSVATGLPASMKIFMYLLTVFLITQMIGSVLFAVYLHRRLDKVEEEVNLH 60

Query:     61   EDFVFMKTIQRCNTGERSLSLLNCEEIKSQFEGFVKDIMLNKEETKKENSFEMQKGDQNP 120
                EDFVF+K ++RCN GE SLSLLNCEE++ QFE  VKDI LNKEE KKENSFEMQ+GD++P
Sbjct:     61   EDFVFIKKLKRCNKGEGSLSLLNCEEMRRQFEDLVKDITLNKEE-KKENSFEMQRGDEDP 119
```

Figure 2.9. *Alignment of human and mouse CD40LG amino acids sequences. This pre-computed alignment is linked from the NCBI HomoloGene page for CD40LG. The human and mouse sequences are 77% identical over their 260 amino acids.*

may be useful in mass spectrometry. The UniProtKB/Swiss-Prot entry page for a protein has links to several tools at the same site, which can analyze the complete amino acid sequence or a feature-defined fragment (Fig. 2.10).

2.4.1 Sequence Similarity Comparisons

The NCBI EntrezGene page usually has a link to a precalculated BLAST alignment of the amino acid sequence of the protein against the NCBInr database (Fig. 2.11). This list can be sorted to determine the most similar sequence in the same species or the most similar sequence in other species. The bl2seq alignment can be

obtained from the results page, as can the protein database page of the related sequence and that sequence's BLINK page. The taxonomic proximity sorting can be used to identify protein that may be a different sequence but that may be a related gene family to the original sequence, and will highlight regions of sequence similarity between gene family members.

2.4.2 Conserved Domains

Several systems can be used to identify conserved protein domains using an amino acid sequence, including the Conserved Domain Database (CDD; Marchler-Bauer et al., 2005) at the NCBI (Fig. 2.12), which is linked from the NCBI pages, and the

ProtParam

TNFL5_HUMAN (P29965)

```
DE    Tumor necrosis factor ligand superfamily member 5 (CD40 ligand) (CD40-
DE    L) (TNF-related activation protein) (TRAP) (T cell antigen Gp39)
DE    (CD154 antigen) [Contains: Tumor necrosis factor ligand superfamily
DE    member 5, membrane form; Tumor necrosis factor ligand superfamily
DE    member 5, soluble form].
```

The computation has been carried out on the complete sequence (**261** amino acids).

Warning: All computation results shown below do **not** take into account any annotated post-translational modification.

References and documentation are available.

```
Number of amino acids: 261
Molecular weight: 29273.5
Theoretical pI: 8.53
Amino acid composition:

Ala (A)    16    6.1%
Arg (R)    11    4.2%
Asn (N)    13    5.0%
Asp (D)     6    2.3%
Cys (C)     5    1.9%
Gln (Q)    16    6.1%
Glu (E)    18    6.9%
Gly (G)    16    6.1%
His (H)     6    2.3%
Ile (I)    15    5.7%
```

Figure 2.10. Section of the Protein Parameters analysis linked from the UniProtKB/Swiss-Prot page for CD40LG. This analysis gives the calculated molecular weight and pI and the amino acid composition of the protein. Other links from the page include peptide fragment predictions, hydrophobicity plots, and secondary structure predictions.

Pfam Protein Families database (Bateman et al., 2004) that is based at the Sanger Centre (Fig. 2.13). The CD-Hub has links to the precalculated domain organizations for the listed proteins. Both of these databases can also be searched with an amino acid sequence to determine whether an amino acid sequence identified experimentally contains any known conserved domains.

2.4.3 Structural Models

Few structural models are available for the CD molecules, and in some cases, the struc-ture of a subset of the domains in the protein have been determined. The structure databases can be accessed through the Research Collaboratory for Structural Bioinformatics (the PDB database; Berman et al., 2000), and the NCBI Entrez databases. It can be difficult to identify the correct structure, as the indexing may not use the same names as other databases. The PDB entries are linked from the Ensembl GeneView page of some proteins. Viewing the structures may require additional soft-ware, which is usually available from the site (Fig. 2.14).

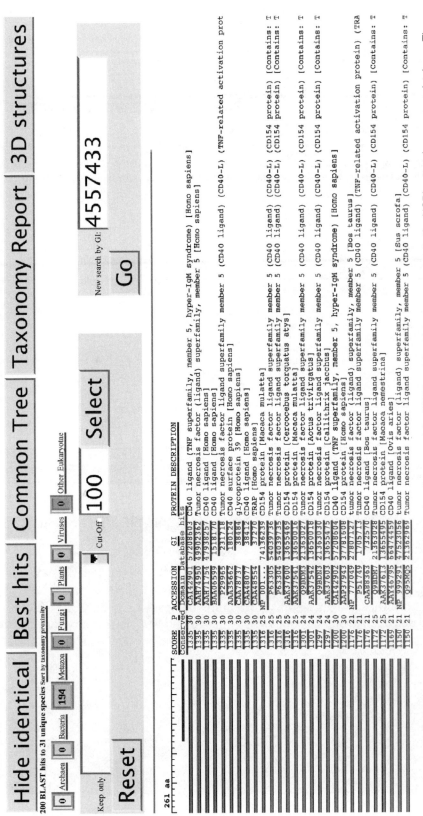

Figure 2.11. Section of the BLINK page for CD40LG showing the alignment of the NCBI protein reference sequence to the NCBInr protein sequence database. There are links to the sequence alignments and protein database entries for each match. The alignments can be sorted by match score or by taxonomic proximity and match score.

Query= gi|4557433|ref|NP_000065.1| CD40 ligand [Homo sapiens]
          (261 letters)
Database: cdd.v2.05

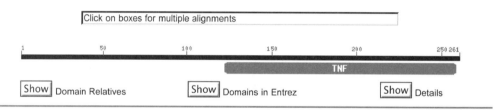

Figure 2.12. *Conserved protein domains' illustration for CD40LG from the NCBI Conserved Domains Database (CDD). The database shows a TNF domain is present in the protein. The domain is linked to support data.*

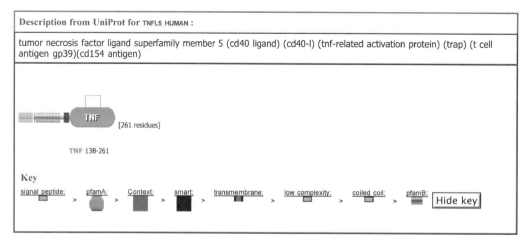

Figure 2.13. *Section of the Pfam database page for CD40LG showing the location of the conserved TNF domain. The page has links to support data for the domain assignments.*

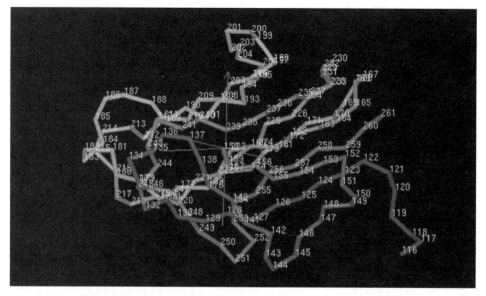

Figure 2.14. *Representation of the structure of CD40LG. The image was prepared with the iMol program using the 1ALY PBD file. The model shows residues 116 to 261 of the extracellular region of the protein.*

2.4.4 Transmembrane Helix Prediction

Most CD molecules are integral membrane proteins that have one or more regions that pass through the plasma membrane. Knowing which regions of a protein are intracellular or extracellular is important in the selection of peptides for immunization, for the expression of domains of the protein, and to understand the interaction of the protein with other proteins in the membrane. Several websites predict the topology and the location of transmembrane helices for a supplied protein sequence. These use different methods and can occasionally give different results. The TMHMM server (Krogh et al., 2001) is capable of using a single sequence or a file containing multiple sequences as the input, and it provides a graphical output of the topology and number of transmembrane helices, as well as the data used for the plot (Fig. 2.15). The HMMTOP server (Tusnady and Simon, 2001) provides a text output of the number and location of the

```
# gi_4557433_ref_NP_000065.1_ Length: 261
# gi_4557433_ref_NP_000065.1_ Number of predicted TMHs:  1
# gi_4557433_ref_NP_000065.1_ Exp number of AAs in TMHs: 22.82637
# gi_4557433_ref_NP_000065.1_ Exp number, first 60 AAs:  22.8084
# gi_4557433_ref_NP_000065.1_ Total prob of N-in:        0.42845
# gi_4557433_ref_NP_000065.1_ POSSIBLE N-term signal sequence
gi_4557433_ref_NP_000065.1_ TMHMM2.0 outside    1    22
gi_4557433_ref_NP_000065.1_ TMHMM2.0 TMhelix    23   45
gi_4557433_ref_NP_000065.1_ TMHMM2.0 inside     46   261
```

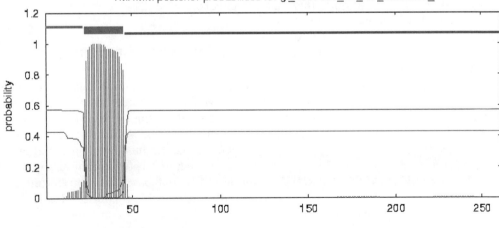

plot in postscript, script for making the plot in gnuplot, data for plot

Figure 2.15. Results of the topology and transmembrane helix prediction for CD40LG. A FASTA format amino acid sequence was used as the input to the TMHMM server. The results indicate that CD40LG is a type 2 transmembrane protein, with an intracellular N-terminal, an extracellular C-terminal, and a transmembrane helix from residues 23 to 45.

predicted transmembrane helices and the topology of the protein. A third option is the SOSUI server (Hirokawa et al., 1998); however, this can produce results that are different from the other servers for some proteins. The Phobius server is an improvement on the TMHMM server (Kall et al., 2004).

2.4.4.1 GPI Anchor Prediction

Plasma membrane proteins may be anchored to the membrane through a glycosylphosphatidylinositol (GPI) anchor, which is added to the protein after the removal of a C-terminal signal sequence (Low, 1989; Fankhauser and Maser, 2005). Several sites can predict whether a protein is likely to be GPI-anchored; however, the prediction may not be conclusive.

2.4.4.2 Glycosylation Prediction

N-linked and O-linked glycosylations are major post-translational modifications of proteins and are present on most CD molecules. For some proteins, the location of any known glycosylated residues is included in the UniProtKB/Swiss-Prot annotation. The residues that may have N-linked and O-linked glycosylations can be predicted at the NetNGlyc and NetOGlyc (Julenius et al., 2005) servers at the Center for Biological Sequence Analysis at the Technical University of Denmark. As these are predictions only, not all sites indicated will necessarily be glycosylated.

2.5   EXPRESSION INFORMATION

Links to the mRNA sequences of each gene can be found at the EntrezGene and Ensembl GeneView pages. Where there are multiple transcripts from a gene, each of these are linked independently. The sequences can be downloaded in various formats for use in local analysis.

The GNF Symatlas is an archive of microarray data that can be searched using gene names or mRNA or protein accession numbers (Fig. 2.16). If the arrays used had multiple probes to a gene, then these are displayed. The location of the microarray probe in the gene sequence can be found using links from the Ensembl GeneView page.

2.6   FUNCTIONAL INFORMATION

The original information about the function of a molecule will be found in the literature. To avoid having to fish through (potentially) thousands of papers, the NCBI EntrezGene page has a one-line digest of more recent papers on each protein and links to the PubMed entry for the paper (Fig. 2.17). A broader look at the role of the protein is available from the Online Mendelian Inheritance in Man (OMIM) page (Fig. 2.18), which reports on the disease associations of the gene in question (Hamosh et al., 2005). Again, there are links to the PubMed entries for the cited papers.

2.7   WEBSITES MENTIONED

It is clear that almost all of the sites described are linked to one another at some level. Within the NCBI, all databases are linked, so it is easy to travel from a gene name to functional information to gene structure to polymorphisms. A map of the NCBI database links can be found at "http://www.ncbi.nlm.nih.gov/Database/". The Ensembl pages are linked to each other and to many external sites, including the UniProtKB/Swiss-Prot, PDB, and NCBI pages for a protein.

The pages for CD40LG that are shown in the figures were accessed between 26 and 28 October 2005.

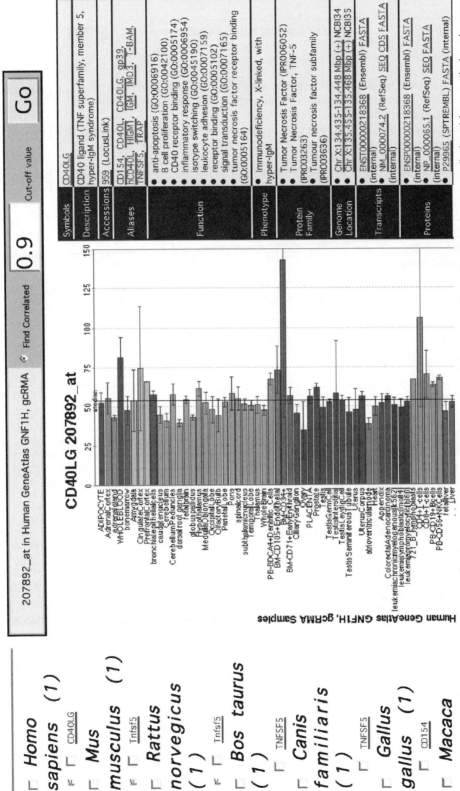

Figure 2.16. Section of the GNF Symatlas page for human CD40LG. The expression data for several cell types and tissues are displayed for a particular microarray platform. The probe accession number (207892_at in this case) can be identified using links from the Ensembl GeneView page.

Bibliography   Gene References into Function (GeneRIF):   **Submit**   ? ↑

PubMed links
GeneRIFs:
1. Ileal pouch mucosa leukocytes presented a significantly higher expression of   PubMed
CD40 and CD40L after proctocolectomy for ulcerative colitis and this alteration
correlated with pouchitis
2. Upregulation of soluble CD40L as a consequence of persistent hyperglycaemia in   PubMed
diabetic patients may contribute to accelerated atherosclerosis development in
diabetes.
3. the majority of thyroid cancers express CD-40 and CD-40 ligand   PubMed
4. TSLP is a major regulatory cytokine for CD40 ligand-induced IL-12 production   PubMed
by DCs, and TSLP-activated DCs could promote the persistence of Th2
inflammation even in the presence of IL-12-inducing signals
5. autocrine VEGF as an important mediator of the antiapoptotic effect of CD40   PubMed
ligation, and thus provide new insights into CLL-cell rescue by CD154 in
lymphoreticular tissues.

Figure 2.17. *A section of the Bibliography from the NCBI EntrezGene entry for CD40LG. A total of 74 references are listed on the page and are linked to the NCBI PubMed entry for the article.*

MOLECULAR GENETICS

Multiple mutations in CD40LG gene have been identified that are associated with hyper-IgM immunodeficiency syndrome type 1.

Allen et al. (1993) demonstrated point mutations in the CD40LG gene in 3 of 4 patients with the syndrome (300386.0003-300386.0005). Recombinant expression of 2 of the mutant CD40LG cDNAs resulted in proteins incapable of binding to CD40 and unable to induce proliferation or IgE secretion from normal B cells. Activated T cells from the 4 affected patients failed to express wildtype CD40LG, although their B cells responded normally to wildtype CD40LG. Patients with the hyper-IgM syndrome type 1 do not express IgE, strongly indicating that CD40LG is required (in conjunction with IL4) for production of IgE in vivo and suggests that it probably helps induce switching to all other isotypes. Korthauer et al. (1993) likewise followed up on the suggestion of a causal relationship of the condition they symbolized HIGM1 and the gene they symbolized TRAP (for TNF-related activation protein) and demonstrated to be the CD40 ligand. They presented evidence that point mutations in the TRAP gene give rise to nonfunctional or defective expression of TRAP on the surface of T cells in patients with this disorder. DiSanto et al. (1993) found a lack of CD40LG in 4 unrelated boys with the hyper-IgM syndrome type 1. Furthermore, CD40LG transcripts in these patients showed either deletions or point mutations clustered within a limited region of the CD40LG extracellular domain. ☺

Figure 2.18. *A section of the OMIM page for CD40LG showing the summary of the identification of CD40LG through the immune changes in hyper-IgM immunodeficiency syndrome type 1 that are caused by gene mutations.*

The CD Hub
Index Page   http://www.hcdm.org/hub_index.htm

Gene Information Pages
NCBI EntrezGene   http://www.ncbi.nlm.nih.gov/entrez/query.fcgi?db=gene
Ensembl search page http://www.ensembl.org/Homo_sapiens/textview

Genomic Context
NCBI MapViewer   http://www.ncbi.nlm.nih.gov/mapview/

Protein-Orientated Sequence Databases
ExPASy UniProtKB/ http://www.expasy.org
 Swiss-Prot
EBI IPI   http://www.ebi.ac.uk/IPI/IPIhelp.html

Structures and Conserved Domains
NCBI CDD   http://www.ncbi.nlm.nih.gov/entrez/query.fcgi?db=cdd
EBI Pfam   http://www.sanger.ac.uk/Software/Pfam/index.shtml
RCBS PDB   http://www.rcsb.org/pdb/index.html

Glycosylation Prediction
CBS NetNGlyc   http://www.cbs.dtu.dk/services/NetNGlyc/
CBS NetOGlyc   http://www.cbs.dtu.dk/services/NetOGlyc/

Transmembrane Helix Prediction
CBS TMHMM   http://www.cbs.dtu.dk/services/TMHMM/
HMMTOP   http://www.enzim.hu/hmmtop/
SOSUI   http://sosui.proteome.bio.tuat.ac.jp/sosuiframe0.html

GPI Anchor Site Prediction
Big-PI Predictor   http://mendel.imp.univie.ac.at/sat/gpi/gpi_server.html
BigGPI Prediction   http://129.194.185.165/dgpi/
GPI Self-Organising Maps http://gpi.unibe.ch/

Disease Association
NCBI OMIM   http://www.ncbi.nlm.nih.gov/entrez/query.fcgi?db=omim

Microarray Expression Database
GNF Symatlas   http://wombat.gnf.org/SymAtlas/

REFERENCES

Bairoch A, Apweiler R, Wu CH, Barker WC, Boeckmann B, Ferro S, et al. The Universal Protein Resource (UniProt). Nucleic Acids Res 2005;33:D154–D159.

Bateman A, Coin L, Durbin R, Finn RD, Hollich V, Griffiths-Jones S, et al. The Pfam protein families database. Nucleic Acids Res 2004;32:D138–D141.

Berman HM, Westbrook J, Feng Z, Gilliland G, Bhat TN, Weissig H, et al. The Protein

Data Bank. Nucleic Acids Res. 2000;28: 235–242.

Fankhauser N, Maser P. Identification of GPI anchor attachment signals by a Kohonen self-organizing map. Bioinformatics 2005;21: 1846–1852.

Hamosh A, Scott AF, Amberger JS, Bocchini CA, McKusick VA. Online Mendelian Inheritance in Man (OMIM), a knowledgebase of human genes and genetic disorders. Nucleic Acids Res 2005;33:D514–D517.

Hirokawa T, Boon-Chieng S, Mitaku S. SOSUI: classification and secondary structure prediction system for membrane proteins. Bioinformatics 1998;14:378–379.

Hubbard T, Andrews D, Caccamo M, Cameron G, Chen Y, Clamp M, et al. Ensembl 2005. Nucleic Acids Res 2005;33:D447–D453.

Julenius K, Molgaard A, Gupta R, Brunak S. Prediction, conservation analysis, and structural characterization of mammalian mucin-type O-glycosylation sites. Glycobiology 2005;15:153–164.

Kall L, Krogh A, Sonnhammer EL. A combined transmembrane topology and signal peptide prediction method. J Mol Biol 2004;338: 1027–1036.

Kersey PJ, Duarte J, Williams A, Karavidopoulou Y, Birney E, Apweiler R. The International Protein Index: an integrated database for proteomics experiments. Proteomics 2004;4:1985–1988.

Krogh A, Larsson B, von Heijne G, Sonnhammer EL. Predicting transmembrane protein topology with a hidden Markov model: application to complete genomes. J Mol Biol 2001;305:567–580.

Low MG. Glycosyl-phosphatidylinositol: a versatile anchor for cell surface proteins. Faseb J 1989;3:1600–1608.

Maglott D, Ostell J, Pruitt KD, Tatusova T. Entrez Gene: gene-centered information at NCBI. Nucleic Acids Res 2005;33:D54–D58.

Marchler-Bauer A, Anderson JB, Cherukuri PF, DeWeese-Scott C, Geer LY, Gwadz M, et al. CDD: a Conserved Domain Database for protein classification. Nucleic Acids Res 2005;33:D192–D196.

Tusnady GE, Simon I. The HMMTOP transmembrane topology prediction server. Bioinformatics 2001;17:849–850.

Wheeler DL, Barrett T, Benson DA, Bryant SH, Canese K, Church DM, et al. Database resources of the National Center for Biotechnology Information. Nucleic Acids Res 2005;33:D39–D45.

Part 2

Molecule Profiles CD1–CD350

How to Use the Molecule Profiles

This book is to be used as a directory, to look up molecules as you come across them in your work. We are assuming no one is likely to read it from cover to cover.

So let's start with an example—you read that CTLA4 may be a useful marker for the T-cell subset that dampens down immune responses, the regulatory T cell (Treg), and you want to know more about CTLA4.

The book is organized by CD number, and you do not know the CD number for CTLA-4. That is why we have an index that includes the more widely used alternative names.

Immunologists can be sloppy with names, so consider CTLA-4 to be synonymous with CTLA4.

The index directs you to CD152. The CD152 profile tells you about the structure and functions of CTLA-4 and tells you what CTL-A stands for. You can find out the physiological ligands for CTLA-4, a brief outline of the function of CTLA-4, and the main cells and tissues that express CTLA-4. There is also a field for "applications," which mentions important potential or actual applications in pathology and medicine for either the gene product or the antibodies against it.

The official gene name is given, as is the NCBI Entrez Gene number. You will probably be aware that several different organizations allocate gene names, and they do not always agree. We have used gene names allocated by the human genome organization, HUGO. A selection of the antibodies officially sanctioned by HLDA as being directed to CTLA-4 is provided. [If you want a more comprehensive list, go to www.hcdm.org, enter, select the "CD1-339" button (which may change to CD1—a higher number in the future), and scroll down to CD152. Click in the CD152, and you will get a table of the full list of antibodies verified by the HLDA.]

Leukocyte and Stromal Cell Molecules: The CD Markers, by Heddy Zola, Bernadette Swart, Ian Nicholson, and Elena Voss
Copyright © 2007 by John Wiley & Sons, Inc.

Our experience suggests that for many purposes, the information provided in the profiles will be enough. However, if you need to know more, the book provides you with an easy entry into World Wide Web information resources for the molecules. Chapter 2 provides a guide to WWW resources for CD and related molecules, and we suggest you start by going to www.hcdm.org, entering, and then going to the "Web Resources" link. Clicking on CD152 will open a page with links to multiple websites with information on the protein and the gene.

Symbols Used to Denote Domains, Motifs, and Repeats

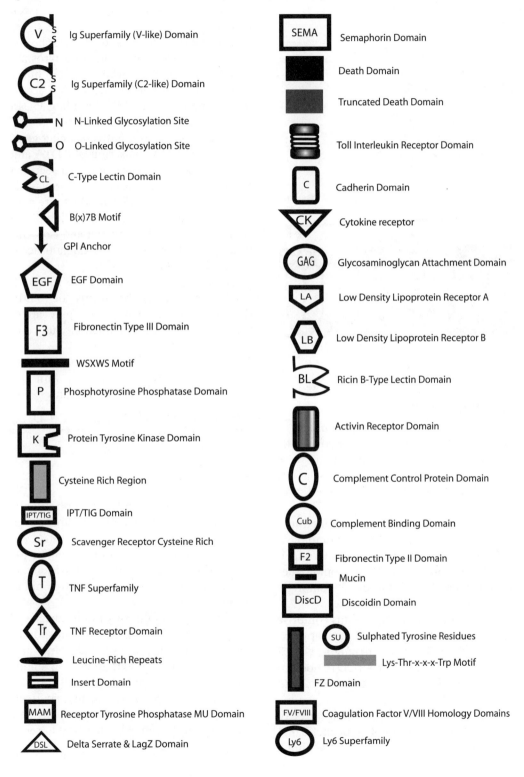

Ig Superfamily (V-like) Domain	Semaphorin Domain
Ig Superfamily (C2-like) Domain	Death Domain
N-Linked Glycosylation Site	Truncated Death Domain
O-Linked Glycosylation Site	Toll Interleukin Receptor Domain
C-Type Lectin Domain	Cadherin Domain
B(x)7B Motif	Cytokine receptor
GPI Anchor	Glycosaminoglycan Attachment Domain
EGF Domain	Low Density Lipoprotein Receptor A
Fibronectin Type III Domain	Low Density Lipoprotein Receptor B
WSXWS Motif	Ricin B-Type Lectin Domain
Phosphotyrosine Phosphatase Domain	Activin Receptor Domain
Protein Tyrosine Kinase Domain	Complement Control Protein Domain
Cysteine Rich Region	Complement Binding Domain
IPT/TIG Domain	Fibronectin Type II Domain
Scavenger Receptor Cysteine Rich	Mucin
TNF Superfamily	Discoidin Domain
TNF Receptor Domain	Sulphated Tyrosine Residues
Leucine-Rich Repeats	Lys-Thr-x-x-x-Trp Motif
Insert Domain	FZ Domain
Receptor Tyrosine Phosphatase MU Domain	Coagulation Factor V/VIII Homology Domains
Delta Serrate & LagZ Domain	Ly6 Superfamily

CD1a–e

Other Names

CD1a: T6/leu-6, R4, HTA1.
CD1b: R1; CD1c: M241, R7.
CD1d: R3; CD1e: R2.

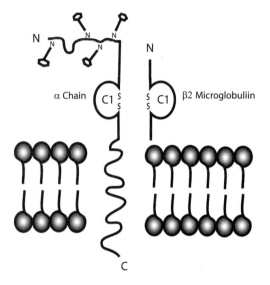

Molecular Structure

Family of Type I integral membrane Ig superfamily glycoproteins, noncovalently associated with ß2-microglobulin, with structural similarities to MHC-class I molecules (Class Ib MHC- related proteins).

CD1 family members are classified into two groups based on sequence homology.

CD1a, CD1b, and CD1c form Group 1; CD1d molecules and their homologues form Group 2; and Group 3 comprises CD1e molecules and homologues.

The CD1 extracellular regions comprise three domains $\alpha1$, $\alpha2$, and $\alpha3$, each approximately 90 amino acids in length, with 2 (CD1e), 3 (CD1a,b,c), or 4 (CD1d) potential N-glycosylation sites in domains $\alpha1$ and $\alpha2$.

The putative antigen-binding groove has two large hydrophobic pockets that hold the fatty-acid tails of the glycolipid, leaving the polar residues protruding and exposed for presentation to the T-cell receptor.

The CD1b, c, d, and e cytoplasmic domains are short and contain a tyrosine-based motif YXXZ (where Z is a bulky hydrophobic residue) essential for access to late endosomes and lipid binding. CD1a lacks this motif.

Tissue-specific alternative splicing gives rise to three RNA transcripts of CD1A and C genes and thus expression of a secreted form, membrane form, or cytoplasmic form. Five possible CD1e products are generated by alternative splicing, with either a short or long cytoplasmic tail and isoforms lacking the transmembrane domain accumulate intracellularly.

Polymorphism restricted to exon 2 results in two allelic forms of CD1a that have characteristics that may affect their interaction with β2-microglobulin and other accessory molecules.

Unlike other CD1 isotypes, CD1d a chain is not always associated with β2-microglobulin at the cell membrane.

Mol Wt: 49 kDa (CD1a), 45 kDa (CD1b), 43 kDa (CD1c), 38 kDa (CD1d), and 36 kDa (CD1e).

Function

CD1 molecules present non-peptide antigens, including lipids and glycolipids to T cells.

CD1-restricted T cells are essential for cell-mediated immunity to intracellular infection and prevention of autoimmune responses.

CD1a is present mostly at the surface of antigen presenting cells, but it can spontaneously enter early/sorting endosomes and then be passed to early/recycling endosomes before returning to the cell surface.

CD1a may play a role in thymic T-cell development, and its presence on activated T cells suggests it may be involved in regulating T cell responses.

Most CD1b molecules are located intra-cellularly in acidic, late endosomes where lipid antigen is loaded onto CD1b.

In mature activated T cells, CD1c expression is low at the cell surface but high in late endosomes.

Antigen presentation by CD1c on T cells seems to be independent of endosomal acidification despite its localization to endosomal compartments and exocytosis is via an atypical pathway that does not require early endosomes.

CD1d$^+$ thymocytes are involved in the positive selection of sublineage of NKT cells.

It is uncertain whether CD1d plays a role in the presentation of microbial lipid antigens during infection.

CD1e molecules accumulate in Golgi of immature dendritic cells; then they transfer to late endosomes in mature dendritic cells where the molecules are cleaved and become soluble.

The function of CD1e remains unknown, but a hypothetical role may be to transport microbial lipids that accumulate in the Golgi and endoplasmic reticulum and transport them to other compartments for processing.

Ligands

Microbial lipids and glycolipids such as mycobacterial mycolic acids and lipoarabinomannan (LAM).

Expression

The CD1 family shows variable expression on leukocytes, including dendritic cells, Langerhans cells, B cells, and T cells in thymocyte differentiation, and on activation. CD1 expression can be regulated by cytokines and activation stimuli.

Outside immune cells, CD1d is expressed by epithelial cells.

Gene Name	Entrez Gene#
CD1e	909
CD1b	910
CD1c	911
CD1d	912
CD1e	913

Selected Monoclonal Antibodies

CD1a: NA1/34 (McMichael; Oxford) T6 (Schlossman; Boston) Leu 6 (Evans; Buffalo).

CD1b: NUT2 (Sagawa; Fukuoka) WM-25 (Bradstock; Sidney) 7C4 (Knapp; Vienna).

CD1c: M241 (Knowles; New York) 7C6 (Knapp; Vienna) L161 (Bernard; Nice).

CD1d: CD1d42 (BD Biosciences).

CD1e: 20.6, VIIC7, 2.9, 1.22 (C. Angenieux; Paris).

CD2

Other Names

T11; Tp50; sheep red blood cell (SRBC) receptor; LFA-2; CD2R refers to cryptic epitopes exposed after activation.

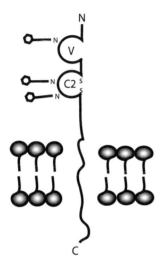

Molecular Structure

A type I transmembrane glycoprotein of 336 amino acids (351 amino acids with leader sequence).

Prototype of the CD2 family of the Ig superfamily (see also CD48, CD58, and CD150).

The extracellular region of 158 amino acids consists of 1 IgV-like and 1 IgC-like domain and has 3 potential N-linked glycosylation sites.

The 124 amino acid cytoplasmic portion is rich in prolines and basic amino acids that are essential for interactions with cytoplasmic signaling molecules.

Mol Wt: 50 kDa.

Function

Adhesion molecule binding LFA-3 (CD58).

Binding to sheep CD58 is the basis of the sheep rosette reaction, formerly used to identify and purify T cells. Binds CD48 with low affinity and possibly CD59 and CD15.

CD2 binding by ligands induces T-cell activation probably by improving adhesion between T cell and antigen-presenting cells but may involve signaling through CD2 cytoplasmic domain.

CD2 has a regulatory role in cytolysis by T cells or NK cells.

Involved in inducing apoptosis in activated peripheral T cells.

Knockout mice have apparently healthy immune systems. Depending on the experimental conditions and antibodies used, CD2 antibodies can activate T cells or inhibit T-cell activation.

Several transmembrane and intracellular molecules associate with CD2, including CD11a/CD18, CD45 (tyrosine phosphatase), CD3 complex components, a-tubulin, and protein tyrosine kinases of scavenger receptor-cysteine (SRC) family p56lck and p59fyn.

Ligands

CD58, CD48, sulfated carbohydrate.

Expression

All T cells, thymocytes, NK cells, and some B cells.

Applications

Original T-cell marker.

Used in typing leukemias and lymphomas.

Therapeutic use in preventing allograft rejection.

Gene Name	Entrez Gene#
CD2	914

Selected Monoclonal Antibodies

9.6. (Hansen; Seattle); T11 (Schlossman; Boston); Leu 5 (Lanier; Mountain View); Some antibodies recognize cryptic epitopes exposed after activation: T11.3 (Reinherz; Boston); VIT13 (Knapp; Vienna); D66 (Bernard; Nice).

CD3

Other Names

CD3 complex, T3, Leu4.

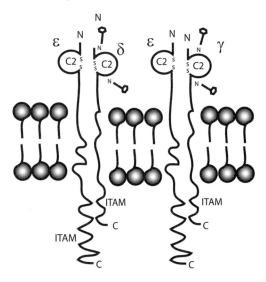

Molecular Structure

CD3 is a multigene cell-surface receptor structure consisting of constant components CD3-γ,δ,ε,ζ (and in mouse η) and variable elements (T-cell receptor [(TCR) α/β or TCR-γ/δ]) depending on the T-cell lineage. CD3ζ has been designated as CD247.

The 6 polypeptides are probably arranged as 3 dimers, i.e., g/ε, δ/εβ, and ζ/ζ.

CD3γ and CD3δ have two glycosylation sites; CD3ε and CD3ζ are unglycosylated.

CD3D,E,G genes are closely linked on human chromosome 11q23 and share significant sequence homology, whereas CD3ζ gene is on chromosome 1.

CD3δ,ε,γ are Ig superfamily members with an Ig-like domain in the extracellular region and transmembrane domains of 26–27 amino acids, and each has 1 immunoreceptor tyrosine-based activation motif (ITAM) in the cytoplasmic domain.

Di-leucine motif present in CD3γ cytoplasmic region is important for internalization of CD3–TCR complex in activated T cells.

CD3ζ differs from the other subunits as it has a short extracellular domain of only 9 amino acids but a intracellular domain that is 112 residues longer than the other subunits and 3 ITAMs.

Mol Wt: CD3γ: 25 kDa; CD3δ: 20 kDa; CD3ε: 20 kDa; CD3ζ: 16 kDa; CD3η: 22 kDa.

Function

Component of the T-cell antigen receptor complex, required for cell surface expression of T-cell receptor and signal transduction.

Intracellular tyrosine kinases, Lck and Fyn phosphorylate ITAMs leading to several signaling pathways being activated.

Depending on experimental conditions, CD3 antibodies activate T cells or inhibit their activation.

CD3ε knockout mice show no development of T cells.

Ligands

CD3–TCR complex interacts with peptide bound to MHC molecules.

Expression

T lineage cells.

Applications

Best marker for mature T cells. Therapeutic antibody (OKT3) used in treating graft rejection and other situations requiring immunosuppression.

Gene Name	Entrez Gene#
CD3D	915
CD3E	916
CD1G	917

Selected Monoclonal Antibodies

T3 (Schlossman; Boston); UCHT1 (Beverley; London); Leu 4 (Evans; Buffalo).

CD4

Other Names

OKT4, Leu 3a, T4.

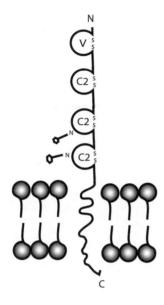

Molecular Structure

A type I transmembrane glycoprotein member of the Ig superfamily.

The extracellular domain has 4 Ig-like domains of 370 amino acids, a transmembrane region of 25 residues, and a cytoplasmic domain of 38 amino acids.

Domains 1, 2, and 4 are stabilized by disulphide bonds.

Two N-linked glycosylation sites on domains 3 and 4.

CD4 has significant structural similarity to LAG-3.

The intracellular domain has a binding motif (CXCP) for the tyrosine kinase Lck.

Mol Wt: 55 kDa.

Function

Coreceptor for MHC class II antigen-restricted T-cell activation that stabilizes the MHC class II/TCR complex.

Involved in thymic differentiation.

Domains 1 and 2 bind MHC class II.

Domains 3 and 4 are involved in interaction with CD3–TCR complex.

CD4 acts as a signal transduction molecule during T-cell activation by its interaction with protein tyrosine kinase Lck.

Serves as receptor for human immunodeficiency virus (HIV) and may play a role in the accelerated level of T-cell apoptosis during HIV infection as in vitro cross-linking of CD4 by HIV protein gp120 or anti-CD4 antibody leads to signaling via TCR-C3 and apoptosis of peripheral blood mononuclear cells from healthy individuals.

Binding of glycoprotein gp17 to CD4 inhibits CD4/TCR-mediated T-cell apoptosis.

CD4 may play a role in regulating helper T-cell recruitment to sites of inflammation as it has been shown to be a receptor for the pro-inflammatory cytokine interleukin-16 (IL-16). IL-16 binding seems to induce a migratory response in CD4$^+$ cells, particularly in the Th1 subset.

Ligands

MHC class II, viral gp120 protein of HIV retroviruses, IL-16, and gp17.

Expression

Thymocyte subsets, T cells that recognize peptide antigen associated with MHC class II (helper T cells), peripheral blood monocytes, tissue macrophages, and granulocytes.

Applications

Marker for helper T cells; CD4 cell counts used in monitoring progression of AIDS.

Therapeutic antibody (Imuclone) for immunosuppression and treatment of psoriasis.

Gene Name

CD4

Entrez Gene#

920

Selected Monoclonal Antibodies

T4 (Schlossman; Boston); Leu3a (Evans; Buffalo); M-T404 (Rieber; Dresden).

CD5

Other Names

Tp67, T1, Ly1, Leu-1.

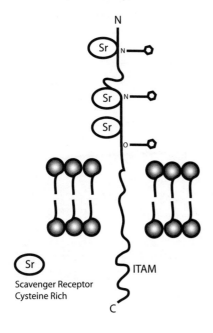

Molecular Structure

A type I transmembrane glycoprotein.

Member of the subgroup B scavenger receptor cysteine-rich (SRCR) family within the scavenger receptor superfamily.

Extracellular region consists of three cysteine-rich scavenger receptor domains.

Domain 1 and Domain 2 separated by Thr and Pro rich connecting peptide, highly conserved phylogeny (74% homology).

Cytoplasmic domain of approximately 90 residues is highly conserved (80% homology).

Cytoplasmic domain has multiple potential Ser/Thr and Tyr phosphorylation sites, some of which are within an ITAM motif.

Mol Wt: Reduced, 67 kDa; unreduced, 58 kDa.

Function

Acts as a dual receptor, sending inhibitory or stimulatory signals depending on the cell type and its maturation stage. Thus, CD5 transmits inhibitory signals in thymocytes and B1a cells but is a costimulatory signal receptor in mature peripheral T cells.

Putative role in thymocyte maturation and selection.

Binding with ligands modulates T–B-cell interactions and thus humoral immune responses.

Regulates responsiveness of human T cells to IL-1.

Binds the antigen-specific receptor complex (T-cell receptor and B-cell receptor) and constitutive B-cell-specific molecule CD72.

Participates in a membrane complex with CD3 or Ig.

Can associate with CD2, CD4, and CD8.

Associates with signaling molecules PTP1C, ZAP-70, p21phospho-ζ, and PI-3K in thymocytes.

Cytplasmic sequence binds PTK p56lck through SH2 domain.

Knockout mice are healthy but show multiple, subtle differences in vitro.

Ligands

CD72 is a putative ligand in humans and gp35–37 in mice.

Expression

Low density expression on early thymocytes.

High density expression on all T cells.

Low density expression on subset of mature B cells (B1a) expanded in neonatal life, several autoimmune disorders, and some B-cell proliferative disorders (B-CLL).

Applications

Widely used as a marker for B-CLL cells, hairy cell leukemia, and for B1a cells in autoimmune disorders.

Increased expression of CD3-positive T cells lacking CD5 expression after bone-marrow transplantation is an indicator of graft-versus-host disease.

Often dysregulated in T-cell malignancies.

Gene Name	Entrez Gene#
CD5	921

Selected Monoclonal Antibodies

T1 (Schlossman; Boston); T101 (Royston; San Diego); UCHT2 (Beverley; London).

CD6

Other Names

T12.

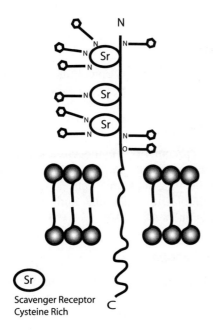

Sr
Scavenger Receptor
Cysteine Rich

Molecular Structure

A type I transmembrane glycoprotein member of the subgroup B scavenger receptor (SRCR) family.

Similar to CD5, the extracellular region consists of three SRCR domains.

Protein predicted to be 668 amino acids in length; however, alternative splicing leads to intracellular tails of either 244, 212, or 171 residues.

CD6 is extensively glycosylated.

Activation of cells via the T-cell receptor complex leads to extensive phosphorylation of intracellular tyrosine and serine residues.

Mol Wt: 105 kDa or 130 kDa.

Function

In vitro studies suggest adhesion function and costimulation of T-cell proliferation and a possible role in regulation of apoptosis of lymphocytes.

Ligands

CD6 binds CD166.

Expression

Thymocytes; T cells; B-cell CLL.

Applications

Can serve as a B-CLL marker.

Anti-CD6 mAb T12 has been used to deplete T cells from bone marrow for allogeneic transplantation to prevent graft-versus host disease (GVHD).

Gene Name	*Entrez Gene#*
CD6	923

Selected Monoclonal Antibodies

T12 (Schlossman; Boston); T411 (Rieber; Dresden); VIT12 (Knapp; Vienna).

CD7

Other Names

Leu 9, 3A1, gp40, T-cell leukemia antigen.

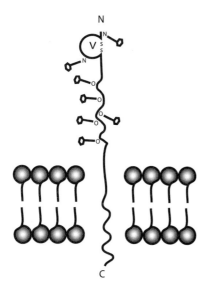

Molecular Structure

A type I integral Ig superfamily membrane glycoprotein. The extracellular region consists of an N-terminal IgV-like domain followed by a putative O-glycosylated extended "stalk" with four consensus repeats containing many Pro, Thr, and Ser residues.

Mol Wt: 40 kDa.

Function

Essential role in T-cell interactions as well as T-cell/B-cell interactions.

In vitro studies suggest CD7 has an important role in regulatory T-cell and NK–T-cell ontogeny and prevention of autoimmune disease.

Costimulatory activity after T-cell activation.

May modulate cell adhesion.

Ligands

Galectin-1, secreted epithelial cell protein K12.

Expression

T-cell precursors, thymocytes, subset of peripheral T cells and NK cells and pre-B lymphocytes, leukemic cells (T-cell acute lymphoblastic leukemia and stem cell leukemia).

Applications

Marker for T-cell ALL (acute lymphoblastic leukemia), pluripotential stem cell leukemia, acute myeloid leukemia (AML), and myelodysplasia.

Potential therapeutic target in the treatment of rheumatoid arthritis and may be a useful target for immunosuppression in transplant patients.

Gene Name	Entrez Gene#
CD7	924

Selected Monoclonal Antibodies

3A1 (Haynes; Durham); WT1 (Tax; Nijmegen); G3-7 (Ledbetter; Seattle).

CD8

Other Names

OKT8, LeuT, LyT2, T8.

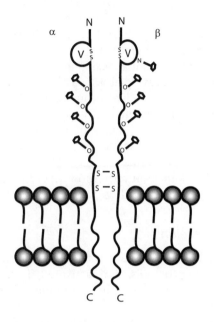

Molecular Structure

Disulfide-linked homodimer of CD8α or heterodimer of CD8α and CD8β. CD8β cannot homodimerize.

Both CD8α and CD8β are members of the Ig superfamily with significant homology to IgV light chains.

The cytoplasmic domain of the α chain contains a binding motif for tyrosine kinase Lck.

In the extracellular domain, the N-terminal IgV-like domain is separated from the transmembrane region by a hinge domain.

Alternative splicing gives rise to a soluble form of CD8α and possibly CD8β.

Mol Wt: Reduced, α 32–34 kDa, β 30–32 kDa; unreduced, 68 kDa or greater in case of multimers.

Function

Coreceptor for MHC class I restricted T-cell activation and selection.

CD8 on T cell binds to MHC class I on an antigen presenting cell enhancing the cognate interaction between the T-cell receptor complex and the antigenic peptide/MHC class I complex.

Anti-CD8 antibodies inhibit cytotoxic T-lymphocytes.

Ligands

MHC class I.

Expression

Thymocyte subset, T cells specific for antigen presented with MHC class I (cytotoxic T cells); some γ/δ T cells and NK cells. α/β T cells express CD8 heterodimer, whereas γ/δ cells express the CD8α homodimer.

Applications

Marker for cytotoxic T-cell subset.

Gene Name	Entrez Gene#
CD8A	925 (CD8α)
CD8B1	926 (CD8β)

Selected Monoclonal Antibodies

T8 (Schlossman; Boston); Leu 2a (Evans; Buffalo); UCHT4 (Beverley; London).

CD9

Other Names

Tetraspanin-29 (Tspan-29), Motility-related protein-1 (MRP-1), p24, leukocyte antigen MIC3, Drap-27 (monkey).

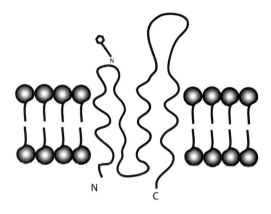

Molecular Structure

A type III membrane protein of 228 amino acids.

Member of the transmembrane 4 superfamily (TM4SF) family with four transmembrane domains and two unequal extracellular loops (EC1 and EC2) (see CD37, CD53, CD63, CD81, CD82, and CD151).

A signature sequence common to tetraspan family members is found between transmembrane domains II and III.

Short N- and C-termini on the cytoplasmic side.

Both 24- and 26-kDa forms of CD9 are acylated and O-glycosylated, but only the 26 kDa form has been shown to be N-glycosylated, and has a single N-glycosylation site in smaller extracellular domain.

Mol Wt: 24 kDa (major band), 26 kDa (minor band).

Function

Forms complexes with integrins and other members of the transmembrane 4 superfamily.

Associates with CD41/CD61 in platelets.

Associates with precursor form of heparin-binding EGF-like growth factor (HB-EGF) in Vero cells.

Modulates cell adhesion and migration.

Can trigger platelet activation and aggregation as well as promote muscle cell fusion and maintenance of myotubes.

Essential component of plasma membrane of mammalian egg required for fusion with sperm.

CD9 knockout mice show severe reduction in female fertility.

Expression

Platelets, early B cells, activated and differentiating B cells, and activated T cells. Lower expression in eosinophils and granulocytes.

Mammalian ova, endothelial and epithelial cells, brain and peripheral nerves, as well as vascular smooth muscle and cardiac muscle.

Applications

Leukemia immunophenotyping, bone marrow purging, and inverse correlation with metastatic potential of leukemic cells.

Gene Name	Entrez Gene#
CD9	928

Selected Monoclonal Antibodies

BA2 (LeBien; Minneapolis); J2 (Ritz; Boston); FMC8 (Zola; Adelaide).

CD10

Other Names

Common acute lymphoblastic leukemia antigen (CALLA), Neutral endopeptidase (NEP), gp100.

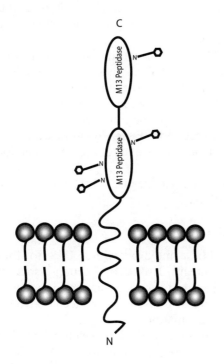

Molecular Structure

A type II transmembrane zinc metalloprotease (metalloendopeptidase) (see also CD13) with varying levels of N-glycosylation.

Extracellular C terminal domain has 4 N-linked glycosylation sites, and 12 cysteines that form disulphide bonds required for enzymatic activity.

A characteristic zinc-binding motif found in several zinc-metalloproteases present in the extracellular domain.

Short N-terminal cytoplasmic tail and a transmembrane domain that acts as a signal peptide.

Mol Wt: 100 kDa.

Function

This neutral endopeptidase (encephalinase) cleaves biologically active peptides (e.g., encephalins, fMLP, substance P) at hydrophobic amino acids.

This activity may dampen responses to peptide hormones by limiting the amount of peptide available for receptor binding.

Inhibition of CD10 activity in vivo enhances B-cell maturation, indicating a regulatory role in B-cell development.

CD10-deficient mice seem normal but are more susceptible to endotoxin.

Expression

Early B lineage cells and again on germinal center B cells; fetal thymocytes, subgroup of parafollicular T cells.

Bone marrow stromal cells and myeloid-lineage cells.

Detectable in several normal tissues but abundant expression in brush border of renal proximal tubules and glomerular epithelium.

Applications

Useful marker for classification of B-lineage leukemias and lymphomas as well as renal and hepatocellular carcinoma and uterine mesenchymal neoplasms.

Prognostic marker of metaplastic breast carcinoma.

Gene Name   Entrez Gene#

MME   4311

Selected Monoclonal Antibodies

J5 (Ritz; Boston); VILA1 (Knapp; Vienna); BA3 (LeBien; Minneapolis).

CD11a

Other Names

α-L integrin chain/subunit, heavy chain of leukocyte function associated antigen-1 (LFA-1), gp180/95.

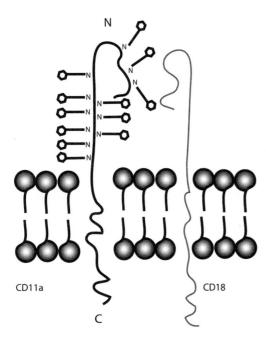

CD11a

CD18

Molecular Structure

A type I integral membrane glycoprotein forming a noncovalently associated heterodimeric complex with CD18 (β-2-integrin).

Member of the integrin α-chain family (see CD11b, CD11c).

Protein of 1145 amino with 1063 amino acid extracellular domain, 29 amino acid transmembrane domain, and 53 amino acid cytoplasmic domain.

Extracellular sequence contains 12 N-glycosylation sites and 7 tandem repeats of about 50 amino acids each.

Repeat domains form a β-propeller-like fold similar to the β subunit of the trimeric G protein.

Three repeats (V, VI and VII) contain EF-hand-like sequences that are putative cation binding sites.

The major ligand binding site is a 200 amino acid inserted/interactive (I) domain found between repeats 2 and 3.

The I domain forms an a-b dinucleotide binding fold and contains a discontinuous metal ion-dependent adhesion site (MIDAS).

The position of the metal ion when bound to MIDAS probably allows it to interact directly with the ligand.

Located between the transmembrane and the cytoplasmic domains is the sequence VGFFKR, required for heterodimerization and regulation of function.

Mol Wt: Reduced, 180 kDa; unreduced, 170 kDa.

Function

CD11a complexes with CD18 to form the integrin leukocyte function-associated antigen-1 (LFA-1), an important adhesion and signal transduction molecule involved in inflammation.

An intact actin cytoskeleton and magnesium are essential for LFA-1 ligand binding, whereas calcium is inhibitory.

T-cell activation alters the conformation and cell-surface distribution but not the level of expression of CD11a/CD18 complexes.

Transient aggregation of CD11a/CD18 complexes leads to increased functional affinity for ligands.

CD11a knockout mice show major deficits in immune reactions.

Patients with leukocyte adhesion deficiency Type 1(LAD-1) do not express CD11a.

Ligands

Ligands of CD11a/CD18 (LFA-1) are CD54 (ICAM-1), CD102 (ICAM-2), CD50 (ICAM-3), ICAM-4 (Landsteiner-Wiener antigen), ICAM-5 (telencephalin), JAM-1 (CD321), and LPS.

Expression

Leukocyte-restricted; highly expressed on lymphocytes (particularly memory T cells), monocytes, macrophages; lower levels on polymorphonuclear cells.

Applications

Useful leukocyte marker in tissue pathology.

Animal models of transplantation, ischemia, and autoimmunity have shown anti-CD11a, anti-CD18, and anti-CD54 antibodies to have therapeutic value as immunosuppressive and anti-inflammatory agents.

Therapeutic use of anti-CD11a in children with bone marrow grafts greatly reduces rate of graft failure.

Antibodies are immunosuppressive in animal models.

Gene Name	Entrez Gene#
ITGAL	3683

Selected Monoclonal Antibodies

TS2/16.1.1 (Springer; Boston); CRIS-3 (Vilella; Barcelona); MHM24 (McMichael; Oxford).

CD11b

Other Names

α-M integrin chain; α-chain of C3biR, CR3 Mac-1, Mo1.

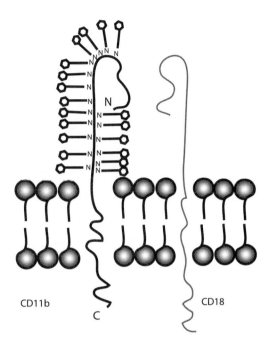

CD11b

C

CD18

Molecular Structure

Type 1 integral membrane glycoprotein and member of the integrin α-chain family.

Some CD11b cDNAs have an extra codon between bp 1580 and 1581, which gives rise to protein of either 1136 or 1137 amino acids with 1092 or 1093 amino acid extracellular domain. No functional difference has been detected between the two forms.

26 amino acid transmembrane region and 19 residue cytoplasmic domain.

The extracellular region has 7 repeating domains (1–7) that may form a β-propeller-like fold and 19 potential N-glycosylation sites.

Major ligand binding site is in an inserted/interactive (I) domain found between repeat domains 2 and 3.

CD11b I domain forms a classic a–b dinucleotide binding fold.

Forms a noncovalently associated heterodimeric complex with the CD18 molecule (β2-integrin).

Mol Wt: Reduced, 170 kDa; unreduced, 165 kDa.

Function

CD11b/CD18 forms the integrin Mac-1, also known as complement receptor 3 (CR3), which binds multiple ligands (see Ligands).

Involved in phagocytosis of opsonized particles.

Indirect role in neutrophil respiratory burst and degranulation, transendothelial migration of monocytes and neutrophils, chemotaxis and apoptosis.

The complex has signaling activity and appears to be involved in inflammation.

The binding site for iC3b, CD54, and CD102 and fibrinogen occurs in the I domain.

CD11b is not detectable in Leukocyte adhesion deficiency-Type 1 (LAD-1) patients.

Ligands

Ligands of CD11b/CD18 (Mac-1, CR3) are iC3b, CD54 (ICAM-1), fibrinogen, kininogen, haptoglobin, Factor X, CD23, CD102 (ICAM-2), heparin, β-glucan, LPS complexed with LPS binding protein (LPS/LPB), Neutrophil inhibitory factor of Ancylostoma caninum, filamentous hemagglutinin from *Bordetella pertussis*, gp63 of *Leishmenia donovani*, and WI-1 antigen of Blastomyces dermatitidis.

Reported to bind denatured proteins.

Expression

Monocytes, granulocytes, and NK cells and some subsets of T and B lymphocytes.

Applications

MAb used to detect monoctyes.

   Target of anti-inflammatory drug therapy.

Selected Monoclonal Antibodies

Mac1 (Springer; Boston); Mo1 (Todd; Ann Arbor); VIM12 (Knapp; Vienna).

Gene Name

ITGAM

Entrez Gene#

3684

CD11c

Other Names

α-X integrin chain; CR4; Leukocyte surface antigen p150, 95; ITGAX.

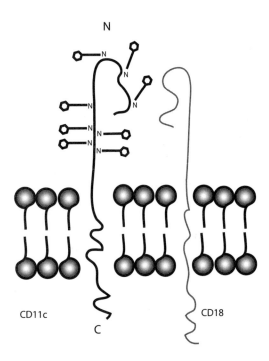

Molecular Structure

A type I integral membrane glycoprotein of 1144 amino acids.

A 1081 amino acid extracellular domain, 26 amino acid transmembrane region, and 29 amino acid cytoplasmic domain.

Member of subclass of integrin α subunits with I-domain near N-terminus.

10 potential N-glycosylation sites and 7 tandem repeats with 3 putative cation-binding motifs.

Repeating integrin domains I-VII reported to form a β-propeller-like fold.

Forms noncovalently associated heterodimeric complex with the CD18 (β2-integrin).

Mol Wt: Reduced, 150 kDa; unreduced, 145 kDa.

Function

CD11c/CD18 forms the integrin p150,95, which is the Type 4 complement receptor (CR4), binding iC3b as well as LPS, ICAM-1, CD23, and fibrinogen.

Mediates cell-to-cell interactions in inflammation.

Required for monocyte adhesion and chemotaxis.

Major CD11/CD18 receptor on macrophages.

Leukocyte adhesion deficiency-type I (LAD-1) patients are CD11c-deficient.

Ligands

Ligands for CD11c/CD18 are iC3b, fibrinogen, ICAM-1(CD54), CD23, and LPS.

Reported to also bind denatured proteins.

Expression

High level expression on monocytes, macrophages, and NK cells.

Moderate expression on granulocytes.

Weakly expressed by CD3[+] T lymphocytes and CD20[+] B lymphocytes.

Used to detect myeloid cells in tissue studies.

Gene Name	Entrez Gene#
ITGAX	3687

Selected Monoclonal Antibodies

Ki-M1 (Radzun; Kiel); 3.9 (Hogg; London).

CDw12

Other Names

p90–120.

Molecular Structure

Protein structure unknown.

CDw12 antibodies detect a carbohydrate epitope on a phosphoprotein of unknown structure (not cloned).

Mol Wt: Reduced, 120 kDa; unreduced, 150–160 kDa.

Expression

Monocytes, granulocytes, NK cells, platelets. Not found on basophils, AML blasts and haemopoetic precursor cells.

Gene Name   Entrez Gene#

23444

Selected Monoclonal Antibodies

M67 (Rieber; Dresden), 20.2.

CD13

Other Names

Aminopeptidase N, APN, ANPEP, gp150, EC3.4.11.2.

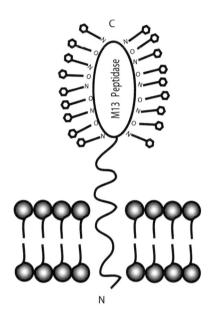

Molecular Structure

A type II transmembrane zinc-metalloprotease of 967 amino acids (see also CD10).

Short N terminus is located in cytoplasm.

Transmembrane domain acts as signal peptide.

Large, highly glycosylated extracellular C terminal region has 10 N-glycosylation sites and numerous O-glycosylation sites. Variations in glycosylation produce different mAb epitopes.

CD13 is expressed on the cell surface as a noncovalently linked homodimer.

Zinc-binding and catalytic activity are associated with pentapeptide motif (His-Glu-Ile/Leu/Met-X-His) common to many zinc-metalloproteases.

Structurally identical to aminopeptidase N, a zinc-metalloprotease that degrades regulatory peptides.

Mol Wt: 150 kDa.

Function

Zinc metalloproteinase that trims peptides bound to MHC class II.

May dampen cellular responses to peptide hormones by lowering the local concentration of peptides available for binding.

Catalyses removal of N-terminal amino acids from small peptides including opioid peptides, fMLP, tuftsin, and brain encephalins.

Requires another metalloprotease CD10 to assist in hydrolysis of peptides.

Has preference for neutral residues.

Cleaves chemokine MIP-1 resulting in a change in target cell specificity from basophils to eosinophils.

CD13 activity is upregulated by IL-4 but inhibited by peptide hormones bradykinin and P.

Antibodies induce oxidative burst in monocytes by cross-linking CD13 molecules with Fcγ receptors.

Receptor for coronaviruses, cytomegalovirus.

CD13 autoantibodies are associated with graft-versus-host disease (GVHD) in bone marrow transplantation.

Ligands

Coronaviruses; Cytomegalovirus.

Expression

CFU-GM (colony-forming units for granulocytes and macrophages), granulocytes, monocytes, bone marrow stroma, osteoclasts, large granular lymphocytes, intestinal brush border epithelium, endothelial cells, renal tubule epithelial cells, fibroblasts, brain cells, and cells lining biliary caniculae.

Applications

Marker for acute myeloid leukemias and some acute lymphoid leukemias.

Presence of CD13 autoantibodies is a strong indicator of graft versus host disease (GVHD) in bone marrow transplantation recipients.

Gene Name	Entrez Gene#
ANPEP	290

Selected Monoclonal Antibodies

My7 (Griffin; Boston); MCS-2 (Sagawa; Fukuoka); MoU28 (Winchester; New York).

CD14

Other Names

LPS receptor, LPS-R.

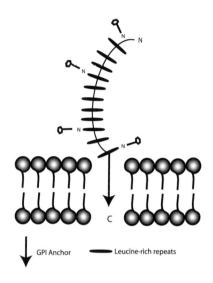

GPI Anchor ━━ Leucine-rich repeats

Molecular Structure

Glycophosphoinositol-linked glycoprotein of 356 amino acids.

A 19 amino acid signal sequence cleaved during processing.

Glycophosphoinositol (GPI) at C terminus anchors protein to the cell surface; however, it can be secreted in soluble forms.

Of two soluble forms described, one retains GPI and is released from the cell surface (48 kDa), whereas the other is released prior to addition of the GPI anchor (>48 kDa).

Contains 11 repeats with similarity to leucine-rich glycoprotein repeats. 4 N-glycosylation sites, unknown number of O-glycosylation sites.

CD14 gene has a single 88 base pair intron after the initiation codon and maps to a chromosomal region with other genes encoding growth factors and receptors.

Mol Wt: Reduced, 55 kDa; unreduced, 53 kDa.

Function

Receptor for the LPS/LPS binding protein (LBP) complex.

LPS/LBP binding to CD14 enables LPS to be transferred to Toll-like receptor-4 (TLR-4)/MD-2 complex on myeloid cells.

Soluble CD14 (sCD14) binds LPS/LBP and mediates LPS-induced activation of endothelial cells and some epithelial cells.

LPS binding activates CD14$^+$ cells resulting in increased cytokine production and expression of cell-surface molecules including adhesion molecules.

Binding of LPS/LBP complex to CD14 enhances binding activity of CR3 (CD11b/CD18 complex) on neutrophils.

Involved in TLR-2 signaling by binding and presenting bacterial antigens such as peptidoglycan and lipoarabinomannan to TLR-2.

Overexpression of human CD14 in transgenic mice results in greater susceptibility to endotoxic shock, but CD14-deficient mice are highly resistant to challenge with live Gram-negative bacteria and LPS.

Ligands

LPS/LBP (lipopolysaccharide/lipopolysaccharide binding protein) complex, Lipoteichoic acid (in vitro), phosphatidyl inositol (in vitro).

Expression

Strong expression on monocytes and osteoclast progenitors.

Weaker expression on tissue macrophages, Langerhans cells, granulocytes, and microglia, not detectable in myeloid progenitors.

Low level expression on B cells.

Soluble forms present in plasma and tissue culture supernatant of CD14-transfected cells.

Applications

CD14 is a marker for monocytes and osteoclast progenitors.

Gene Name	Entrez Gene#
CD14	929

Selected Monoclonal Antibodies

UCHM1 (Beverley; London); Mo2 (Todd; Ann Arbor); MEM18 (Horejsi; Prague).

CD15

Other Names

Lewis X, Le-X, X-Hapten. CD15u indicates 3′ sulfo Lewis X; CD 15s indicates sialyl Lewis X, and CD15su is 6′ sulfo-sialyl Lewis X.

$$\text{Gal } \beta 1 \longrightarrow 4\text{Glc NAc-R}$$
$$\overset{3}{\underset{\uparrow}{}}$$
$$\text{Fuc } \alpha 1$$

Molecular Structure

Cluster of cell-surface glycoproteins and glycolipids with terminal trisaccharide epitope 3-FAL (Gal-β1-4 [Fuc-α1-3]GlcNAc) also known as Lewis X (Le-X) antigen.

Epitope can be sialylated and/or sulphated, and the core protein or lipid may vary depending on the cell type.

Function

An important role in adhesion as leukocyte adhesion deficiency type II (LAD-2) is associated with low levels of CD15 and CD15s and impaired selectin-mediated adhesion.

Not all glycoproteins carrying CD15s bind selectins, but the basis for this restricted binding is not yet understood.

Ligands

CD15s binds the selectins CD62P and CD62E.

CD15su appears to act as a coreceptor for L-selectin (CD62L).

Helicobacter pylori blood group antigen adhesin (BabA) selectively adheres to CD15.

Expression

All forms of CD15 are expressed on granulocytes.

Also expressed on monocytes, macrophages, eosinophils, mast cells, Langerhans cells, activated.

T4 cells and activated B cells.

Reed–Sternberg cell of Hodgkin's lymphoma.

Expressed in various epithelia including secretory epithelium of breast, collecting tubules of kidney, lung, and intestinal tract.

Constitutively expressed by astrocytes and variably by oligodendrocytes and neurons.

Applications

Used as a granulocyte marker.

Important marker for diagnosis of Hodgkin's lymphoma and in the differentiation of mesothelioma from adenocarcinoma, and anaplastic gliomas versus normal glial cells. Prognostic marker for hepatocellular, gastric, colonic, and thyroid medullary carcinomas as well as achievement of remission in acute myeloid leukemias.

Histopathologic grading of gliomas.

Selected Monoclonal Antibodies

My1 (Civin; Baltimore); VIMD5 (Knapp; Vienna); 1G10 (Bernstein; Seattle); FMC10 (Zola, Adelaide).

CD16

Other Names

CD16a: FcγRIIIa, FCRIIIA; CD16b: FcγRIIIb, FCRIIIB.

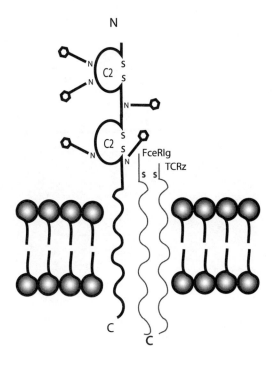

Molecular Structure

Member of the Fcγ receptor family within the immunoglobulin (Ig) superfamily.

Two genes and two transcripts have been described for CD16, and both receptors bind IgG complexes.

Two forms of human CD16 are a type I transmembrane protein (CD16a) and a glycosyl-phosphotidylinositol (GPI)-linked form (CD16b) that lacks a cytoplasmic domain.

Extracellular region consists of two IgC-like domains.

Horizontal configuration of the membrane-proximal Ig-like domain exposes its ligand binding site.

CD16a describes the FcγRIII-unique ligand binding α chain, which associates with the FcεRI-γ chain or the T-cell receptor ζ-chain to transduce signals.

Mol Wt: 50–60 kDa.

Function

Binds constant region of IgG1 and IgG3 with low affinity.

CD16a associates with FcεRγ-chain on human phagocytes and mast cells and the TCR ζ-chain in NK cells.

CD16a triggering in NK cells leads to antibody-dependent cellular cytotoxicity (ADCC) and lymphokine production, indicating a role in defence against viral infection and neoplasms.

CD16a-dependent but antibody-independent lysis of tumor cells and virus-infected cells has also been demonstrated.

CD16b has no intrinsic signaling function, does not associate with other signaling subunits, but is capable of inducing ADCC of erythrocytes and phagocytosis by neutrophils.

Ligands

IgG immune complexes and aggregates.

Expression

CD16a found on NK cells, macrophages, activated monocytes, mast cells, and γ/δ T cells.

CD16b constitutively expressed on neutrophils and expression can be induced in eosinophils by IFN-γ.

Applications

Phenotypic marker in leukemia and in HIV-1. Used to purify bone marrow and germinal center subsets.

CD16 alleles (and CD32 alleles) can be used as risk markers for systemic lupus erythematosus (SLE).

Gene Name	Entrez Gene#
FCGR3A	2214 (CD16a)
FCGR3B	2215 (CD16b)

Selected Monoclonal Antibodies

Bw209/2 (Kurrle; Marburg); VEP13 (Rumpold; Vienna); CLB/Fc Gran1(von dem Borne; Amsterdam).

CD17

Other Names

LacCer, lactosylceramide.

$$Glu\ \beta1 \longrightarrow 4Gal1-Ceramide$$

Molecular Structure

Glycosphingolipid lactosylceramide with lactosyl disaccharide group (LacCer or $Gal\beta1\text{-}4Glc\beta1\text{-}1$ceramide).

The epitope is not known to be found on glycoproteins.

Function

Mediates homotypic adhesion.

Binds to bacteria and may function in phagocytosis.

May be involved in intracellular trafficking.

Surface expression is downregulated after cell activation and is associated with membrane internalization and granule exocytosis.

Ligands

GM3 gangliosides.

Expression

Most abundant in neutrophils (both on the surface and as cytoplasmic granules). Also found in monocytes, basophils, platelets, subset of B cells, and tonsillar dendritic cells.

Selected Monoclonal Antibodies

GO35 (Thompson; Lexington); Hulym13 (McKenzie; Melbourne); T5A7 (Bernstein; Seattle).

CD18

Other Names

β2-Integrin, β2-Integrin chain, CD11a β subunit, CD11b β subunit, CD11c β subunit.

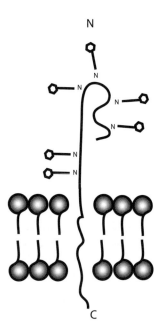

Molecular Structure

A type I transmembrane glycoprotein noncovalently linked to either CD11a, CD11b, or CD11c molecules (integrin α chains).

Member of the integrin β-chain family.

A 678 amino acid extracellular domain, 23 amino acid transmembrane domain, and 46 amino acid cytoplasmic domain.

The extracellular region has 6 potential N-linked glycosylation sites and is heavily internally cross-linked, with 28 potential disulphide links.

Mol Wt: Reduced, 95 kDa; unreduced, >120 kDa.

Function

Essential for correct leukocyte adhesion and signaling.

Interacts noncovalently with CD11a, b, c, or d to form the adhesion molecule complexes LFA-1, Mac-1, p150, 95, and aDb2, respectively.

Knockout mice show marked defects in leukocyte function. CD18 deficiency results in leukocyte adhesion deficiency type I (LAD-1). LAD-1 patients have recurrent infections.

CD18 antibodies inhibit cell–cell interactions and consequently activation and effector functions.

Ligands

The complexes of CD18 with CD11a, CD11b, and CD11c have different ligands—refer to the CD11 individual entries.

Expression

Expressed on all leukocytes.

Gene Name   Entrez Gene#

ITGB2   3689

Selected Monoclonal Antibodies

TS1/18.1 (Springer; Boston); MHM23 (McMichael; Oxford); M232 (Bernard; Nice).

CD19

Other Names

Bgp95, B4.

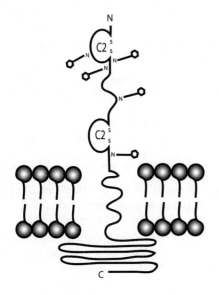

Molecular Structure

A type I transmembrane glycoprotein member of the Ig-gene superfamily.

A 288 amino acid extracellular region is heavily glycosylated and has two IgC-like domains separated by a small potentially disulphide-linked domain.

Extracellular domain has extensive sequence similarity to the β-subunits of Shiga-like toxin of *E. coli* and potentially binds CD77 (Shiga-toxin receptor and marker for germinal center B cells).

A 240 amino acid cytoplasmic domain is related to Epstein–Barr virus proteins and has multiple tyrosine phosphorylation sites.

Mol Wt: Reduced, 95 kDa; unreduced, 90 kDa.

Function

Interaction with CD77 plays a role in germinal center formation, B-cell homing, and apoptosis.

Involved in signal transduction and has a regulatory role in setting signaling thresholds for antigen receptors and other B lymphocyte surface receptors.

Forms part of B-cell receptor complex with CD21 and CD81.

Leu13 associates directly with CD81 and therefore indirectly with CD19.

CD19 null mice have decreased numbers of B cells, decreased mitogenic responses, low germinal center formation, and decreased humoral immune responses to T-cell-independent type 1 and T-cell-dependent antigens. CD19 antibodies increase cytoplasmic calcium levels in B cells and block proliferation of resting B cells in response to various stimuli except PMA.

Cytoplasmic domain can associate with PI-3K, Vav, and Src family kinases Lyn and Fyn.

Ligands

CD77

Expression

Expression is found in the earliest B-lineage cells up to B-cell blasts but is lost on maturation to plasma cells.

Also expressed in malignant B cells and follicular dendritic cells.

Applications

Major B lineage marker.

Therapeutic antibody for lymphoma (e.g., Bexxar).

Gene Name   Entrez Gene#

CD19   930

Selected Monoclonal Antibodies

B4 (Nadler; Boston); HD37 (Dörken; Berlin); SJ25-C1 (Peiper; Memphis).

CD20

Other Names

B1, Bgp35, Leu-16.

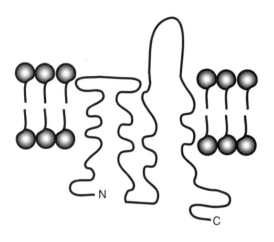

Molecular Structure

Phosphoprotein expressed on B cells in three forms depending on extent of phosphorylation.

When activated, B cells have increased levels of the 37-kDa and 35-kDa forms.

Member of MS4A family, with four membrane-spanning regions.

Both the N-terminus and the C-terminus are cytoplasmic.

One extracellular region detectable with antibodies, the other possibly buried.

Mol Wt: 33, 35, 37 kDa.

Function

Forms homo-oligomeric complexes thought to act as calcium channels. Is associated with membrane rafts.

Regulator of cell-cycle progression.

Regulator of B-cell activation and proliferation.

Involved in differentiation of B cells into plasma cells.

Functionally associates with B-cell receptor (BCR) on stimulated B lymphocytes and then rapidly dissociates prior to internalization.

Can form complexes with Src family of tyrosine kinases Lyn, Fyn, and Lck.

Associates with MHC class I and II molecules as well as CD53, CD81, and CD82.

CD20 null mice have normal B-cell function.

Most anti-CD20 mAb are effective at recruiting complement and causing cell lysis as binding to CD20 enhances localization of CD20 into membrane rafts that are more susceptible to complement. Nevertheless, the therapeutic action of anti-CD20 antibodies seems to be complex and to depend on features additional to complement-mediated lysis of malignant cells.

Expression

Mature B cells.

Low level expression on peripheral blood T lymphocytes.

Applications

Marker for follicular B-cell non-Hodgkins lymphoma.

Therapeutic antibody for lymphoma (e.g., Rituximab).

L26 (antibody against intracellular region) widely used for immunohistochemistry.

Gene Name   Entrez Gene#

MS4A1   931

Selected Monoclonal Antibodies

B1 (Nadler; Boston); 1F5 (Clark; Seattle); 2H7 (Clark; Seattle).

CD21

Other Names

C3d receptor, complement receptor type 2 (CR2), gp140; EBV receptor.

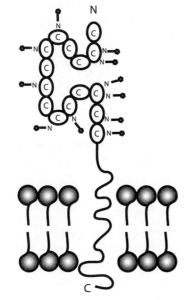

© Complement Control Protein

Molecular Structure

A type I transmembrane glycoprotein consisting of 15 or 16 complement control protein domains.

It is a member of the regulator of complement activation (RCA) gene family (see also CD35, CD46, and CD55).

The extracellular region has 15 to 16 short consensus repeats (SCR), tightly folded units of 60 amino acids arranged in at least five groups that form a minimum of 6 epitopes.

The transmembrane domain consists of 28 residues, and the 34 amino acid cytoplasmic region has potential protein kinase C and tyrosine kinase sites.

SCR 1 and 2 have binding sites for C3 fragments and EBV that although distinct probably overlap.

SCR 3 and 4 bind soluble cross-linked C3dg with high affinity.

SCR 5 to 8 have two distinct epitopes recognized by different mAb.

Mol Wt: 130 kDa (soluble); 145 kDa.

Function

Receptor for C3d (CR2) and Epstein–Barr virus (EBV), through distinct binding sites.

It forms part of the B-cell antigen receptor complex, with CD19, CD81, and leu 13, involved in signal transduction.

IgM acts synergistically with CD21 in B-cell activation.

High density CD21 expression on marginal B cells enables a rapid primary immune response, in particular to T-cell-independent antigens.

The inability of infants below the age of two to make adequate antibody responses to polysaccharides is associated with the lack of CD21$^+$ marginal zone B cells.

Association of CD21 with CD23 may be involved in T–B-cell interaction and in regulating IgE production.

CD21 knockout mice have impaired IgM-mediated induction of primary antibody responses.

Ligands

The ligands for CD21 are C3d, C3dg, iC3b, CD23, EBV, and CD35.

Expression

Found on mature B cells with strong expression in marginal zone cells after the age of two (in humans), moderate expression by mantle zone B cells, and no expression by germinal centre B cells.

CD21 is strongly expressed by follicular dendritic cells (FDC).

Low density expression of CD21 is detectable on pharyngeal and cervical epithelial cells, fetal astrocytes, subsets of immature and normal thymocytes, T cells, and T-ALL.

Applications

CD21 is a surface marker useful in phenotyping malignant B-cell lymphoma.

It is a useful marker for immunohistologic study of FDC patterns.

The combined demonstration of EBV and CD21 is used in the diagnosis of posttransplant lymphoproliferative disease.

Gene Name	Entrez Gene#
CR2	1380

Selected Monoclonal Antibodies

B2 (Nadler; Boston); HB-5 (Cooper; Birmingham); F74 (LeBien; Minneapolis); Bly4 (Poppema; Groningen); BL13 (Brochier; Montpellier).

CD22

Other Names

Bgp135, BL-CAM, Siglec2, Lyb8, LPAP.

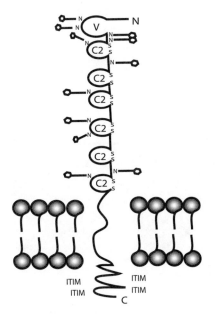

Molecular Structure

Member of the Ig gene superfamily with significant homologies to sialoadhesin, the myelin-associated glycoprotein (MAG), and CD33 (sialoadhesin family).

It is a single-chain type I integral membrane glycoprotein with 6 IgC2-like and 1 IgV domain and is both N- and O-glycosylated.

Variable splicing of exon 6 or exons 6 and 7 give rise to different isoforms.

The 140-kDa molecule is the major form found on the B-cell surface, but low level expression of a 130-kDa isoform (lacking the fourth Ig-like domain) is also detectable on most B cells.

The 140 amino acid cytoplasmic tail contains four immunoreceptor tyrosine-based inhibition (ITIM) motifs.

A sialic acid binding region is located in domain 1; however, the presence of domain 2 is essential for ligand binding.

CD22 antibodies may recognize carbohydrate determinants on the CD22 molecule because all three so far known epitopes are destroyed by treatment with endoglycosidase F.

Mol Wt: 140 kDa. 130-kDa isoform.

Function

Functions as an adhesion and signaling molecule that regulates B-cell function.

It binds sialylated ligands of erythrocytes, all leukocytes, and endothelial cells but predominantly recognizes the sialylated glycoconjugate NeuAca2,6Galβ1-4GlcNAcβ1.

CD22 binds numerous glycoproteins, including all isoforms of CD45, IgM, and haptoglobin; however, physiologically active ligands have not been identified.

Cross-linking of CD22 and BCR leads to rapid tyrosine phosphorylation, enabling binding of several kinases and phosphatases involved in signal effector functions, including tyrosine phosphatase SHP1, p72sky, p53/56lyn, phosphatidylinositol-3 kinase, and phospholipase Cg (PLCg).

Knockout mice have normal B-cell development but fewer mature B cells, less suface Ig and are more sensitive to triggering through the B-cell receptor.

Ligands

CD22 binds sialylated glycoproteins.

Expression

Expressed by mature B cells and corresponding malignancies. Earlier B cells have cytoplasmic CD22.

Applications

CD22 is useful for the diagnosis and experimental therapy of mature B-cell malignancies.

Selected Monoclonal Antibodies

HD39 (Dörken; Berlin); To15 (Mason; Oxford).

Gene Name   Entrez Gene#

CD22   933

CD23

Other Names

Low affinity IgE receptor, FcεRII, gp50-45, Blast-2.

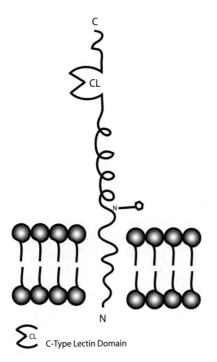

C-Type Lectin Domain

Molecular Structure

A type II integral membrane glycoprotein.

Shares significant homologies with human, rat, and chicken asialoglycoprotein receptors but not with rat IgE-binding factors.

The extracellular region contains a C-type lectin domain (see CD69, CD72, CD94, and CD161) with three repeats of 21 amino acids.

CD21 forms trimers in the cell membrane, with an α-helical coiled-coil structure.

Alternative splicing of exon 2 gives rise to two forms (FcεRIIa and FcεRIIb), which differ only by six amino acids at the NH2-terminal cytoplasmic region and are found in different cell types (see Expression).

Continuous proteolytic cleavage of membrane-bound CD23 results in soluble CD23 molecules of varying size (all of which retain the lectin domain).

Mol Wt: 45 kDa; soluble CD23: 37 kDa, 29 kDa, 25 kDa, and 16 kDa.

Function

CD23 is involved in negative feedback regulation of IgE synthesis.

It also plays a role in inflammation by triggering release of TNF, IL-1, IL-6, and GM-CSF by monocytes.

The two forms of CD23 are thought to have different signaling roles and functions. FcεRIIa seems to play a role in endocytosis, whereas FcεRIIb has some function in phagocytosis.

Soluble CD23 has an autocrine-like B-cell growth factor (BCGF) activity and is identical to the IgE binding factor.

CD23 knockout mice have elevated levels of IgE and impaired IgE-mediated antigen presentation.

Ligands

CD23 binds IgE with low affinity.

Expression

Resting B cells express only FcεRIIa, whereas FcεRIIb is expressed by activated B cells and other cell types, including monocytes, FDC, T cells, eosinophils, neutrophils, Langerhans cells, platelets, and thymic epithelium.

Applications

Serum CD23 is elevated in chronic lymphocytic leukemia (CLL) and is an indicator of poor prognosis.

CD23 is a useful marker in differentiation of small lymphocytic lymphomas and mantle cell lymphomas.

Gene Name	Entrez Gene#
FCER2	2208

Selected Monoclonal Antibodies

MHM6 (McMichael; Oxford); Blast-2 (Thorley-Lawson; Boston); HD50 (Dörken; Berlin).

CD24

Other Names

Heat stable antigen homologue (HSA), BA-1.

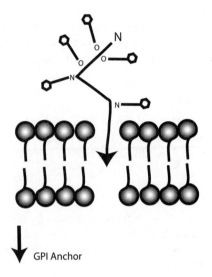

GPI Anchor

Molecular Structure

CD24 is a highly glycosylated sialoprotein linked to the cell membrane by glycophosphoinositol (GPI).

It has a small protein core of 27 amino acids.

Almost half of the amino acid residues are Ser and Thr residues that are potential O-linked glycosylation sites.

Extensive N- and O-linked glycosylation gives rise to molecules of varying molecular weight, and the extent of glycosylation is cell-type dependent.

Three different epitopes that are of a carbohydrate nature have been described.

Mol Wt: 35–70 kDa.

Function

CD24 is involved in regulating the binding capacity of VLA-4 (CD49d/CD29).

It may play a role in B-cell differentiation as pre-treatment of B cells with mAb blocks this process and knockout mice have mildly affected B-cell maturation.

Cross-linking of CD24 by mAb also induces a rapid rise in Ca^{++} levels.

P-selectin ligand (CD62P) binds a carbohydrate of CD24.

CD24 has a signal transduction role in granulocytes as some antibodies (VIBE3) induce an oxidative burst response and co-stimulate B cells to proliferate with PMA.

CD24 may play a role in memory cell formation and is thought to be involved in the adhesion and spread of metastatic tumors.

Ligands

P-selectin (CD62P).

Expression

Expressed by all B lineage cells (except plasma cells), mature granulocytes, and non-T-cell acute lymphoblastic leukemia (ALL).

High level expression of CD24 is found in pancreatic, ovarian, breast, prostate, and small cell lung cancer.

Applications

Marker for staging B-cell development.

Diagnostic and prognostic marker in acute myelogenous leukemia, B-cell malignancies, and Sezary syndrome.

Presence correlates with aggressive progression of breast, ovarian, prostate, and non-small cell lung cancer.

Gene Name	Entrez Gene#
CD24	934

Selected Monoclonal Antibodies

BA1 (LeBien; Minneapolis); VIBC5 (Knapp; Vienna); HB8 (Cooper; Birmingham).

CD25

Other Names

Interleukin (IL)-2 receptor α-chain, Tac-antigen.

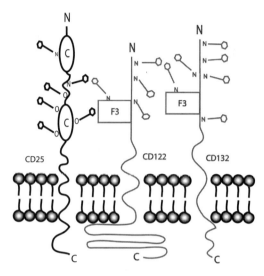

Ⓒ Complement Control Protein Domain

Molecular Structure

A type I integral membrane glycoprotein.

The extracellular region contains two Complement Control Protein (CCP) domains and is extensively N- and O-linked glycosylated.

The protein has a short cytoplasmic tail.

Alternative spliced forms are detectable as mRNA, but the significance of each is not known.

Soluble CD25 is formed by proteolytic cleavage.

Mol Wt: 55 kDa.

Function

CD25 has low affinity IL-2 binding capacity.

By noncovalently associating with CD122 and CD132 (which can also combine with CD124 and CD127 to form the IL4 and IL7 receptors), it forms the high affinity IL-2 receptor complex.

$CD4^+CD25^+$ regulatory T cells (Treg) seem to regulate other T cells and play a role in limiting inflammatory responses and preventing autoimmunity as knockout mice develop autoimmune diseases.

Ligands

CD25 is the α-chain of a three-chain receptor for IL-2. CD25 does bind IL-2 by itself but with low affinity.

Expression

CD25 is constitutively expressed by natural $CD4^+CD25^+$ regulatory T cells and is expressed by activated T and B cells, monocytes, and macrophages.

Low level CD25 expression is detectable on a subset of resting T cells.

CD25 is proteolytically released from lymphoid cells and found in serum.

Applications

Membrane-bound and soluble CD25 are used to monitor cell activation in immune response.

Gene Name	Entrez Gene#
IL2RA	3559

Selected Monoclonal Antibodies

TAC (Waldmann; Bethesda); 7G7/B6 (Nelson; Bethesda); 2A3 (Maino; Mountain View).

CD26

Other Names

EC3.4.14.5, Dipeptidyl peptidase IV; DPP IV ectoenzyme, adenosine deaminase-binding protein, Tp103.

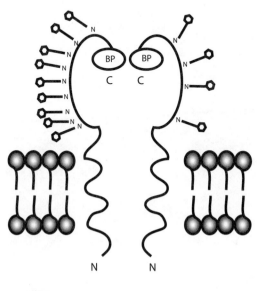

BP 8 Bladed β Propeller

Molecular Structure

CD26 is a 766 amino acid, single-chain, type II transmembrane glycoprotein and a member of the poly-oligopeptidase family.

The C-terminal 260 residue extracellular domain has a membrane proximal region with 9 N-glycosylation sites and contains dipeptidyl peptidase IV activity with serine proteinase conserved sequence Gly-X-Ser-X-Gly.

The three residues Ser630, Asp708, and His740 form the catalytic triad located in the α/β hydrolase fold in the C-terminus. The remaining N-terminal amino acids form an eight-bladed β-propeller.

The hydrolase and propeller domains are required for dimerization.

CD26 forms noncovalently linked homodimer in the membrane or is released as a truncated soluble form.

Mol Wt: Reduced, 120 kDa, 110 kDa; unreduced, 110 kDa.

Function

Serine-type exopeptidase, which cleaves dipeptides (X-proline or X-alanine) from the N-termini of proteins. Independent of its enzymatic activity, CD26 plays a role in lymphocyte proliferation probably via binding of adenosine deaminase (ADA) and possibly via its association with CD45.

Binds collagen in the extracellular matrix with possible role in tissue restructuring in tumors and liver disease.

Can also bind fibroblast activation protein (FAP); however, the effects of this interaction have yet to be elucidated.

Knockout mice demonstrate a role for CD26 in regulating blood glucose levels probably by inactivating incretins such as glucagon-like peptide-1 (GLP-1), which are responsible for about 50% of nutrient-induced insulin secretion and have other roles in glucose homeostasis.

Immunosuppression during human immunodeficiency virus (HIV) infection may be mediated by inactivation of CD26 by binding of HIV protein Tat to the ADA binding site.

Ligands

CD26 binds collagen, fibroblast activation protein (FAP), and the Tat protein of HIV. Also binds adenosine deaminase.

Expression

Constitutively expressed on mature thymocytes, T cells, B cells, NK cells, macrophages epithelial cells and monocytes, epithelial cells in intestine, kidney, prostate, and bile duct and lining cells of the spleen.

Applications

Human studies support a role for CD26 as a potential therapeutic agent in control of type II diabetes.

Marker of autoimmune disease, HIV disease progression, and adenosine deaminase deficiency.

Gene Name	Entrez Gene#
DPPA	1803

Selected Monoclonal Antibodies

134-2C2 (Vilella; Barcelona); TS145 (Ueda; Nagoya); 4ELIC7 (Reinherz; Boston).

CD27

Other Names

T14, S152, Tp55, TNFRSF7.

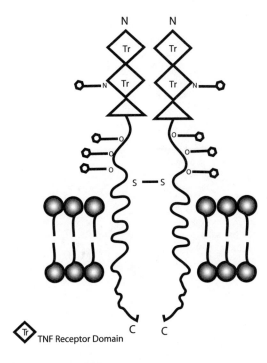

Tr TNF Receptor Domain

Molecular Structure

A 240 amino acid, type I transmembrane protein.

Member of the tumor necrosis factor (TNF)/nerve growth factor (NGF) receptor family (see CD30, CD40, CD95, CD120a, CD120b, CD134, and CDw137).

Forms disulfide-linked homodimers.

The 171 amino acid extracellular domain consists of two cysteine-rich repeats (TNF receptor domains) and a membrane-proximal half-TNF receptor domain, and it contains one N- and extensive O-glycosylation sites.

21 amino acid hydrophobic transmembrane domain.

48 amino acid C-terminal cytoplasmic domain has a serine phosphorylation site but does not contain any known signaling motif.

PIQEDYR motif in cytoplasmic domain is essential for binding of TNF receptor associated factors (TRAF) 2 and TRAF 5.

Soluble form is released by activated lymphocytes.

Mol Wt: Reduced, 55 kDa: unreduced, 110–120 kDa.

Function

Triggering on murine hematopoietic stem cells and early progenitors by CD70 inhibits differentiation to leukocytes.

In both primary and secondary T-cell responses, CD27 is a co-stimulatory molecule that on binding of CD70 regulates expansion and differentiation of effector cells.

Knockout mice have normal overall hematopoiesis but have increased numbers of leukocytes (particularly B cells) and display impaired T-cell responses after antigenic challenge.

Involved in activation of NF-κB and stress-activated protein kinase (SAPK)/c-Jun N-terminal kinase (JNK).

Ligands

CD70.

Expression

Found on hemopoetic stem cells and early progenitor cells, medullary thymocytes, activated B cells, and NK cells. Constitutively expressed on T cells with expression elevated on activated CD45RA$^+$ T cells.

Soluble form found in serum.

Applications

Marker for naive T cells and memory B cells.

Increased serum CD27 in inflammatory conditions.

Gene Name

TNFRSF7

Entrez Gene#

939

Selected Monoclonal Antibodies

VIT14 (Knapp; Vienna); CLB-9F4 (Tetteroo; Leiden); S152 (Bigler; New York).

CD28

Other Names

Tp44, T44.

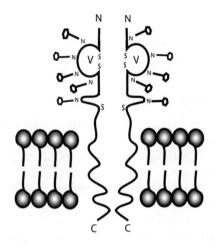

Molecular Structure

CD28 is a disulfide-linked homodimeric type I transmembrane glycoprotein structurally related to CD152 (CTLA-4) and a member of the Ig gene superfamily.

The 202 amino acid protein has a 134 residue extracellular region containing a single IgV-like domain, 27 amino acid transmembrane region, and 41 amino acid cytoplasmic domain.

Four transcripts are detectable in T cells. The longer transcripts of 3.5 kb/3.7 kb result from the use of an alternative polyadenylation signal. The other two transcripts (1.3 kb/1.5 kb) arise from alternative splicing within exon 2 of the extracellular domain.

The extracellular domain has 5 potential N-linked glycosylation sites, and the cytoplasmic domain has a tyrosine-containing motif.

Mol Wt: Reduced, ~44 kDa; unreduced, ~90 kDa.

Function

CD28 is the ligand for CD80/CD86 (B7-1, B7-2) and is involved in co-stimulation of T-cell effector function and T-cell-dependent antibody production.

Blocking CD28 interaction with CD80/CD86 causes functional inactivation of T cells.

Knockout mice display effective T-cell responses but are defective in mounting T-cell-dependent antibody responses.

The cytoplasmic region binds intracellular signaling molecules phosphatidylinositol 3-kinase (PI-3 kinase) and guanine nucleotide exchange protein (GRB-2-SOS) via the PYMNM motif and binds tyrosine kinase ITK.

Binding to PYMNM motif requires phosphorylation by Lck and Fyn.

CD28 antibodies augment T-cell proliferation after suboptimal doses of PHA, PMA, CD3 antibodies, or CD2 antibodies.

Ligands

Binds CD80 and CD86.

Expression

Constitutively expressed on most T-cell lineages with the exception of a small subset of CD8[+] cells. Mature thymocytes have higher level of CD28 expression than immature cells.

CD28 is also expressed by plasma cells.

Applications

CD28 is a potential target for immunosuppression.

Gene Name

Gene Name	Entrez Gene#
CD28	940

Selected Monoclonal Antibodies

9.3 (Hansen; Seattle); Kolt2 (Sagawa; Kurume).

CD29

Other Names

Integrin β1-chain, platelet GPIIa, VLA (CD49) β-chain.

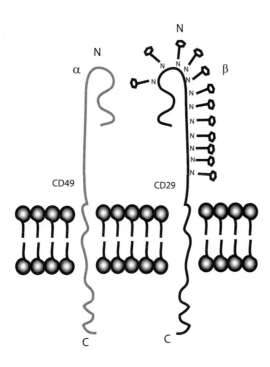

Molecular Structure

Transmembrane glycoprotein representing the major β-chain of the VLA protein family (CD49 molecule family).

Associates with integrin α-chains (see CD49 and CD51) to form a variety of heterodimeric adhesion molecules (see Ligands).

Four isoforms with different cytoplasmic domains are generated by alternative splicing. Expression seems to be tissue dependent.

Mol Wt: Reduced, 130 kDa; unreduced, 115 kDa.

Function

Adhesion to ligands such as VCAM-1 and MAdCAM-1, and adhesion to matrix proteins collagen, laminin, and fibronectin.

Critical for embryogenesis and development.

Essential for hematopoietic stem cell differentiation.

B1-integrins play a role in metastasis of tumor cells.

Ligands

CD29/CD49a complex binds type IV collagen and laminin.

CD29/CD49b complex binds type I collagen.

CD29/CD49c complex binds fibronectin, laminin-V, laminin-1, entactin, and collagen.

CD29/CD49d complex binds VCAM-1 (CD106), connecting segment-1 (CS-1, isoform of fibronectin), microbial ligand invasin, and thrombospondin.

CD29/CD49e complex binds fibronectin and neural adhesion molecule L1.

CD29/CD49f complex binds laminin, invasin, and merosin.

CD29/CD51 complexes bind fibronectin and vitronectin.

Expression

Broadly expressed on most cells and all leukocytes with higher expression on memory T cells than naive cells and low levels on granulocytes.

Not expressed on RBC.

Gene Name

ITGB1

Entrez Gene# 3688

Selected Monoclonal Antibodies

4B4 (Schlossman; Boston); K20 (Boumsell; Paris); A-1A5 (Hemler; Boston).

CD30

Other Names

Ki-1 antigen, Ber-H2 antigen, TNFRSF8.

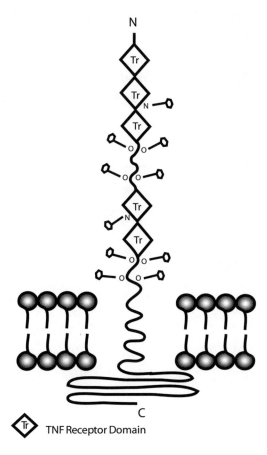

TNF Receptor Domain

Molecular Structure

A type I transmembrane glycoprotein and member of the tumor necrosis factor (TNF)/nerve growth factor (NGF) receptor family (see CD27, CD40, CD95, CD120a, CD120b, CD134, and CD137).

The extracellular domain consists of five cysteine-rich repeats with a central hinge sequence with two N-linked glycosylation sites in cysteine repeats.

The hinge region and the area proximal to the membrane are probably O-glycosylated.

Soluble form of CD30 is released by metalloproteinase.

A variant form of CD30 (CD30v) with only the cytoplasmic domain is expressed in alveolar macrophages and is derived from an alternative promoter located in the intron.

Mol Wt: Reduced, 105 kDa; unreduced, 120 kDa.

Function

CD30 binds CD153, a TNF-family member.

It is involved in negative selection of T cells in the thymus.

CD30 plays a role in TCR-mediated cell death and reduction in cytolytic activity.

CD30 null mice have increased numbers of thymocytes, whereas CD30 overexpression in mice results in increased thymocyte apoptosis following TCR binding.

CD30 activates NF-κB, Jun N-terminal kinase (JNK), and p38 via its interaction with TRAFs1,2,3 and 5 although TRAF-independent activation of NF-κB has also been demonstrated. It also activates extracellular-regulated kinase (ERK) by an as yet unknown mechanism.

Soluble CD30 interferes with CD30 signaling by binding CD153 and preventing its interaction with the membrane CD30. Alternatively, it may form complexes with the membrane form that have greater negative influence on the cell.

Poxviruses encode soluble truncated homologues of CD30 that are capable of binding CD153.

The CD30/CD153 complex may play a role in autoimmune disease and graft versus host disease (GVHD) in transplantation recipients.

Ligands

CD30 binds CD153 (also known as CD30 ligand).

Expression

Expressed by activated B, T, and NK cells and by monocytes, Reed–Sternberg cells in Hodgkin's lymphoma, non-Hodgkin's lymphoma cells, and many other malignant cell lines.

Expression of CD30 is also detectable in the large lymphoid cells of lymph node, tonsil, thymus, deciduas, and endometrial cells with decidual cells.

Applications

CD30 is a marker of infection of lymphocytes with HIV, HTLV-1, and EBV.

Elevated soluble CD30 correlates with activity of Hepatitis B infection.

CD30$^+$ lymphoma has a better prognosis.

Gene Name	Entrez Gene#
TNFRSF8	943

Selected Monoclonal Antibodies

Ki-1 (Stein; Berlin); HRS-4 (Pfreundschuh; Cologne).

CD31

Other Names

Platelet endothelial cell adhesion molecule (PECAM-1); platelet GPIIa; endocam.

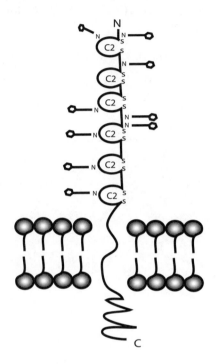

Molecular Structure

A type I integral membrane protein, a member of the Ig gene superfamily, and is related to Fcγ receptors and cytoadhesion molecules.

The 574 amino acid extracellular region consists of 6 IgC-like domains with 9 N-glycosylation sites.

N-linked glycosylation accounts for up to 20% of the molecular weight.

Domains 1 and 2 are required for homophilic binding.

The 118-residue cytoplasmic tail contains an ITIM-like sequence and is serine and tyrosine phosphorylated after activation creating docking sites for SHP-2 and possibly other signaling molecules.

The cytoplasmic domain may be palmitoylated on cysteine residue 595.

Alternative splicing leading to the omission of exon 9 (transmembrane region) occurs to varying degrees depending on the cell type and results in a soluble form.

Mol Wt: 130–140 kDa.

Function

CD31 is an adhesion molecule with no known enzymatic function and is involved in leukocyte trans-endothelial migration to sites of acute inflammation.

Cell-to-cell adhesion occurs via homophilic and heterophilic binding, but ligands other than CD31 and CD38 have not been demonstrated.

Homophilic binding may play a role in maintaining vascular integrity and permeability. CD31 has a signaling function in an adhesion cascade as CD31 ligation leads to activation of β-1, β-2, and β-3 integrins depending on the cell type.

It may be a regulator of cell survival and apoptosis as the cytoplasmic region binds β- and γ-catenin, SHP-2, and STAT3 and 5, all of which are involved in apoptopic and cell survival pathways.

CD31 knockout mice show defective transendothelial leukocyte migration as well as increased apoptopic cell death in liver, kidney, and spleen, and elevated levels of TNF-α, IFN-γ, MCP-1, MCP-2, TNF receptors, and IL-6.

Decreased levels of phosphorylated transcription factor STAT3 in CD31 knockout mice lead to greater susceptibility to endotoxic shock.

Ligands

CD31, CD38.

Expression

High level expression of CD31 is detectable on all continuous endothelium such as vascular endothelium and is concentrated in junctions between the endothelial cells in vitro.

It is expressed on polymorphonuclear cells, platelets, and T-cell subsets but not circulating B cells.

Soluble forms are found in serum.

Applications

Minor histocompatibility antigen associated with graft versus host disease (GVHD) in bone marrow transplantation.

Gene Name	Entrez Gene#
PECAM1	5175

Selected Monoclonal Antibodies

SG134 (Goyert; New York); TM3 (Ohto; Saitama); CLB-HEC/75 (von dem Borne; Amsterdam).

CD32

Other Names

Fcγ receptor type II (FcγRII), gp40.

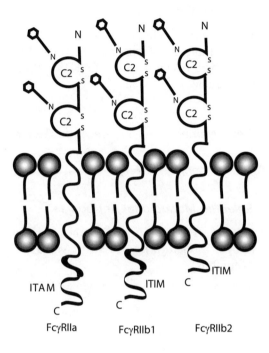

FcγRIIa   FcγRIIb1   FcγRIIb2

Molecular Structure

The extracellular region consists of two IgC-like domains each with a single N-glycosylation site.

At least 9 isoforms are known that originate from alternative splicing of three genes on chromosome 1q23-24 (FcγRIIA, -B, and -C).

Major differences between the isoforms are in the cytoplasmic domains, but minor extracellular domain differences also occur.

Intracellular region has ITAM ("a" and "c" isoforms) or ITIM ("b" isoform).

FcγRIIc has high homology with the extracellular domain of FcγRIIb and with the intracellular region of the FcγRIIa.

Alternative splicing of FcγRIIa gives rise to two products, one of which lacks a membrane anchor (FcγRIIa2).

Three splicing variants of FcγRIIb occur. FcγRIIb1 has a 19 amino acid insert in the cytoplasmic domain.

FcγRIIb3 lacks L2 exon in the extracellular region but otherwise is identical to FcγRIIb1.

Four isoforms of FcγRIIc have been described in NK cells. FcγRIIc1 is a functional membrane-bound molecule, FcγRIIc2 and c3 lack the ITAM sequence, and FcγRIIc4 is a soluble form.

Isoform expression is cell-type dependent.

FcγRIIa displays a functionally distinct polymorphism. A G to A point mutation in the ligand-binding domain causes an arginine (R) to histidine (H) substitution and results in two phenotypes FcγRIIa-R131 and FcγRIIa-H131.

Mol Wt: Reduced, 40 kDa.

Function

FcγRII molecules have low affinity for monomeric IgG but bind immune complexes efficiently.

ITAM-bearing isoforms mediate activation and ITIM-bearing FcγRII downregulate responses.

Present on platelets where it can trigger aggregation and granule release.

FcγRIIa is a potent inducer of phagocytosis and degranulation.

Heterotypic linking of FcγRIIa and FcγRIIIb triggers synergistic responses and may be important for regulation and induction of select leukocyte functions.

FcγRIIa-H131 is the only receptor that interacts with IgG2 and is probably involved in clearing of encapsulated bacteria.

FcγRIIb isoforms mediate feedback inhibition of B-cell responses and inhibition of antibody uptake and presentation to T cells.

Murine studies demonstrate FcγRIIb regulates inflammatory responses.

FcγRIIc expression on NK cells varies between individuals due to polymorphisms in the FcγRIIc gene.

In vivo function of FcγRIIc has yet to be determined, but in vitro studies show that triggering with antigen-antibody complexes results in cell activation and triggering of antibody-dependent cellular cytotoxicity (ADCC).

Ligands

CD32 binds IgG aggregates or complexes with antigen.

Expression

Different cell types express different isoforms.

FcγRIIa is expressed on all myeloid cells, platelets, epithelial cells, dendritic cells, and Langerhans cells, with low expression on a T-cell subset.

FcγRIIb is found on B cells, monocytes, and macrophages.

FcγRIIc is expresssed on NK cells.

Applications

A polymorphism in the extracellular region of the a and c isoforms may be related to pathology, because only the H131 allele binds IgG2.

Gene Name	Entrez Gene#
FCGR2A	2212 (FcγRIIa)

Selected Monoclonal Antibodies

CIKM5 (Pilkington; Melbourne); 41H16 (Boyd; Victoria); IV.3 (Anderson; Columbus).

CD33

Other Names

My9, gp67, p67, Siglec3.

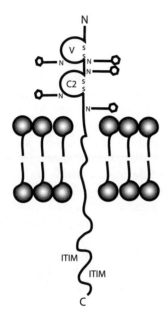

Molecular Structure

A type I transmembrane glycoprotein of 364 amino acids and smallest member of the sialoadhesin family or sialic acid-binding Ig-like lectin (Siglec) subgroup within the Ig supergene family (see also CD22).

The extracellular region of 241 amino acids consists of one IgV- and one IgC-like domain with 5 sites for N-glycosylation.

The transmembrane domain consists of 22 amino acids and the cytoplasmic domain of 81 residues has 2 immunoreceptor tyrosine-based inhibitory motifs (ITIMs).

CD33 is expressed on the cell surface as both monomers and homodimers.

Amino terminal V domain interacts with sialic acid, but the IgC-like domain is also required for binding.

Mol Wt: Reduced, 67 kDa; unreduced, 150 kDa.

Function

Lectin that binds α-2, 3- and α-2, 6-linked sialic acid bearing proteins and mediates intercellular adhesion.

Intracellular ITIM sequence serves as binding site for Src homology 2 domain-containing protein tyrosine phosphatase (SHP)-1 that in turn has an inhibitory effect on signal transduction.

Although in vivo function is unknown, in vitro studies suggest CD33 plays a negative regulatory role in myeloid hematopoiesis.

Ligands

Binds α2,3- and α2,6-linked sialic acid bearing glycans.

Expression

Principally restricted to cells of myeloid lineage with decreasing expression on maturation and differentiation.

Strong on monocytes, macrophages, dendritic cells, and Langerhans cells but weak on polymorphonuclear cells.

Found on hematopoietic progenitor cells but not on the earliest stem cells.

Applications

Phenotypic marker in acute myeloid leukemia (AML) particularly types M1-5 (FAB classification).

Target in treatment of CD33$^+$ AML patients, with a humanised CD33 antibody (Myelotarg) conjugated to a cytotoxic drug approved for clinical use.

Gene Name   Entrez Gene#

CD33   945

Selected Monoclonal Antibodies

My9 (Griffin; Boston); L4F3 (Bernstein; Seattle); H153 (Herrmann; Freiburg).

CD34

Other Names

My10, gp105-120.

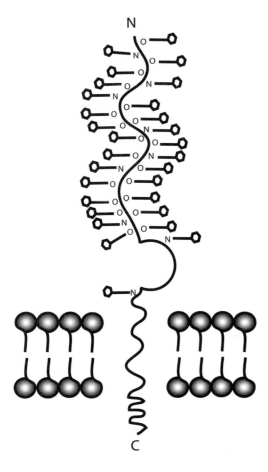

Molecular Structure

CD34 is a sialomucin-like (see CD43, CD68, CD164) type I transmembrane glycophosphoprotein of either 385 or 328 amino acids.

A cysteine-rich Ig-like domain is present in the 258-residue extracellular region.

The 73 amino acid cytoplasmic region has consensus sites for protein kinase C (PKC) phosphorylation, serine and threonine phosphorylation by other kinases, and tyrosine phosphorylation. Only serine phosphorylation has been demonstrated.

Two spliced forms exist; the shorter form lacks most of the cytoplasmic region (only 16 residues remain) including the potential phosphorylation sites.

The protein core is highly N- and O-glycosylated.

Mol Wt: 40 kDa.

Function

CD34 is a potential cytoadhesion molecule probably interacting with CD62E and CD62L molecules.

Knockout mice have no defect in leukocyte trafficking, but in one study have shown decreased progenitors.

More recently a study of mast cell adhesion in CD34-deficient mice found increased mast cell aggregation and an inability to repopulate with mast cells and hematopoietic precursors in the absence of CD34 suggesting a role for CD34 as a negative regulator of cell adhesion.

Antibodies recognize at least three different epitopes, some can induce integrin dependent cell adhesion.

Ligands

Binds CD62L (L-selectin) and CD62E (E-selectin).

Expression

Expressed by hematopoietic precursor cells, bone marrow stromal cells, capillary endothelium, embryonic fibroblasts, and some cells in fetal and adult nervous tissue.

Applications

CD34 is a marker for stem cells and is used in stem cell enrichment.

Gene Name	Entrez Gene#
CD34	947

Selected Monoclonal Antibodies

My10 (Civin; Baltimore); BI-3C5 (Tindle; Brisbane); ICH3 (Levinsky; London).

CD35

Other Names

C3b/C4b receptor; complement receptor type 1 (CR1), Immune adherence receptor.

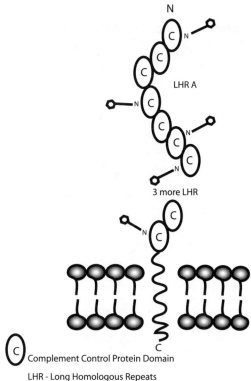

3 more LHR

Complement Control Protein Domain

LHR - Long Homologous Repeats

Molecular Structure

CD35 is a 998 amino acid, type 1, single-chain polymorphic glycoprotein existing in four allelic forms. The A allotype occurs at a frequency of 80%, B at 18%, and the others are rare.

It is a member of the regulators of complement activation (RCA) gene family consisting of 3 to 6 homologous repeats (allotype dependent), each of which contains 7 complement control protein (CCP) repeats also known as short consensus repeats (SCRs) of about 65 amino acids (see CD21, CD46, CD55).

Each repeat has four conserved cysteines and a tryptophan.

The high sequence homology between every seventh repeat enables grouping of SCRs into long homologous repeats (LHRs) A, B, C, and D.

The extracellular domain (for the most common allotype, A) consists of 930 amino acids and has 24 potential N-linked glycosylation sites.

The transmembrane domain consists of 25 amino acids, and the cytoplasmic domain has 43 amino acids.

Molecular mass polymorphism is due to the variable number of SCRs encoded by different alleles.

The functional domains map to the first three SCRs of LHRs A, B, and C.

Mol Wt: (for the common A allotype): In erythrocytes: Reduced, 190, 220, 250, 280 kDa; unreduced, 160, 190, 220, 250 kDa. In leukocytes: Reduced, 195, 225, 255, 285 kDa; unreduced, 165, 195, 225, 255 kDa.

Function

The major role of CD35 is the removal and processing of immune complexes and facilitating transport to lymphoid follicles.

It binds C3b, iC3b, C3dg, and C4b complement fragments and is the receptor for C3b and C4b bound to immune complexes.

CD35 limits complement activation and creates ligands for complement receptors by accelerating the decay of C3 and C5 convertases and acting as a cofactor to plasma serine protease factor 1, which cleaves C3b and C4b.

CD35 mediates adherence of C4b/C3b coated particles in preparation for phagocytosis.

All four allotypes of CD35 carry the Knops blood group antigen polymorphism, with one allele more common in individuals of African origin reported to confer some protection against severe malaria.

Invasion by a number of bacterial and protozoan pathogens is facilitated by CD35.

Ligands

CD35 binds C3b, iC3b, C3dg, C4b, iC3, and iC4.

Expression

Expressed on erythrocytes, neutrophils, monocytes, eosinophils, B lymphocytes, and 10–15% T cells.

Applications

Soluble CD35 is currently undergoing clinical trials as a complement inhibitor.

Gene Name	Entrez Gene#
CR1	1378

Selected Monoclonal Antibodies

TO5 (Mason; Oxford); J3B11 (Kazatchkine; Paris); CB04C (Malavasi; Torino).

CD36

Other Names

Platelet GPIV, GPIIIb, OKM-5 antigen, PASIV.

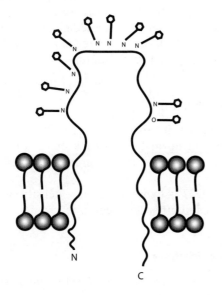

Molecular Structure

A transmembrane glycoprotein and a member of the SR-B subgroup of the scavenger receptor superfamily.

The protein consists of 471 amino acids and contains two hydrophobic segments that are thought to be two transmembrane domains resulting in N- and C-terminal cytoplasmic tails.

The extracellular region is heavily glycosylated with 10 N-linked and 1 O-linked glycosylation sites.

CD36 is palmitoylated on both cytoplasmic tails.

Threonine 92 is phosphorylated.

Mol Wt: Reduced, 85 kDa; unreduced (platelets), 88–113 kDa.

Function

Scavenger receptor for oxidized low density lipoproteins (LDL).

Binds thrombospondin, collagen I, IV, and V.

Recognition and phagocytosis of apoptotic cells, including shed photoreceptor outer segments cells of the eye.

Adherence of *Plasmodium falciparum*-infected erythrocytes to microvascular endothelial cells.

Acts as a cell adhesion molecule involved in platelet adhesion and aggregation as well as platelet-monocyte adhesion and platelet–tumor cell interaction.

Interacts with fatty acid translocase (FAT) of pancreatic β cells and mediates fatty acid effects on insulin secretion.

In patients with type 1 and type 2 diabetes, CD36 expression is upregulated on macrophages during hyperglycemia and is associated with atherosclerotic lesions. Murine model of diabetes suggests increased expression of CD36 in renal proximal tubular cells renders them more susceptible to apoptosis.

CD36 also has a role in the innate immune system, binding bacterial diacyl glycerides and presenting them to Toll-like receptor (TLR) 2 and TLR6.

Ligands

CD36 binds oxidized LDL, long chain fatty acids, anionic phospholipids, collagen types I, IV, and V, thrombospondin, *Plasmodium falciparum*-infected erythrocytes, and bacterial diacyl glycerides.

Expression

Expressed by platelets, mature monocytes, macrophages, microvascular endothelial cells, mammary endothelial cells, and pancreatic β cells.

Gene Name	Entrez Gene#
CD36	948

Selected Monoclonal Antibodies

5F1 (Bernstein; Seattle); CIMeg1 (Pilkington; Melbourne); SMO (Hogg; London).

CD37

Other Names

gp52-40, Tspan-26.

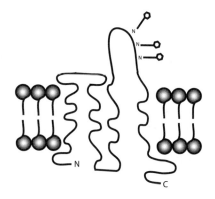

Molecular Structure

A glycoprotein member of the TM4SF (Tetraspanin) family, with both termini cytoplasmic and two extracellular loops (see also CD9).

The 281 amino acid protein core of 26 kDa contains 3 N-glycosylation sites, with generally only 2 sites occupied.

Mol Wt: 40–64 kDa.

Function

CD37 Forms complexes in the B-cell membrane with CD53, CD81, CD82, and MHC class II, which may be involved in antigen transport and processing.

Knockout mice show normal hematopoietic cell development but have impaired T-cell-dependent B-cell responses. These mice have altered TCR signaling, increased T-cell proliferation, increased IL-2 production, as well as increased kinase activity of Lck, which suggests a regulatory role for CD37 in T-cell proliferation.

Expression

High density expression of CD37 is present on normal and neoplastic mature B cells but is lost on maturation to plasma cells.

CD37 is expressed at low density on T cells and other leukocytes.

Applications

CD37 is a marker of B cells and B-cell malignancies.

Gene Name	Entrez Gene#
CD37	951

Selected Monoclonal Antibodies

HD28 (Dörken; Berlin); HH-1 (Funderud; Oslo); G28-1 (Clark; Seattle).

CD38

Other Names

T10, gp45, ADP-ribosyl cyclase.

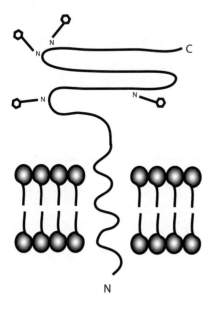

Molecular Structure

A single-chain, type II, transmembrane glycoprotein of 300 amino acids with 4 N-glycosylation sites and 6 disulphide bridges.

256 amino acid extracellular domain has the catalytic domain, 2 hyaluronic acid binding sites, and 11 conserved cysteines. Four cysteines (119, 160, 173, and 201) are esssential for synthesis and hydrolysis of cADPR.

Several leucines distributed in the extracellular and transmembrane regions can potentially form leucine zipper motifs that may allow interaction of CD38 with other molecules.

21-residue transmembrane domain.

23 amino acid N-terminal cytoplasmic domain does not contain any motifs known to associate with signaling molecules.

Post-translational modification on myeloid leukemic cells leads to expression of 190-kDa oligomeric form.

Soluble form found in serum exists as either a monomer or dimer, both of which have normal enzymatic activity.

Mol Wt: 45 kDa; soluble form, 39 kDa.

Function

CD38 is a multifunctional molecule that can act as an ectoenzyme and cytosolic enzyme, adhesion molecule, and has regulatory functions.

It can act as a NAD^+ glycohydrolase, ADP-ribosyl cyclase, and ADP-ribose hydrolase.

It is able to bind CD31 enabling adherence of lymphocytes to endothelial cell and can bind hyaluronic acid in extracellular matrix.

CD38 appears to act as a channel that allows activation signals to enter monocytes, NK, T, and B cells resulting in synthesis and release of cytokine and cytoplasmic calcium fluxes.

CD38 signaling requires involvement of B-cell receptor (BCR) or T-cell receptor (TCR).

CD38 regulates T-cell-mediated cytotoxicity.

Ligation of CD38 induces cell activation and proliferation or death depending on the cellular environment.

Knockout mice show deficiencies in enzyme activities.

Ligands

CD31, hyaluronic acid.

Expression

Early stages of maturation of CD34+ progenitor into commited erythroid, lymphoid, and myeloid precursors.

Early B and T cells, activated T cells, germinal center B cells, plasma cells, and NK cells.

50–80% mononuclear cells in the first 3 years of life with gradual decline thereafter. Tissues with high glucose metabolism.

Applications

CD38 is a phenotypic and prognostic marker in leukemia and in HIV-1. It is used to purify bone marrow and germinal center subsets and is a target of immunotherapy in myeloma treatment.

Anti-CD38 antibodies are found in patients in type I and II diabetes mellitus.

Gene Name	Entrez Gene#
CD38	952

Selected Monoclonal Antibodies

T10 (Schlossman; Boston); HB7 (Tedder; Boston); GR7A4 (Garrido; Granada).

CD39

Other Names

gp80, E-ATPDase, NTPDase-1, ecto-apyrase, ecto-diphosphohydrolase; EC 3.6.1.5.

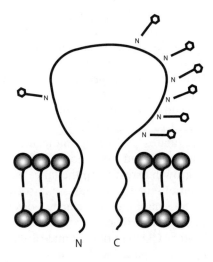

Molecular Structure

A member of the ecto-apyrase family.

Based on its primary structure, CD39 is predicted to have two transmembrane domains near the N- and C- terminal ends, short N and C terminal cytoplasmic tails, and a large extracellular domain that contains the enzymatic site.

Seven potential N-glycosylation sites at Asn 73, 226, 291, 333, 375, 429, and 458. Mutations of these sites indicate glycosylation is important for formation of a functional molecule.

CD39 has five highly conserved regions characteristic of the ecto-apyrase family called apyrase conserved regions (ACR) 1-5.

ACR1 and 4 share similarity with the β- and γ-phosphate binding domains of cytoplasmic ATPase superfamily.

Mutations in ACRs lead to the loss of enzymatic activity, whereas mutations in other residues can change the nucleotide specificity of the isoform.

The formation of oligomers in the plasma membrane is essential for enzyme activity.

Transmembrane regions TM1 and TM2 are helical and appear to interact with each other and with TM regions of other CD39 molecules.

Mol Wt: 78 kDa.

Function

CD39 is a cation-dependent enzyme that hydrolyses ATP and ADP equally and other di- and tri-phosphate nucleosides.

Hydrolysis of ATP and ADP inhibits inflammatory and thrombotic responses.

Soluble CD39 can also prevent ADP-induced platelet aggregation.

Thrombin deactivates CD39 on endothelial cells.

In the nervous system, CD39 hydrolyzes ATP and other nucleotides to regulate purinergic neurotransmission.

Knockout mice have prolonged bleeding times.

Expression

Expressed by mantle zone B cells, activated T cells, NK cells, macrophages, Langerhans cells, dendritic cells, neurons, platelets, and endothelial cells.

Gene Name	Entrez Gene#
ENTPD1	953

Selected Monoclonal Antibodies

G28-10 (Ledbetter; Seattle); AC2 (Rowe; Birmingham); R22 (Hekman; Amsterdam).

CD40

Other Names

Bp50, TNF receptor 5.

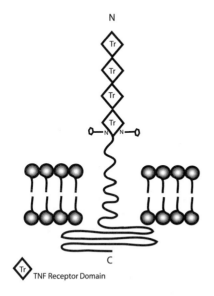

TNF Receptor Domain

Molecular Structure

A type I integral membrane glycoprotein.

Member of the tumor necrosis factor (TNF)/nerve growth factor (NGF) receptor family (see CD27, CD30, CD95, CD120a, CD120b, CD134, and CDw137).

The 193 amino acid extracellular domain consists of four cysteine-rich repeats.

A 22 hydrophobic amino acid transmembrane region.

The 42 amino acid cytoplasmic region contains two distinct functional domains.

Phosphorylated on serine and threonine residues but not on tyrosines.

Two alternatively spliced transcript variants encoding distinct isoforms have been reported.

The overall polypeptide portion is about 28 kDa, indicating that about 20 kDa of the glycoprotein may consist of carbohydrate.

Mol Wt: Reduced, 48 kDa; unreduced, 85 kDa (dimers).

Function

Receptor for CD154 (CD40L) providing a costimulatory signal to B cells, which influences their growth, differentiation and isotype switching. Can provide rescue signal preventing apoptosis of germinal center B cells, therefore, influencing B-cell selection.

Promotes cytokine production by monocytes and dendritic cells.

Involved in cognate T–B interaction and is central to T-cell-dependent responses.

Upregulates adhesion molecules on dendritic cells and keratinocytes and promotes growth arrest in epithelial cells.

Mutations in the ligand are associated with the immune deficiency disorder Hyper-IgM syndrome.

CD40 or CD50 knockout mice are more susceptible to parasitic infection.

CD40 antibodies can deliver progression signals that augment the proliferation of activated B cells. CD40 antibodies are costimulatory with competence signals, including anti-IgM, CD20 antibodies, and PMA, but are not costimulatory with IL-4, or low-molecular-weight B-cell growth factor.

Ligands

CD154 (CD40L).

Expression

B cells (pro-B through to plasma cells), monocytes, follicular dendritic cells, basal epithelial cells, endothelial cells, fibroblasts, keratinocytes, interdigitating cells, and CD34+ hematopoietic progenitor cells.

Applications

The CD40 antibody can substitute for CD40 ligand in activating B cells.

Potential therapeutic target in treatment of autoimmunity, allograft rejection, and atherosclerosis.

Gene Name	Entrez Gene#
TNFRSF5	958

Selected Monoclonal Antibodies

G28-5 (Ledbetter; Seattle); EA-5 (LeBien; Minneapolis); BE-1 (LeBien; Minneapolis).

CD41

Other Names

Platelet glycoprotein GPIIb, α IIb integrin chain.

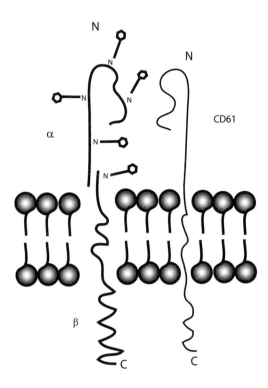

Molecular Structure

CD41 is a member of the integrin α-chain family (see CD11a, b, c).

A 140-kDa transmembrane glycoprotein post-translationally cleaved into a disulfide-linked 120-kDa α-chain (GPIIba) and a 22-kDa β-chain (GPIIbb), which forms a calcium-dependent complex with platelet glycoprotein GPIIIa (CD61).

GPIIba is extracellular and has four repeated sequences with similarity to the calcium-binding repeats of other proteins, which may be involved in binding of divalent cations.

GPIIbb is the membrane bound portion of GPIIb and has a 91 amino acid extracellular domain, 26-residue transmembrane region, and 20 amino acid C-terminal cytoplasmic domain.

CD41 has five potential N-linked glycosylation sites and is O-glycosylated on serine residues.

Alternatively spliced form lacking exon 28 has been described.

CD41 antibodies react with that complex but not with the isolated subunits.

Mol Wt: Reduced, 135 kDa; unreduced, 120 kDa (GPIIba), 23 kDa (GPIIbb).

Function

CD41/CD61 complex is involved in platelet activation and aggregation and platelet binding to extracellular matrix proteins.

This complex functions as an activation-dependent receptor for fibrinogen, fibronectin, and von Willebrand factor (vWF) and binds to RGD-containing sequences in adhesion molecules.

Mutations in CD41 that give rise to a dysfunctional CD41/CD61 complex result in the development of Glanzmann's thrombasthenia (GT).

Several alloantigenic polymorphisms of CD41 have been identified, of which at least two are involved in alloimmune thrombocytopenia.

Ligands

CD41/CD61 complex binds soluble fibrinogen and many other RGD-containing proteins such as vWF and fibronectin.

Expression

Platelets and platelet precursors (megakaryocytes).

Applications

Marker for GT and megakaryoblastic leukemias.

Target in anti-thrombotic therapy.

Selected Monoclonal Antibodies

CLB-thromb/7 (Tetteroo; Leiden); VIPL1 (Knapp; Vienna); J15 (McMichael; Oxford).

Gene Name	Entrez Gene#
ITGA2B	3674

CD42a

Other Names

Platelet glycoprotein GPIX, gp9.

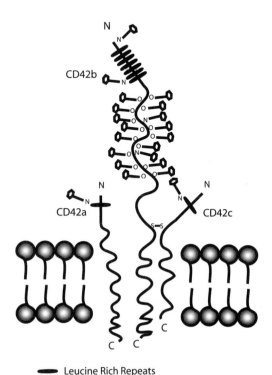

— Leucine Rich Repeats

Molecular Structure

CD42a is a type I membrane protein that forms a noncovalent complex (CD42 complex) with platelet glycoproteins GPIba (CD42b), GPIbb (CD42c), and GPV (CD42c). It has one leucine-rich repeat at the N-terminus.

CD42a consists of a 134 amino acid N-terminal extracellular domain, 20 amino acid transmembrane region, and 6-residue cytoplasmic domain.

The extracellular domain contains one N-glycosylation site and may be myristoylated.

See also CD42b, CD42c, and CD42d.

Mol Wt: Reduced, 17–22 kDa; unreduced, 22 kDa.

Function

CD42a combines with CD42b, CD42c, and CD42d to form the CD42 complex.

The CD42 complex functions as a receptor for the von Willebrand factor (vWF) and as a vWF-dependent adhesion receptor, thus mediating adhesion of platelets at high shear rates to vWF in the sub-endothelial matrices that are exposed when damage to endothelium occurs.

When thrombin is present, the CD42 complex amplifies the response to thrombin during platelet activation.

Mutations in CD42a (and/or other CD42 molecules) can give rise to the bleeding disorder Bernard–Soulier syndrome.

Ligands

CD42 complex binds von Willebrand factor and thrombin.

Expression

CD42a is expressed by platelets and megakaryocytes.

Gene Name	Entrez Gene#
GP9	2815

Selected Monoclonal Antibodies

FMC25 (Zola; Adelaide); BL-H6 (Fiebig; Leipzig); GR-P (Garrido; Granada).

CD42b

Other Names

Platelet glycoprotein GPIb-α, Glycocalicin.

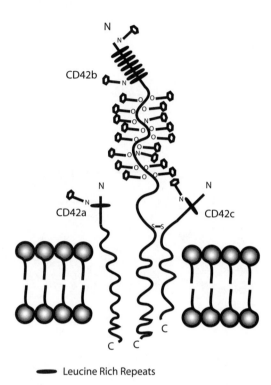

— Leucine Rich Repeats

Molecular Structure

CD42b is a mucin that belongs to the leucine-rich repeat family.

It is the α chain (GPIbα) of a 160-kDa heterodimer complex known as platelet glycoprotein Ib (GPIb) and is disulfide linked with the β chain (CD42c).

GPIb noncovalently associates with CD42a and CD42d.

CD42b has 481 amino acid N-terminal extracellular domain, 29-residue transmembrane region, and 100 amino acid cytoplasmic domain.

The extracellular domain has seven tandem leucine rich repeats of 24 amino acids flanked by 22 amino acid consensus sequences.

Two hydrophilic regions, one of which is extensively O-glycosylated.

Two possible N-glycosylation sites and three sulfated tyrosine residues (Tyr276, 278, 279).

Size polymorphisms occur where between one and four copies of a 13 amino acid sequence occurs in the highly O-glycosylated region.

A single amino acid polymorphism (Met145-Thr) gives rise to the Ko (Syp, HPA-2) alloantigen system.

Acylation, primarily palmitoylation of GPIb, has been described.

See also CD42a, CD42c, and CD42d.

Mol Wt: Reduced, 145 kDa; unreduced, 160 kDa (heterodimer).

Function

CD42b combines with CD42a, CD42c, and CD42d to form the CD42 complex.

The CD42 complex functions as a receptor for von Willebrand factor (vWF) and as a vWF-dependent adhesion receptor.

The CD42 complex mediates adhesion of platelets at high shear rates to vWF present in the subendothelial matrix, which becomes accessible following damage to the endothelium.

This complex also amplifies the response of platelets to thrombin during platelet activation.

The CD42b cytoplasmic domain associates via actin-binding protein filamin with the cytoskeleton and is the binding site in the CD42 complex for the 14-3-3 ζ protein.

The binding site for vWF and thrombin is on CD42b.

Mutations in CD42b (and/or other CD42 molecules) can give rise to the bleeding disorder Bernard–Soulier syndrome.

Ligands

The CD42 complex binds von Willebrand factor and thrombin.

Expression

CD42b is expressed by platelets and megakaryocytes.

Selected Monoclonal Antibodies

AN51 (McMichael; Oxford); PHN89 (Bai; Beijing); MB45 (von dem Borne; Amsterdam).

Gene Name	Entrez Gene#
GP1BA	2811

CD42c

Other Names

Platelet glycoprotein GPIb-β.

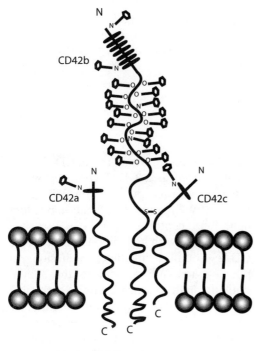

— Leucine Rich Repeats

Molecular Structure

CD42c is a member of the leucine-rich repeat family (see CD42a, CD42b, and CD42d).

CD42c is the 22-kDa β-chain of platelet glycoprotein GPIb; the other component of this disulphide linked heterodimer being CD42b (the α-chain).

A 122 amino acid extracellular region followed by a 25 amino acid transmembrane region and a 34 amino acid cytoplasmic domain.

The extracellular domain has one tandem leucine-rich repeat sequence of 24 amino acids flanked by consensus sequences of 22 amino acids.

One potential N-glycosylation site and a phosphorylation site at Ser166.

Mol Wt: Reduced, 24 kDa; unreduced, 160 kDa (heterodimer).

Function

CD42c combines with CD42b, CD42a, and CD42d to form a CD42 complex, which functions as a receptor for von Willebrand factor (vWF) and as a vWF-dependent adhesion receptor.

The CD42 complex mediates adhesion of platelets at high shear rates to vWF present in subendothelial matrix, which becomes accessible following damage to the endothelium.

This complex also amplifies the response of platelets to thrombin during platelet activation.

Cytoskeletal interactions may be regulated by phosphorylation of Ser166. Mutations in CD42c (and/or other CD42 molecules) can give rise to the bleeding disorder Bernard–Soulier syndrome.

Ligands

CD42 complex binds von Willebrand factor and thrombin.

Expression

CD42c is expressed by platelets and megakaryocytes.

Gene Name	Entrez Gene#
GP1BB	2812

Selected Monoclonal Antibodies

GI27 (Santoso; Giessen).

CD42d

Other Names

Platelet glycoprotein GPV.

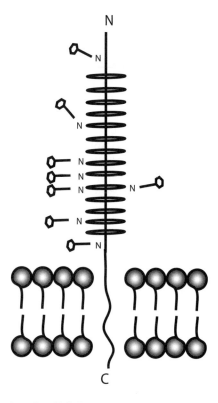

━━━ Leucine Rich Repeats

Molecular Structure

CD42d is a single-chain, type 1, transmembrane glycoprotein and subunit of the CD42 complex (see also CD42a, b, and c).

It forms a noncovalent complex with CD42a, b, and c.

CD42d consists of a N-terminal extracytoplasmic region of 504 amino acids, a transmembrane domain of 24 amino acids, and a short cytoplasmic region of 16 amino acids.

The extracellular domain contains 14 leucine-rich glycoprotein repeat sequences of 24 amino acids, flanked by consensus flanking sequences of 22 amino acids as well as a thrombin cleavage site and cleavage sites for other physiologically relevant proteases such as calpain.

The protein has eight potential N-glycosylation sites and may have two to three O-glycosylation sites in a region close to the membrane.

Mol Wt: 82 kDa.

Function

CD42d combines with CD42a, CD42b, and CD42c to form a CD42 complex, which functions as a receptor for von Willebrand factor (vWF) and as a vWF-dependent adhesion receptor.

In regions with high blood flow rates, the CD42 complex mediates adhesion of platelets to vWF present in the subendothelial matrix, which becomes accessible following damage to the endothelium. This complex also amplifies the response of platelets to thrombin during platelet activation.

Ligands

CD42 complex binds von Willebrand factor and thrombin.

Expression

CD42d is expressed by platelets and megakaryocytes.

Gene Name	Entrez Gene#
GP5	2814

Selected Monoclonal Antibodies

SW16 (von dem Borne; Amsterdam).

CD43

Other Names

Leukosialin; gp95; sialophorin; leukocyte sialoglycoprotein, gpL115.

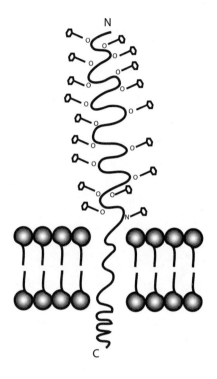

Molecular Structure

CD43 is a highly O-sialylated type I integral membrane protein and a member of the cell surface mucin family (see CD34, CD68, and CD164).

CD43 is a single-chain molecule of 385 amino acids with a 245 amino acid extracellular domain made up of 5 repeats of an 18 amino acid sequence rich in serine and threonine residues.

It is predicted to form an extended rod-like structure of 45 nm in length.

The whole of the extracellular domain is highly serine and threonine glycosylated and has one N-linked glycosylation site in the membrane-proximal region.

Serine residues of the cytoplasmic domain are constitutively phosphorylated to a low level and superphosphorylated upon activation.

A soluble form known as galactoglycoprotein is shed into serum.

Mol Wt: Resting lymphocytes, 95–115 kDa; activated lymphocytes and neutrophils, 115–135 kDa.

Function

CD43 possibly acts to inhibit cell-to-cell adhesion of leukocytes due to its long rod-like structure and several negatively charged residues.

Under other conditions, CD43 is possibly involved in adhesion via its interaction with CD54. In migrating lymphocytes, CD43 via its intracellular domain interacts with actin-binding proteins moesin and ezrin and is subsequently redistributed to uropods, which the cell uses for traction during migration.

CD43 promotes T-cell activation and proliferation by inducing IL-2 and CD69 expression. IL-2 production is dependent on a functional intracellular domain.

It acts as a T-cell counter-receptor for the macrophage-adhesion receptor CD169 (sialoadhesin/Siglec-1).

Knockout mice show increased T-cell adhesion and easier activation.

Ligands

CD43 binds CD54, MHC class I, CD62P, and hyaluronic acid and acts as a T-cell counter-receptor for CD169.

Expression

High level expression of CD43 is found on all leukocytes except resting B cells.

The extent of sialylation of CD43 varies between cell types.

Activation of lymphocytes and neu-trophils leads to rapid shedding of CD43 molecules from the cell surface.

Applications

CD43 is a histopathological marker for the identification of normal and malignant T cells in tissue section.

It is a useful marker for leukemia and lymphoma phenotyping.

Gene Name	Entrez Gene#
SPN	6693

Selected Monoclonal Antibodies

G10-2 (Ledbetter; Seattle); L60 (Buck; Mountain View); MEM-59 (Horejsi; Prague).

CD44

Other Names

Phagocyte glycoprotein 1 (Pgp-1); gp80-95; Hermes antigen, ECMR-III, HUTCH-I, H-CAM.

Variant forms are known as CD44R or CD44v1-10.

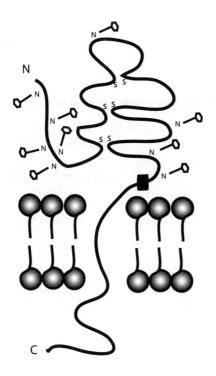

■ Splice Insertion Site

Molecular Structure

CD44 is a member of the cartilage link protein (hyaladhesin) family.

The standard CD44 molecule (CD44s) is a 341 amino acid molecule with a 248 amino acid extracellular domain, 21 amino acid transmembrane region, and 72-residue intracellular domain.

A large number of CD44 isoforms arise from complex alternative splicing of 19 exons in the gene.

Exons 1-5, 16, and 17 form the invariant extracellular portion of CD44s.

Alternative splicing can insert 10 variant exons either individually or in multiple combinations within the invariant region.

Ligand binding specificity is regulated by alternative splicing probably by altering the structure of the CD44 molecule.

The CD44s extracellular domain has six cysteine residues that have the potential to form a globular domain.

The protein has multiple potential N- and O-linked glycosylation sites as well as several sites for the addition of chondroitin or heparin sulfate. Post-translational modifications at these sites results in even greater diversity of isoforms. Exon 8-containing isoforms can also be modified by heparan sulfate.

The cytoplasmic domain has six serine residues, which are potential phosphorylation sites. The N terminus has significant homology with cartilage link and proteoglycan core proteins that bind hyaluronan.

Mol Wt: 90 kDa when glycosylated; 180–200 kDa after glycosaminoglycan modification.

Function

CD44 maintains polar orientation of epithelial cells by binding to hyaluronan in the basement membrane.

The activity of the many isoforms of CD44R remains to be clarified. The expression of variant isoforms of CD44 appears to correlate with hyaluronan-binding.

Binding to hyaluronic acids results in suppression of apoptosis during hematopoiesis.

CD44R and, in particular, CD44v6-containing isoforms may be involved in leukocyte attachment to and rolling on endothelial cells, homing to peripheral lymphoid organs and to sites of inflammation.

CD44v6 isoforms have been implicated in tumor metastasis.

CD44 signaling induces cytokine release and T-cell activation.

The glycosylation pattern determines the ability of the molecule to bind ligands and growth factors.

Streptococcus pyogenes produces a hyaluronic acid that can bind CD44, thus enabling the organism to adhere to and invade tissues.

Ligands

CD44 binds hyaluronan, osteopontin, MIP1b, E-selectin, MIF, MIP1b, and CD74.

Expression

CD44 is expressed on leukocytes and erythrocytes, whereas CD44R encompasses a diverse group of CD44 variant isoforms constitutively expressed in epithelial cells and monocyte-lineage cells, whose expression is upregulated in activated lymphocytes.

Applications

CD44 variants are useful phenotypic and prognostic markers in non-Hodgkin's lymphoma, gastric and colonic tumors, and breast cancer.

Gene Name	Entrez Gene#
CD44	960

Selected Monoclonal Antibodies

F-10-44-2 (Dalchau; East Grinstead); GRHL1 (Garrido; Granada); BRIC35 (Anstee; Oxford).

CD44R: FW11.24 (Mackay; Baltimore).

CD45

Other Names

Leukocyte common antigen, LCA, B220, CD45R, RA, RO, RC, RB isoforms, Ly5, T200, EC 3.1.34.

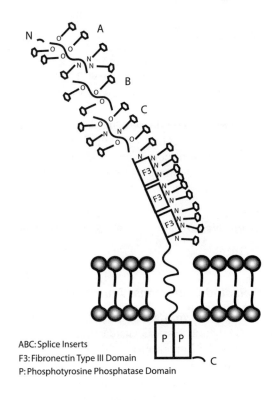

ABC: Splice Inserts
F3: Fibronectin Type III Domain
P: Phosphotyrosine Phosphatase Domain

Molecular Structure

CD45 is a type I transmembrane glycoprotein and a receptor-like protein tyrosine phosphatase (PTP).

Exons 4, 5, and 6 encode extracellular regions referred to as A, B, and C inserts, respectively. Alternative splicing of these regions results in multiple isoforms of CD45 that range in size from 1120 to 1281 amino acids.

A, B, and C regions have multiple O-linked glycosylation sites and are variably modified by sialic acid leading to further size variation between CD45 molecules.

The 220-kDa isoform has all three inserts, the 210-kDa isoforms have either the A and B or the B and C determinants, the 200-kDa isoform has the B determinant, and the 180-kDa isoform lacks A, B, and C.

CD45RA descibes isoforms of CD45 sharing the exon 4 (A) sequence.

CD45RO is a 180-kDa isoform of the CD45 molecule family and does not contain A, B, or C inserts.

CD45RB describes isoforms sharing exon 5 (B) inserts.

CD45RC describes isoforms of CD45 sharing exon 6 (C) sequences.

The extracellular domain has three potential fibronectin type III (FNIII) domains that are extensively N-glycosylated. The membrane proximal FNIII domain is more glycosylated than the other two domains.

The 707 amino acid cytoplasmic tail has two phosphatase domains, but only the first has significant phosphatase activity as the second domain lacks an amino acid essential for catalytic activity. Membrane modeling predicts that the membrane proximal region of the cytoplasmic domain forms a structural wedge.

Mol Wt: 180 kDa, 200 kDa, 210 kDa, 220 kDa.

Function

The CD45 molecule has intrinsic cytoplasmic protein tyrosine phosphatase activity and probably functions in specific signal transduction pathways via protein tyrosine dephosphorylation.

It is essential for T- and B-cell antigen receptor-mediated activation and may be required for receptor-mediated activation in other leukocytes.

Cross-linking of CD45 induces apoptosis of lymphocytes.

CD45 regulates Src-kinases such as p56lck and p59fyn, which are required for T- and B-cell receptor signal transduction.

CD2, CD3, and CD4 associate with the CD45 extracellular domain.

All isoforms of CD45 associate non-covalently with lymphocyte phosphatase-associated phosphoprotein (LPAP), i.e., CD22.

Knockout mice have defective thymocyte development, reduced numbers of mature T cells, and lack responses to T- and B-cell antigen receptor-mediated activation.

The functional differences between the isoforms are not understood.

Ligands

CD45 and its isoforms bind galectin-1.

CD45RO interacts via carbohydrate residues with the CD22 molecule.

Glycoforms of CD45 bind CD206.

Expression

High level expression of CD45 is found on all nucleated hematopoietic cells but is highest on lymphocytes.

Isoform expression is characteristic of differentiated subsets of leukocytes and can change with activation.

Multiple isoforms are co-expressed on a single cell type.

CD45RA is expressed on naive T cells and B cells.

CD45RO is expressed by memory T cells and monocytes. The proportion of CD45RO$^+$ cells increases with age to ultimately 40–60% of total T-cell population in adults.

CD45RB is expressed at high levels by peripheral CD4$^+$ T cells and CD8$^+$ T cells and at moderate levels by thymic CD4$^+$ T cells and CD4$^+$CD8$^+$ T cells. It is also expressed on B cells, granulocytes, and monocytes.

CD45RC is expressed on a subset of T cells, B cells, and NK cells.

Applications

CD45RO is widely used as a marker of previously activated or "memory" T cells.

CD45RA is used as a marker of "naive" lymphocytes.

CD45 is a leukocyte marker used, for example, in "gating" for flow cytometric analysis of leukocyte subpopulations.

Target for immunosuppressive antibody treatment.

Gene Name	Entrez Gene#
PTPRC	5788

Selected Monoclonal Antibodies

T29/33 (Trowbridge; San Diego); BMAC1 (Dalchau; East Grinstead); 124-2H12B (Vilella; Barcelona).

CD45RA: 2H4 (Schlossman; Boston); G1-15 (Ledbetter; Seattle); F8-11-13 (Dalchau; East Grinstead).

CD45RB: PD-7/26/16 (Mason; Oxford).

CD45RC: OTH75E4 (Hadam; Hannover); 11G8 (Vanlier/Voom; Rotterdam).

CD45R0: UCHL1 (Beverley; Oxford); 2CH-6-33A4 (Tang; Hangzhou); IPO-51 (Mikhalap; Kiev).

CD46

Other Names

Membrane cofactor protein (MCP).

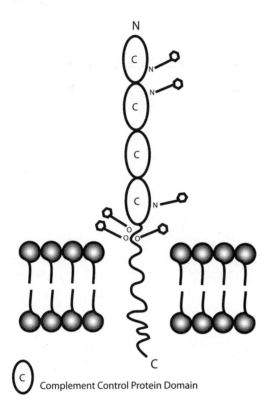

Complement Control Protein Domain

Molecular Structure

A type I transmembrane glycoprotein with four N-terminal complement control protein domains.

Member of the regulators of complement activation (RCA) gene cluster (see CD21, CD35, and CD55).

Four main isoforms (C1, C2, BC1, and BC2) and two other isoforms (ABC1 and ABC2) occur due to alternative splicing of predominantly exons 7, 8, 9, and 13 and glycoslyation.

C1: 238 amino acids; C2: 335 amino acids; BC1: 343 amino acids; BC2: 350 amino acids; ABC1: 358 amino acids; ABC2: 365 amino acids.

CD46 isoform found on sperm acrosome is probably due to different exon splicing and glycosylation.

Four N-terminal short consensus repeat (SCR) domains.

SCR domains 2, 3, and 4 have C3b/C4b binding site.

Three N-glycosylation sites in SCRs 1, 2, and 4 and various degrees of O-glycosylation adjacent to the SCR modules.

Two possible cytoplasmic tails Cyt-1 and Cyt-2 arise from alternative splicing of exon 13.

Mol Wt: Reduced, 64–68 kDa/72–78 kDa; unreduced, 52–58 kDa (except sperm form 35–40 kDa).

Function

Inhibits complement activation by inhibition of C3 convertase formation. Cofactor for factor I proteolytic cleavage of C3b and C4b, thereby protecting host tissues from complement-mediated damage.

Regulates T-cell inflammatory responses and contact hypersensitivity reaction with different effects depending on the cytoplasmic tail. Cyt-1 engagement suppresses inflammation, whereas Cyt-2 promotes inflammation.

Implicated as a ligand and protective molecule in fertilization possibly by protecting acrosome-reacted sperm and fetus from the maternal immune system; however, male CD46 knockout mice demonstrate an increased rate of acrosomal reaction and higher fertility rate compared with wild type, suggesting a regulatory role for CD46.

Associates with β1-integrins and tetraspanins.

Serves as receptor for a number of pathogens, including measles virus, Herpes virus, *Streptococcus pyogenes*, and pathogenic *Neisseria* sp.

Ligands

Complement components C3b and C4b.

Host cell receptor for many pathogens, including measles virus, Herpes virus, *Streptococcus pyogenes*, and pathogenic *Neisseria* sp.

β1-integrins and tetraspanin molecules.

Expression

Variable level of expression and co-expression of isoforms on all nucleated cells except unfertilized oocytes.

High level expression at blood-brain barrier, salivary gland ducts, and kidney ducts.

Moderate expression on lymphocytes and endothelium.

Expression is often increased on tumor cells.

Gene Name	Entrez Gene#
MCP	4179

Selected Monoclonal Antibodies

Hulym5 (E4.3) (McKenzie; Melbourne); J48 (Pesando; Seattle); 122-2 (Vilella; Barcelona).

CD47

Other Names

Integrin-associated protein (IAP), Ovarian carcinoma antigen (OA3), neutrophilin, gp42, Rh-associated protein, MEM-133, CDw149.

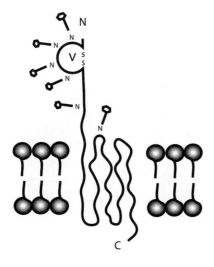

Molecular Structure

A member of the immunoglobulin (Ig) gene superfamily.

Glycoprotein with an extracellular N-terminal IgV-like domain of approximately 120 amino acids, 5 transmembrane segments of approximately 152 amino acids, and a short (~30 amino acid) C-terminal cytoplasmic domain.

Tissue-specific expression of four isoforms resulting from alternative splicing at the C terminus.

Six potential N-glycosylation sites in the extracellular domain.

The SIRPα-binding site is the IgV-like domain.

Mol Wt: Reduced, 50–55 kDa; unreduced, 45–60 kDa.

Function

Binds and activates the leukocyte inhibitory receptor signal regulatory protein α (SIRPα) on phagocytic cells, thereby preventing phagocytosis of self blood cells.

Physically and functionally associated with the integrins αII/β-b3 (CD41/CD61), αv/β3 (CD51/CD61), and α2/β1 (CD49b/CD29) integrins.

Ligand binding to the integrin/CD47 complex can lead to either cell activation or apoptosis via a heterotrimeric Gi-protein signaling pathway.

Receptor for thrombospondin-1 (TS1) that upon binding possibly changes the conformation of TS1 allowing it to bind CD47-associated integrins and modulate their function.

In vitro studies have demonstrated TS1/CD47 interaction modulates αv/β3 integrin function during cell spreading on vitronectin, stimulates chemotaxis of endothelial cells and smooth muscle cells on collagen coated filters, and activates platelet aggregation via α2/β1 integrin.

TS1/CD47 interaction can mediate caspase-independent cell death in a number of cell types, including activated T cells, macrophages, dendritic cells, and various tumor cells.

CD47 null mice have a defect in host defense and are sensitive to autoimmune hemolytic anemia.

Ligands

SIRPα, thrombospondin-1 (TS1).

Expression

Broadly expressed on all human cells so far tested with the notable exception of Rh-negative red blood cells.

Strong expression in brain.

Antibodies previously assigned CD149 are now called CD47R. Their reactivity is similar to CD47, but they do not react with any erythrocytes.

Gene Name	Entrez Gene#
CD47	961

Selected Monoclonal Antibodies

BRIC126 (Anstee; Bristol); CIKM1 (Pilkington; Melbourne); BRIC125 (Anstee; Bristol).

Antibodies previously assigned CD149 are now called CD47R: MEM-120 (Horejsi, Prague); MEM-133 (Horejsi, Prague); N-L159 (Shen, Tianjin).

CD48

Other Names

BLAST-1, Hulym3, OX45, BCM1.

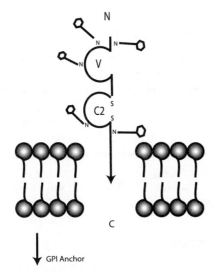

GPI Anchor

Molecular Structure

Mannose containing glycophosphatidyli-nositol (GPI)-linked surface glycoprotein of 194 amino acids.

Member of the CD2 family (see CD2, CD58, and CDw150) within the immuno-globulin (Ig) gene superfamily.

The extracellular region consists of one IgV- and one IgC-like domain.

Mol Wt: 45 kDa.

Function

Ligand for CD2 in the rat and mouse; in the human system, this interaction has a very low affinity and may promote IL-2 and IFN-γ production by T cells.

Ligand of the natural killer cell inhibitory receptor 2B4 (CD244).

CD48/CD244 interaction between homotypic cells augments the immune response; otherwise, this interaction inhibits NK effector functions.

Mast cell receptor for fimbrial adhesion molecule Fim H of *E. coli* and critical mediator of mast cell activation following exposure to mycobacteria.

Ligands

CD48 displays high affinity binding to CD244 (2B4) and low affinity binding to CD2.

Expression

Pan-lymphocyte; not neutrophils or platelets.

Expression is increased in activated lymphocytes.

Applications

Fewer CD48[+] lymphocytes in patients with paroxysmal nocturnal hemoglobulinuria (PNH).

Gene Name   Entrez Gene#

CD48   962

Selected Monoclonal Antibodies

WM68 (Henniker; Sydney); LO-MN25 (Ravoet; Brussels); J4–57 (Pesando; Seattle).

CD49a

Other Names

Integrin α1-chain, very late antigen, VLA 1α.

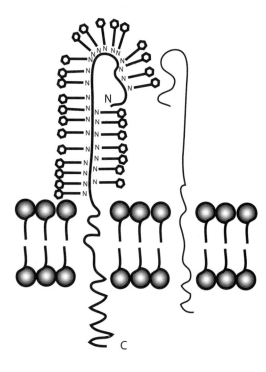

Molecular Structure

A type I transmembrane glycoprotein of the integrin α subclass.

A 1152 amino acid protein with large N-terminal extracellular region containing an I-domain and 26 potential N-glycosylation sites, followed by a transmembrane region and a short 15 amino acid C-terminal cytoplasmic domain.

All integrin α chains have a conserved sequence found in the cytoplasmic domain immediately following the transmembrane domain ([FYWS]-[RK]-x-G-F-F-x-R) that may be the motif involved in heterodimer formation.

Noncovalently associates with the CD29 molecule to form the VLA-1 (integrin α1β1) complex.

Mol Wt: Reduced, 210 kDa; unreduced, 200 kDa.

Function

VLA-1 acts as an adhesion receptor for collagen IV and laminin-1.

Involved in leukocyte migration into tissues.

In vitro studies have shown enhancement of effector T-cell proliferation and cytokine production when bound to collagen via VLA-1.

Modulates effector inflammatory responses in vivo.

Ligands

CD29/CD49a complex binds type IV collagen and laminin-1.

Expression

Activated T cells, monocytes, NK cells, cultured neuronal cells, melanoma cells, mesenchymal cells including smooth muscle cells, fibroblasts, hepatocytes, and microvascular endothelium.

Applications

Upregulated in several inflammatory diseases of human intestine.

Gene Name	Entrez Gene#
ITGA1	3672

Selected Monoclonal Antibodies

IB3.1 (Bank; Ramat Gan); SR84 (Rettig; New York).

CD49b

Other Names

Integrin α2-chain, VLA-2-α-chain, platelet GPIa.

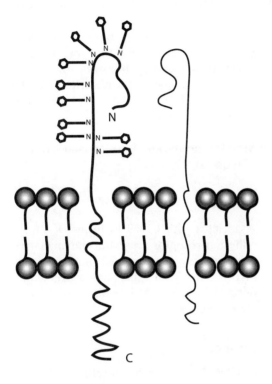

Molecular Structure

A type I transmembrane glycoprotein of the integrin α subclass. Noncovalently associates with the CD29 molecule to form the VLA-2 (integrin α2/β1) complex.

A 1152 amino acid protein with a large N-terminal extracellular region containing an I-domain and 10 potential N-glycosylation sites followed by a transmembrane region and a 27 amino acid C-terminal cytoplasmic domain.

All integrin α chains have a conserved sequence found in the cytoplasmic domain immediately following the transmembrane domain ([FYWS]-[RK]-x-G-F-F-x-R), which may be the motif involved in heterodimer formation.

Mol Wt: Reduced, 165 kDa; unreduced, 160 kDa.

Function

VLA-2 mediates cell adhesion to collagen and laminin.

In vitro studies have shown enhancement of effector T-cell proliferation and cytokine production when bound to collagen via VLA-2.

Modulates effector inflammatory responses in vivo. Promotes wound healing by collagen contraction.

Ligands

CD29/CD49b complex binds type I collagen, VLA-3, E-cahedrin, and is a receptor for echovirus.

Expression

Platelets, megakaryocytes, activated T cells, B lymphocytes, monocytes, epithelial cells, endothelial cells, and fibroblasts.

Gene Name	Entrez Gene#
ITGA2	3673

Selected Monoclonal Antibodies

CLB-thromb/4 (von dem Borne; Amsterdam); Gi44 (Santoso; Giessen).

CD49c

Other Names

Integrin α3-chain, VLA-3-α-chain.

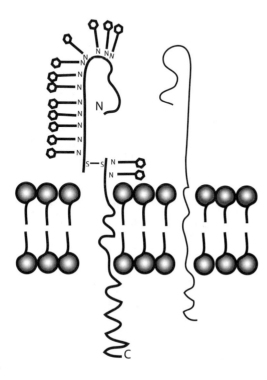

Molecular Structure

A type I transmembrane glycoprotein of the integrin α subclass.

Noncovalently associates with the CD29 molecule to form the VLA-3 (integrin α3/β1) complex.

A 1019 amino acid protein proteolytically cleaved into two disulfide linked fragments of 125 kDa and 30 kDa.

N-terminal large extracellular domain consists of seven-fold repeat structures with putative cation-binding motifs in 3 of 4 C-terminal repeats and 14 potential N-glycosylation sites.

Single transmembrane region followed by a short cytoplasmic domain.

Two alternatively spliced forms of the CD49c molecule known as A and B isoforms differ only in the cytoplasmic domain.

All integrin α-chains have a conserved sequence found in the cytoplasmic domain immediately following the transmembrane domain ([FYWS]-[RK]-x-G-F-F-x-R), which may be the motif involved in heterodimer formation.

Mol Wt: Reduced, 125 kDa and 30 kDa; unreduced, 150 kDa.

Function

Associates with CD29 to form VLA3, an adhesion receptor for extracellular matrix components (see ligands) and may be involved in signal transduction. Knockout mice show prenatal lethality and kidney abnormalities.

Ligands

CD29/CD49c binds fibronectin, laminin-V, laminin-1, entactin, and collagen.

Expression

T and B lymphocytes, monocytes, and adherent cell lines.

Gene Name	Entrez Gene#
ITGA3	3675

Selected Monoclonal Antibodies

A3-IIF5 (Hemler; Boston); 10.1.2 (Cort; Bethesda).

CD49d

Other Names

Integrin α4-chain, VLA-4-α-chain.

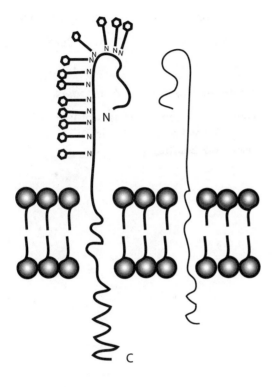

Molecular Structure

A type I transmembrane glycoprotein, differing structurally from α integrin subclass proteins.

Noncovalently associates with CD29 molecules to form VLA-4 (integrin α4/β1) complexes and with β7 integrin subunit to form the α4/β7 integrin.

A 999 amino acid protein that is sometimes post-translationally cleaved to 80-kDa and 70-kDa fragments.

Extracellular region has more than 3 EF-hand-like divalent cation binding sites and 11 N-glycosylation sites.

Cys278 and Cys717 are required for optimal binding to connecting segment-1

(fibronectin isoform) as is the region containing Arg89–Arg90.

Tyr187 and Gly190 are essential for CS-1 and VCAM-1 binding.

Homotypic cell aggregation requires the region encompassing Arg89–Arg90.

A 32 amino acid cytoplasmic domain.

All integrin α chains have a conserved sequence found in the cytoplasmic domain immediately following the transmembrane domain ([FYWS]-[RK]-x-G-F-F-x-R), which may be the motif involved in heterodimer formation.

Multiple stimuli are able to induce the adhesive conformation, including divalent cations, chemokines, and some mAb.

Mol Wt: Reduced, 145 kDa (180 kDa); unreduced, 150 kDa. A 180-kDa isoform called α4/180 also occurs.

Function

Associates with either β1 or β7 integrin chains to provide cell adhesion to VCAM-1, MAdCAM-1, fibronectin, and thrombospondin.

Regulates multiple inflammatory responses by enhancing adhesion to and rolling of lymphocytes on vascular endothelium via binding to VCAM-1, thereby promoting lymphocyte migration from circulation into tissue.

Involved in homing of T-cell subsets to Peyer's patches via interaction with MadCAM-1.

Essential to differentiation and migration of hemopoietic stem cells by their adhesion to bone marrow stromal cells.

Provides a costimulatory signal with TCR-CD3 mediated signaling by inducing tyrosine phosphorylation of some focal adhesion proteins.

Has a role in tumor progression and metastases that bind fibronectin, thrombospondin, and CD106 molecules.

Integrin α4/β1 assists entry if invasive bacteria through binding of microbial protein invasin.

Knockout mice show embryonic lethality and abnormal formation of heart and placenta.

Ligands

VLA-4 binds VCAM-1 (CD106), connecting segment-1 (CS-1, isoform of fibronectin), microbial ligand invasin, and thrombospondin.

Integrin α4/β7 (CD49d/β7 complex) binds MadCAM-1, VCAM-1, CS-1, and invasin.

Expression

Broad, including B cells, monocytes, T cells, eosinophils, basophils, NK cells, and dendritic cells but not platelets.

Gene Name	Entrez Gene#
ITGA4	3676

Selected Monoclonal Antibodies

B-5G10 (Hemler; Boston); HP2/1 (Sanchez-Madrid; Madrid); JH136 (Pesando; Seattle).

CD49e

Other Names

Integrin α5-chain, VLA-5-α-chain.

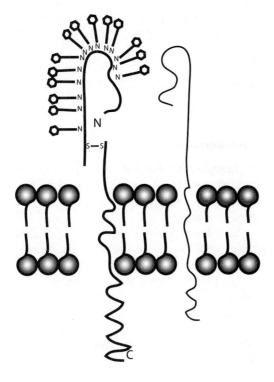

Molecular Structure

A type I transmembrane glycoprotein of the integrin α subclass.

Noncovalently associates with the CD29 molecule to form the VLA-5 (integrin α5/β1) complex.

A 1008 amino acid protein that is post-translationally cleaved into two disulfide linked units of 135 kDa and 25 kDa.

Large N-terminal extracellular domain consists of a seven-fold repeated structure with putative cation binding motifs in four C-terminal repeats.

Fourteen potential N-glycosylation sites.

A 28 amino acid transmembrane domain.

All integrin α chains have a conserved sequence found in the cytoplasmic domain immediately following the transmembrane domain ([FYWS]-[RK]-x-G-F-F-x-R), which may be the motif involved in heterodimer formation.

Mol Wt: Reduced, 135 kDa, 25 kDa; unreduced, 155 kDa.

Function

VLA-5 binds to RGD sequence in fibronectin and binds to neural adhesion molecule L1.

Important in maintaining the integrity of the endothelial monolayer as well as adhesion of cells to fibronectin.

Involved in monocyte migration into the extracellular tissues.

Role in regulation of the cell survival and apoptosis.

VLA-5 mediated binding to fibronectin provides a co-stimulatory signal to T cells and enhances receptor and complement receptor-mediated phagocytosis.

Null mutation is embryonic lethal with mesodermal abnormalities.

Ligands

Fibronectin, neural adhesion molecule L1.

Expression

Expressed on thymocytes, activated and memory T cells, early and activated B cells, monoctyes NK cells, dendritic cells, osteoblasts, and endothelia.

Gene Name   *Entrez Gene#*

ITGA5   3678

Selected Monoclonal Antibodies

2H6 (Morimoto; Boston); SAM-1 (Figdor; Amsterdam).

CD49f

Other Names

Integrin α6-chain, VLA-6-α-chain, platelet gpIc.

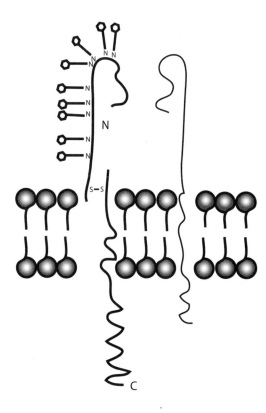

Molecular Structure

A type I transmembrane glycoprotein of the integrin α subclass.

Noncovalently associates with the CD29 molecule to form the VLA-6 (integrin α6/β1) complex and with CD104 to form the integrin α6/β4 complex.

Two spliced forms A and B that differ in the cytoplasmic domain occur and have tissue-specific expression.

A 1050 or 1068 amino acid protein post-translationally cleaved into two disulfide-linked units of 120 kDa and 30 kDa.

Nine N-glycosylation sites and three putative cation-binding motifs.

A 36 or 54 amino acid cytoplasmic domain.

All integrin α chains have a conserved sequence found in the cytoplasmic domain immediately following the transmembrane domain ([FYWS]-[RK]-x-G-F-F-x-R), which may be the motif involved in heterodimer formation.

Mol Wt: Reduced, 120 kDa and 30 kDa; unreduced, 140 kDa.

Function

Adhesion receptor for laminins, invasin, merosin involved in cell adhesion and migration, embryogenesis, and cell-surface mediated signaling.

Enables interaction between epithelial cells and basement membrane during wound healing.

Important for the formation of hemidesmosomes of stratified squamous and transitional epithelia.

CD49f/CD2-mediated T-cell binding to laminin provides a costimulatory signal to T cells for activation and proliferation.

Involved in tumor metastasis.

Candidate receptor for papilloma virus.

Knockout mice show perinatal lethality with blistering of the skin, which is the same phenotype seen in integrin β4 (CD104) knockout mice.

Ligands

CD29/CD49f complex binds laminin, invasin, and merosin.

CD104/CD49f complex binds laminins (especially laminin-5).

Expression

Platelets, megakaryocytes, monocytes, T cells, and thymocytes. Widely expressed on many cultured adherent cell lines and on epithelia in non-lymphoid tissues.

   Only the A isoform is expressed in lung, liver, spleen, and cervix, whereas only the B isoform is found in brain, ovary, and kidney.

Gene Name	Entrez Gene#
ITGA6	3655

Selected Monoclonal Antibodies

GoH3 (Sonnenberg; Amsterdam).

CD50

Other Names

ICAM-3, intercellular adhesion molecule 3.

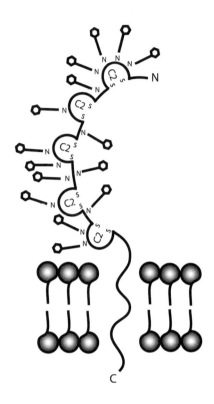

Molecular Structure

A 518 amino acid, type I integral membrane glycoprotein and member of the Ig superfamily.

Structurally homologous to ICAM-1 (CD54) and ICAM-2 (CD102).

The 456 amino acid extracellular region consists of 5 IgC-like domains, which have 15 potential N-glycosylation sites (but only half are thought to be glycosylated at any one time).

The extracellular domain is proteolytically cleaved when leukocytes are activated and soluble forms are found in the blood.

The 25 amino acid transmembrane domain is followed by a 37 amino acid cytoplasmic domain that is tyrosine and serine phosphorylated in activated cells and is associated with tyrosine kinase activity.

Electron microscopy studies have shown CD50 to be a straight rod of approximately 15 nm long.

Mol Wt: Unreduced ranges from 110 kDa to 170 kDa depending on the cell type and extent of glycosylation.

Function

Functions as ligand for $\alpha D/\beta 2$ ($\alpha D/CD18$) and LFA-1 (CD11a/CD18) integrins on activated cells.

Regulates LFA-1/ICAM1 and integrin $\beta 1$-dependent adhesion.

Functions as a primary adhesion molecule during initial contact between T cell and antigen presenting cells prior to antigen recognition.

Provides costimulatory signal during immune response that leads to polarization of the microtubular cytoskeleton.

Redistributes to leukocyte uropods during cell migration and plays a role in cell recruitment.

DC-SIGN, a C-lectin expressed by dendritic cells, is a high affinity ligand for dendritic cell-specific ICAM-3 and may therefore play a role in primary immune responses.

Ligands

LFA-1 (CD11a/CD18), integrin $\alpha D\beta 2$ ($\alpha D/CD18$), DC-SIGN (CD209).

Expression

Leukocytes, Langerhans cells, and endothelial cells.

Gene Name	Entrez Gene#
ICAM3	3385

Selected Monoclonal Antibodies

101–1D2 (Vilella; Barcelona); CBR-IC3/1 (De Fougerolles; Boston); RAT1.7, (Balogh; Pecs).

CD51

Other Names

Integrin α-chain, vitronectin receptor α chain, integrin αV-subunit.

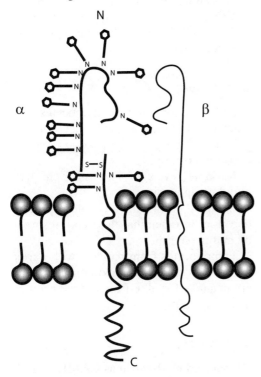

Molecular Structure

A type I integral membrane glycoprotein of the integrin α subclass. Forms noncovalent heterodimeric complexes with several β integrins: CD29, CD61, β5, β6, and β8.

Does not have an I domain and is post-translationally cleaved into two disulfide-linked subunits of 125 kDa and 25 kDa.

A 1018 amino acid protein with 13 N-glycosylation sites and 18 conserved cysteines.

Four cation binding sites.

A 32 amino acid cytoplasmic domain.

Integrin α chains all share a conserved sequence found at the beginning of the cytoplasmic domain just after the trans-membrane region. This motif may be involved in heterodimer formation.

Mol Wt: Reduced, 125 kDa and 24 kDa; unreduced, 150 kDa.

Function

Can noncovalently associate with β1 (CD29), β3 (CD61), β5, β6, or β8 integrins.

Complex of CD51/CD61 acts as an adhesin by binding RGD motifs in extracellular matrix proteins to act as an activation-independent receptor for platelet attachment.

CD51/C61 mediates leukocyte-endothelial cell adhesion via interaction with CD31, initiates bone resorption by mediating adhesion of osteoclasts to osteopontin, and possibly has a role in angiogenesis.

Ligands

CD51/CD29 (αVβ1) and CD51/β6 (αVβ6) integrins bind fibronectin. CD51/β5 binds vitronectin.

CD51/CD61 complex binds vitronectin, fibrinogen, fibronectin, von Willebrand factor, laminin and thrombospondin, bone sialoprotein (Bsp1), osteopontin, and neural adhesion molecule L1.

Expression

CD51/CD29 complex is found on fibroblasts and neuroblastoma cells.

CD51/CD61 complex is expressed on endothelial cells; cultured/activated monocytes and macrophages, platelets, some B cells, and osteoclasts,

CD51/β5 complex is expressed on hepatoma cells, carcinoma cells, and fibroblasts.

Gene Name	Entrez Gene#
ITGAV	3685

Selected Monoclonal Antibodies

13C2 (Horton; London); NKI-M7 (Hogervorst; Amsterdam); 23C6 (Horton; London).

CD52

Other Names

Campath-1, HE5.

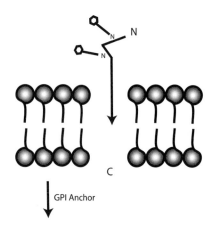

GPI Anchor

Molecular Structure

Highly N-glycosylated protein, C-terminally anchored in the membrane via glycophosphatidylinositol.

Belongs to a family, which includes CD24 and murine heat stable antigen (HSA).

A complex carbohydrate consisting of a tetra-antennary fucosylated mannose core containing sialylated polylactosamine units is attached to Asn-3.

Very short protein backbone consists of 12–18 amino acids.

Sperm CD52 differs from lymphocyte CD52 in its carbohydrate structure with more than 50 glycoforms and up to 6 sialic acid residues.

Mol Wt: 25–29 kDa.

Function

Function remains unknown.

Present at high concentrations (5×10^5 molecules per lymphocyte).

Upon cross-linking and in the presence of appropriate costimulatory factors, antibodies induce proliferation and lymphokine production in T cells.

CD52-negative cells (in patients treated with anti-CD52 antibody) appear to function normally.

Expression

High level expression on thymocytes, lymphocytes, monocytes, and macrophages. Also found on peripheral blood dendritic cells and eosinophils.

Variable levels of expression in lymphoid malignancies.

Shed by epithelium of male reproductive tract into seminal fluid and absorbed by mature sperm.

Lymphocytes from patients with paroxysmal nocturnal hemoglobinuria (PNH) are negative for all GPI-anchored proteins including CD52.

Applications

Humanized mAbs such as CAMPATH-1H (alemtuzumab) are lytic for CD52$^+$ target cells and are used to treat lymphoproliferative disorders as well as to reduce lymphocyte numbers and function in autoimmune diseases and organ or bone marrow transplantation.

Gene Name   Entrez Gene#

CDW52   1043

Selected Monoclonal Antibodies

Campath-1 (Hale, Cambridge) (097 (Bernard; Nice); YTH66.9; (Hale; Durham); YTH34.5 (Hale; Durham).

CD53

Other Names

MRC OX-44 (rat), tetraspanin-25, Tspan-25.

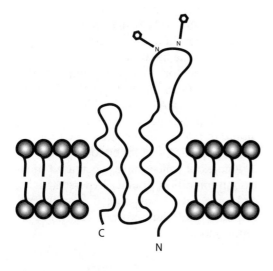

Molecular Structure

Member of the tetraspan family, associated in several cells with other members of this family (CD37, CD81, CD82).

A 219 amino acid, type III membrane protein, with four putative transmembrane domains and two unequal extracellular loops.

A Tetraspan family signature sequence is found between the transmembrane domains II and III.

Two N-glycosylation sites in the large extracellular loop.

The short ends are located in the cytoplasm.

Mol Wt: Unreduced, 32–42 kDa.

Function

Function has not yet been elucidated.

Decreased expression of CD53 is found in activated and migrating leukocytes.

CD53 cross-linking induces calcium mobilization, signal transduction, and oxidative burst formation in monocytes, and promotes activation of human B cells and rat macrophages.

Associates with other tetraspan molecules, VLA-4 and HLA-DR, and may form part of a large complex of integrins, tetraspans, and MHC class II molecules.

In rat, CD53 is associated with CD2 and signal transduction via tyrosine phosphatase activity.

Expression

Highest expression on monocytes and B cells but also expressed on thymocytes, T cells, granulocytes, osteoblasts, and osteoclasts.

Not present on erythrocytes, platelets, and non-hemopoietic cells.

Gene Name   Entrez Gene#

CD53   963

Selected Monoclonal Antibodies

MEM-53 (Horejsi; Prague); HD77 (Moldenhauer; Heidelberg); HI29 (Chen; Tiajin).

CD54

Other Names

ICAM-1, intercellular adhesion molecule 1.

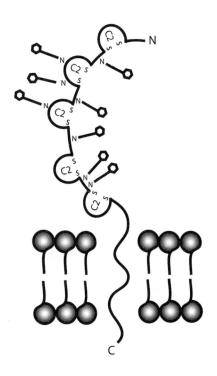

Molecular Structure

A 500 amino acid, type I, integral membrane glycoprotein.

Member of the Ig supergene family.

Heavily glycosylated.

Extracellular region is an 18.7-nm bent rod with five IgC-like domains.

A short cytoplasmic domain follows a single transmembrane region.

Soluble form in serum.

Mol Wt: 80–114 kDa.

Function

Major signaling adhesion molecule in inflammatory and immune reactions.

Adhesion molecule binding to LFA-I, Mac-I, fibrinogen, hyaluronan, and CD43.

ICAM-1/LFA interaction is required for effective antibody responses, T-cell proliferation, and IL-2 secretion and plays a role in allograft rejection.

Expression of ICAM-1 on endothelium enables migration of activated leukocytes to sites of inflammation.

Receptor for a major group of rhinoviruses. The binding site for these viruses overlaps the LFA-1 binding site.

In vitro can act as receptor for *Plasmodium falciparum*-infected erythrocytes to postcapillary venular endothelium.

Knockout mice have decreased neutrophil migration, contact hypersensitivity, and generation of mixed lymphocyte response and demonstrate resistance to septic shock.

Ligands

LFA1 (CD11a/CD18), Mac-1 (CD11b/CD18), fibrinogen, hyaluronan, rhinoviruses, and unknown molecule on *Plasmodium falciparum*-infected erythrocytes.

Expression

Absent from resting leukocytes but moderate expression on activated T cells, activated B cells, and monocytes.

Constitutively expressed at low level on certain endothelia and epithelia but is inducible on epithelial, endothelial, and fibroblastic cells.

High level expression on endothelia activated by pro-inflammatory cytokines.

Applications

Potential target for immunosuppression in transplantation.

Serum level of soluble CD54 is a potentially useful indicator of inflammation, infection, and a variety of tumors.

Gene Name	Entrez Gene#
ICAM1	3383

Selected Monoclonal Antibodies

RR1/1 (Springer; Boston); LB-2 (Clark; Seattle); My13 (Civin; Baltimore).

CD55

Other Names

DAF, decay accelerating factor.

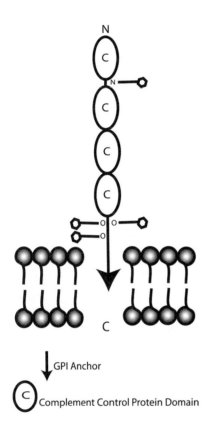

Molecular Structure

Single-chain, glycophosphatidylinositol (GPI)-linked, type 1 membrane glycoprotein.

Member of the regulator of complement activation (RCA) gene family (see CD21, CD35, and CD46).

The extracellular region contains four N-terminal complement control protein (CCP) domains also known as short consensus repeat (SCR) domains.

C3b/C4b binding and regulatory activity is found in SCR 2, 3, and 4 but not in SCR1.

Membrane proximal extracellular region is heavily glycosylated, but there is one N-linked glycosylation site at the C-terminal end of SCR1.

The difference in molecular weight between CD55 found on erythrocytes and that of lymphocytes is due to glycosylation differences.

Two alternatively spliced isoforms of CD55 are expressed as DAF-A and DAF-B. DAF-A lacks the GPI-anchor and is secreted, whereas DAF-B is the membrane anchored form. Both of these isoforms can be further modified by varying glycosylation patterns.

Mol Wt: Reduced, 80 kDa; unreduced, 70 kDa (lymphocytes) or 50 kDa (erythrocytes).

Function

Protects against inappropriate complement activation and deposition on plasma membranes by binding C3b and C4b to inhibit C3 convertase formation.

Binds C3bBb and C4b2a to accelerate decay of C3 convertases.

Ligand of the CD97 molecule.

May act as a ligand or as a protective molecule in fertilization by protecting sperm from complement deposition in the female reproductive system.

Serves as receptor for coxsackie B viruses, echoviruses and enterovirus, and *E.coli* Dr-adhesins.

Shown in vitro to act as a signal transduction molecule as mAb directed against CD55 can activate monocytes.

CD55 loss is associated with paroxysmal nocturnal hemoglobinuria (see also CD59).

Ligands

C3b/C3bBb convertase, C4b/C4b2a convertase, CD97, coxsackie viruses (B1, B3, B5), echoviruses (type7), *E.coli* Dr-adhesins, and enterovirus 70.

Expression

Wide expression on cells throughout the body including erythrocytes.

Low level expression on NK cells.

Overexpressed on various tumors, including breast, colon, and stomach.

Applications

Possible target for tumor therapy.

Potential use in xenotransplantation to protect against inappropriate complement activation.

Gene Name	Entrez Gene#
DAF	1604

Selected Monoclonal Antibodies

143-30 (Vilella; Barcelona); BRIC110 (Anstee; Bristol); F2B-7.2 (Poncelet; Marseille).

CD56

Other Names

NKHI, neural cell adhesion molecule (NCAM).

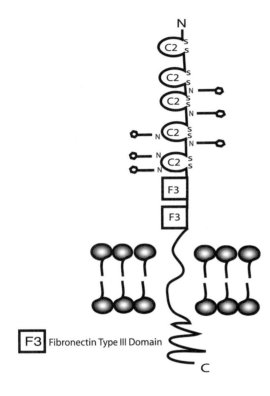

F3 Fibronectin Type III Domain

Molecular Structure

A member of the Ig supergene family.

Heavily glycosylated isoform of N-CAM.

Three forms and 20–30 splice variants.

All neurons express the largest form (180 kDa), which has a long cytoplasmic tail; a hemopoietic form (140 kDa) has a shorter cytoplasmic tail; and a GPI-linked form (120 kDa) is found in muscle.

The 689 amino acid extracellular domain consists of 5 IgC-like domains and 2 fibronectin type III domains and 6 potential N-glycosylation sites.

Electron microscopy shows that the IgC-like domains are arranged to form a flexible rod-like structure projecting from the cell surface.

All 5 IgC-like domains appear to be required for homotypic binding, with domain 1 binding domain 5, domain 2 binding domain 4, and domain 3 binding domain 3.

The three-dimensional structure of the N terminal IgC-like domain has great similarity to domain 1 of VCAM-1.

CD56 is extensively modified with polysialic acid on NK and T cells.

Variable glycosylation depending on the tissue, which includes the CD57 epitope (see CD57).

Mol Wt: 180 kDa (long cytoplasmic domain), 140 kDa (short cytoplasmic domain), 120 kDa (GPI-linked form).

Function

Homophilic and heterophilic adhesion molecule in neuronal tissue, implicated in control of neural development by regulating cell migration, neurite outgrowth, selective fasciculation and axon sorting, target recognition, and synaptic plasticity.

Binding of CD56 to chondroitin sulphate proteoglycans of the cell matrix inhibits outgrowth of neuronal cells.

Function on T cells and NK cells not known although some evidence that CD56 is involved in homophilic adhesion of these cells.

Some CD56 antibodies inhibit NK-target cell interactions in certain systems.

Knockout mice show neurologic abnormalities, but NK- and T-cell development appear normal.

Ligands

NCAM-1 (homotypic adhesion), heparin sulphate, and chondroitin sulphate proteoglycans.

Expression

Isoforms on neural cells (NCAM), muscle cells, and embryonic tissue and tumors.

In hemopoietic cells, restricted to NK cells and a subset of T cells. The level of CD56 expression defines subsets of NK cells such that the highest expression is by NK cells of the liver and decidua, and CD56^{dim} cells are found in the peripheral blood and spleen. CD56$^+$ T cells are concentrated in the liver.

Applications

Marker of NK cell subsets.
   Identification of various solid tumors.

Gene Name   Entrez Gene#

NCAM1   4684

Selected Monoclonal Antibodies

NKH1A (Ritz; Boston); NKH1 (Griffin; Boston); Leu19 (Lanier; Mountain View).

CD57

Other Names

HNK1.

Glucuronic acid β - 1 ⟶ 3 Gal β1 - 4 GlcNAc

     |

  3 - SO$_4$

Molecular Structure

A carbohydrate structure consisting of a sulphated trisaccharide 3-O-sulfoglucuronic acid β1-3Gal β1-4GlcNAc.

Probably attached to several glycoproteins, including CD56, myelin glycoprotein PO, and neural cell adhesion molecule L1.

Present on glycolipids and chondroitin sulphate proteoglycans in the nervous system.

Function

Adhesion reaction via laminin and L- and P-selectin binding.

As part of myelin glycoprotein PO, CD57 probably maintains the structural integrity of myelin by homophilic adhesion.

IL-1-activated brain microvascular endothelial cells collect a CD57-bearing glycolipid that has been implicated in the L-selectin-dependent binding of lymphocytes.

CD57$^+$ T cells are implicated as suppressors of T-cell responses.

In vitro, CD4$^+$ CD57$^+$ T cells do not promote differentiation of B cells into antibody-producing cells, and both CD4$^+$CD57$^+$ and CD8$^+$CD57$^+$ T cells display poor proliferative responses.

Function of CD57 on NK cells has not been determined.

Ligands

G2 domain of laminin and P- and L-selectins.

Expression

Subsets of NK and T cells, neural tissue.

Applications

NK-cell marker.

Target of auto-antibodies in peripheral neuropathy.

Expressed on some solid tumors such as well-differentiated prostate cancers and uveal and cutaneous melanoma.

Gene Name	Entrez Gene#
CD57	964

Selected Monoclonal Antibodies

HNK-1 (Abo; Birmingham); L186 (Maino; Mountain View); Leu-7 (Maino; Mountain View).

CD58

Other Names

LFA-3, lymphocyte function associated antigen-3.

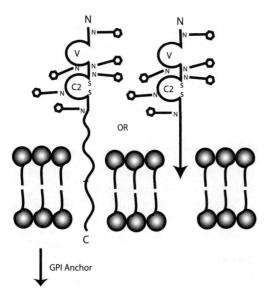

Molecular Structure

Occurs as glycophosphatidylinositol (GPI)-anchored and type I integral membrane protein on all cells except erythrocytes, which express the GPI-linked form only. A member of the CD2 family (see CD2, CD48, and CD150) within the Ig supergene family.

The 188 amino acid extracellular region consists of one IgV-and one IgC-like domain.

The IgC domain but not the IgV domain has a disulphide bond.

A 12 amino acid cytoplasmic domain.

Alternative splicing gives rise to either the transmembrane form or the GPI-anchored form.

Six potential N-glycosylation sites in the extracellular domain.

Mol Wt: 40–70 kDa depending on the cell type.

Function

Ligand for CD2, providing a costimulatory signal in immune responses.

CD58/CD2 binding mediates adhesion between killer and target cells and thus plays a role in cell-mediated cytotoxicity.

Adhesion via CD2 occurs between APC and T cells as well as between thymocytes and thymic epithelial cells and in T-cell–erythrocyte interactions.

CD2/CD58 molecule interaction may prime cellular responses by both the CD2-positive and the CD58-positive cells as both forms of CD58 have signaling activity.

The sheep homologue binds human CD2 and mediates the phenomenon of sheep erythrocyte rosetting on T cells. CD58 antibodies can inhibit CD2/CD58 interactions.

Absent from erythrocytes of patients with paroxysmal nocturnal hemoglobinuria.

Ligands

CD2.

Expression

Leukocytes, erythrocytes, endothelial and epithelial cells, fibroblasts, and smooth muscle.

Gene Name	Entrez Gene#
CD58	965

Selected Monoclonal Antibodies

TS2/9 (Springer; Boston); BRIC5 (Anstee; Bristol); MEM-63 (Horejsi, Prague).

CD59

Other Names

MACIF, MIRL, P-18, protectin.

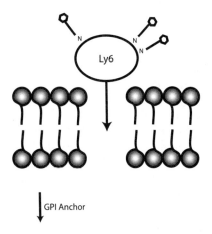

GPI Anchor

Molecular Structure

A single-chain glycophosphatidylinositol (GPI)-linked glycoprotein. Member of the Ly-6 superfamily (see CD87) containing one cysteine-rich Ly-6 domain. The murine homologue is known as Ly6C.

NMR studies reveal the molecule to be relatively flat, disk-shaped, with a two-stranded β-sheet finger loosely packed against a core formed by a three-stranded β-sheet and a short helix.

N-glycanation site at residue 18; however, this site is not essential for function.

Structurally related to snake venom neurotoxins.

Mol Wt: Reduced, 19–25 kDa; unreduced, 18–25 kDa.

Function

Binding to C9 inhibits its incorporation into C5b-8, thereby blocking the terminal steps of polymerization of the complement membrane attack complex (MAC) on the plasma membrane, thus protecting cells from complement-mediated lysis.

Human immunodeficiency virus (HIV) incorporates CD59 into its envelope protecting virus and infected cells from complement deposition.

CD59 has signaling activity and plays a role in T-cell activation.

CD59 expression is essential for erythrocyte survival.

Paroxysmal nocturnal hemoglobinuria is partially caused by a reduction in or loss of CD59 expression (see also CD55).

Some antibodies enhance lytic activity and stimulate NK activity.

Ligands

Complement proteins C8-a and C9.

Expression

Widely expressed on cells in all tissues.

Applications

CD59 transgenic pigs are being studied for use of their tissues in xenotransplantation.

Gene Name	Entrez Gene#
CD59	966

Selected Monoclonal Antibodies

MEM-43 (Horejsi; Prague); YTH53.1 (Waldmann; Cambridge).

CD60

Other Names

GD3 (CD60a), 9-0-acetyl GD3 (CD60b), 7-0-acetyl GD3 (CD60c).

Molecular Structure

Comprises three subgroups, CD60a, CD60b, and CD60c, which define the oligosaccharide sequence of ganglioside GD3.

CD60a has the oligosaccharide NeuAc-α2-8NeuAc-α2-3Gal-β1-4Glc-β1-Cer of ganglioside G3.

CD60b is the 9-O-acetyl-GD3 and related structures.

CD60c is the 7-O-acetyl-GD3 and related structures.

It may also be expressed on a 90-kDa T-cell glycoprotein.

Function

CD60a is involved in regulation of apoptosis and induction of mitochondrial permeability during apoptosis. CD60 antibodies provide costimulatory signals for T cells.

CD60$^+$ T cells within CD4$^+$ and CD8$^+$ subsets act as helper cells to B cells and secrete greater levels of IL-4.

Expression

CD60a: melanocytes, adrenal medullary cells, glial cells, neurons and pancreatic islet cells, and thymocytes; subset of peripheral T cells; weakly expressed on B cells, granulocytes, and platelets.

CD60b: T-cell subsets, activated B cells, and neuroectodermal cells in thymus epithelium and the skin; CD60 expression may correlate with CD4 Th2-type cytokine profile, melanomas, and breast carcinomas.

CD60c: T cells.

Applications

Strong marker for malignant melanoma.

High frequency of CD60$^+$ T cells in synovial fluid of normal and arthritic patients and in cutaneous psoriatic lesions.

Selected Monoclonal Antibodies

M-T32 (Rieber; Dresden); UM4D4 (Fox; Ann Arbor); M-T41 (Rieber; Dresden).

CD61

Other Names

Glycoprotein IIIa, β3 integrin.

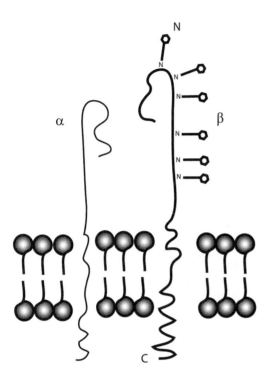

Molecular Structure

A type I integral glycoprotein, member of the β integrin family that forms a calcium-dependent complex with platelet glycoprotein GPIIb (complex recognized by CD41 antibodies).

The CD61 molecule can also associate with integrin αV (CD51) forming the αVβ3 integrin and vitronectin receptor.

Cysteine-rich single-chain protein with an 856 amino acid extracellular domain, 26 amino acid transmembrane region, and 41 amino acid cytoplasmic domain.

Potentially has two large loops extending from Cys5-Cys435 and Cys405-Cys655.

At least six CD61 polymorphisms have been identified with one (Arg636-Cys) shown to induce an alloimmune response.

Mol Wt: Reduced, 110 kDa; unreduced, 90 kDa.

Function

CD41/CD61 complex involved in platelet activation and aggregation. This complex functions as an activation-dependent receptor for fibrinogen, fibronectin, and von Willebrand factor (vWF) and binds to RGD-containing sequences in adhesion molecules. Complex of CD51/CD61 binds RGD motifs in ECM proteins such as vitronectin and vWF and plays a role in tumor metastasis and in adenovirus infection.

Absent or dysfunctional CD41/CD61 complex on platelets leads to the bleeding disorder Glanzmann's Thrombasthenia (GT).

Ligands

CD41/CD61 only binds fibronectin in resting cells; however, upon activation, the complex becomes a receptor for soluble fibrinogen, fibronectin, vWF, and other RGD-containing adhesive proteins.

CD51/CD61 binds vitronectin, fibronectin, vWF, and other RGD-containing adhesive proteins.

Expression

CD41/CD61 is expressed on platelets and megakaryocytes.

CD51/CD61 is found on a wide variety of cells including endothelium, smooth muscle, some B cells, monocytes, macrophages, platelets, osteoclasts, some mast cells, fibroblasts, and tumor cells.

Gene Name   Entrez Gene#

ITGB3   3690

Selected Monoclonal Antibodies

VIPL2 (Knapp; Vienna); Y2/51 (Cordell; Oxford); CLB-thromb/1 (v.d.Borne; Amsterdam).

CD62E

Other Names

E-selectin, LECAM-2, ELAM-1.

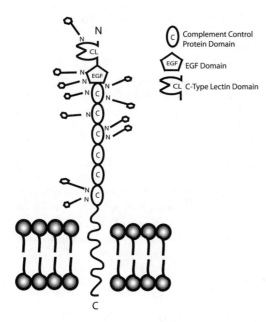

Complement Control Protein Domain

EGF Domain

C-Type Lectin Domain

Molecular Structure

Type I transmembrane glycoprotein that contains in the 585 amino acid extracellular region an N-terminal C-type lectin-like domain, followed by an epidermal growth factor-like domain and six complement control binding protein domains. The extracellular region contains 11 potential N-linked glycosylation sites.

A 32 amino acid cytoplasmic domain follows a 22 amino acid transmembrane sequence.

CD62E is structurally related to CD62L and CD62P molecules (selectin family).

Mol Wt: Reduced, 97 kDa; unreduced, 107–115 kDa.

Function

Recognizes carbohydrate ligands (e.g., sialyl Lewis X (CD15s)) on various molecules, including GlyCAM1, CD34, CD107a, CD162, and ESL-1 (mouse).

Promotes leukocyte extravasation by mediating leukocyte rolling on activated endothelia during inflammation.

Reported to support tumor cell adhesion during metastasis as well as play a role in angiogenesis.

CD62E knockout mice show no major changes to leukocyte recruitment in various models of inflammation. However, mice deficient in both CD62E and CD62P do have reduced leukocyte recruitment to inflammatory sites and are less resistant to opportunistic infections.

Ligands

Carbohydrate ligands including sialyl Lewis X, sialyl Lewis a, cutaneous leukocyte antigen, CD66a, CD162, and ESL-1 (mouse).

Expression

Activated endothelial cells in both acute and chronic inflammatory conditions.

Expressed in non-inflammatory state in skin, placenta, and bone marrow endothelium.

Gene Name · Entrez Gene#

SELE · 6401

Selected Monoclonal Antibodies

CL-3 (Anderson; Houston); ENA1 (Leeuwenher; Maastricht).

CD62L

Other Names

L-selectin, LAM-1, Mel-14.

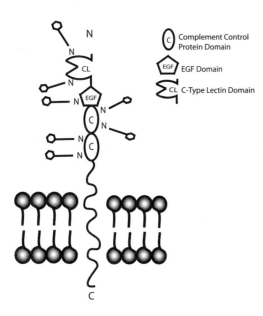

Molecular Structure

A type I transmembrane glycoprotein of 334 amino acids.

Structural organization similar to the CD62E molecule. The 279 amino acid extracellular region consists of a N-terminal C-type lectin—like domain followed by an epidermal growth factor like domain and two complement control binding protein (CCP) domains.

There is 15 amino acid spacer between the membrane proximal CCP domain and the transmembrane region, which contains the proteolytic cleavage site (Lys283-Ser284).

A 17 amino acid cytoplasmic domain follows the 23 amino acid transmembrane region.

Mol Wt: Reduced, 74–94 kDa; unreduced, 65 kDa.

Function

Recognizes carbohydrate ligands (e.g., CD15s) on various molecules (see Ligands).

Involved in "rolling" of leukocytes on activated endothelium, a precursor to extravasation during inflammation.

Mediates lymphocyte homing to high endothelial venules of peripheral lymphoid tissue.

$CD62L^{-/-}$ mice cannot be tolerized, and adoptive transfer of their cells prevents tolerization in wild-type mice. This effect is due to the inability of CD62- T cells to reach lymph nodes and other lymphoid organs that are tolerogenic environments.

Ligands

Several extensively glycosylated, fucosylated, sulfated, sialylated glycoproteins including CD34, GlyCAM-1, MAdCAM-1, sulfated glycolipids, and polyanionic molecules such as heparin sulphate.

Expression

Most T and B lymphocytes, granulocytes, monocytes, and some NK cells. Among T cells, memory cells express CD62L preferentially.

Expressed on certain hemopoietic malignant cells.

High levels of the soluble form of CD62L are detectable in the blood.

Applications

Potential target for the treatment of chronic inflammatory diseases such as asthma.

Soluble CD62L is released by proteolysis during inflammation, and serum CD62L is thus an indicator of inflammation.

Gene Name	Entrez Gene#
SELL	6402

Selected Monoclonal Antibodies

DREG56 (van Agthoven; Marseille); LAM1-3 (Tedder; Boston); SK11 (Warner; San José).

CD62P

Other Names

P-selectin, granule membrane protein-140 (GMP-140), platelet activation-dependent granule-external membrane protein (PADGEM).

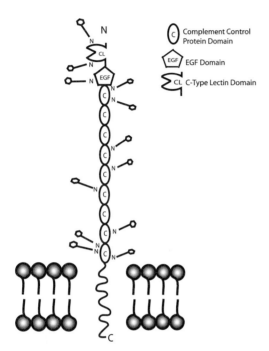

Molecular Structure

A 789 amino acid, type I transmembrane glycoprotein.

Structural organization similar to the CD62E molecule. The 730 amino acid extracellular region consists of a N-terminal C-type lectin-like domain followed by an epidermal growth factor (EGF)-like domain and nine complement control binding protein (CCP) domains.

The extracellular domain forms an approximately 48 nm long rod-like structure.

Extensive N-linked glycosylation.

A 24 amino acid transmembrane region and 35 amino acid cytoplasmic domain that

has no homology to the CD62E or CD62L domains.

Alternative splicing gives rise to molecules that lack the exon 11 (encoding the seventh CCP domain) or lack exon 14 resulting in a soluble CD62P detectable in the blood.

Transient phosphorylation of CD62P Ser, Thr, Tyr, and His residues occurs when platelets are activated.

Cys 766 is acylated with palmitic and stearic acid.

Mol Wt: Reduced, 140 kDa; unreduced, 120 kDa.

Function

Binds glycoproteins with CD15s (Sialyl Lewis X) epitopes, including CD162 [P-selectin glycoprotein ligand-1, (PSGL-1)].

Also binds unrelated polyanions.

Endothelial CD62P binding to CD162 enables tethering and rolling of leukocytes that precedes leukocyte extravasation and migration toward sites of inflammation.

Mediates rolling of platelets on endothelial cells and assists platelet-mediated delivery of leukocytes to high endothelial venules.

Implicated in the metastasis of various carcinomas as CD24-expressing tumor cells bind P-selectin on platelets and form thrombi, which protect tumor cells from immune destruction while circulating.

Binding of CD62P to CD24 enables rolling of tumor cells on vascular endothelium in the process of extravasation and tissue penetration during metastasis.

Constitutive CD62P expression during inflammation can result in thrombosis, atherogenesis, and tissue destruction.

CD62P knockout mice display reduced leukocyte rolling on endothelium and migration to sites of inflammation. CD62P and CD62E double knockout mice demonstrate that the roles of CD62P and CD62E overlap, as the inflammation defects are much more severe. These mice also have severe leukocytosis, altered hematopoiesis, and greater susceptibility to infection.

Ligands

CD162, CD24.

Expression

Megakaryocytes, activated platelets, and activated endothelium.

Applications

Potential target for the treatment of chronic inflammatory diseases such as asthma.

Gene Name   Entrez Gene#

SELP   6403

Selected Monoclonal Antibodies

G1 (McEver; Oklahoma City); AC1.2 (Warner; San José).

CD63

Other Names

LIMP, gp55, LAMP-3, neuroglandular antigen, melanoma-associated antigen ME 491, Pltgr40, granulophysin.

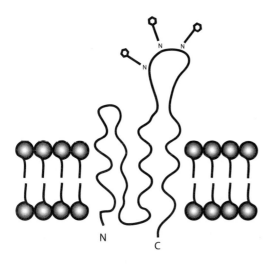

Molecular Structure

A heavily glycosylated lysosmal protein belonging to the TM4SF tetraspanin family (see CD9).

Has four hydrophobic transmembrane domains with a larger, heavily glycosylated extracellular domain of 95 amino acids between transmembrane segments 3 and 4 and a smaller extracellular domain between transmembrane domains 1 and 2.

Three potential N-glycosylation sites are glycosylated in a cell-type specific manner, and the N-glycans are characteristic of those found on lysosomal membrane proteins.

The C-terminal SGYEVM sequence acts as lysosomal targeting sequence.

Mol Wt: 40–60 kDa.

Function

Associated on the cell surface with VLA3, 4, and 6 and with CD11/CD18 integrin as well as other TM4SF molecules CD9 and CD81. Probably forms large complexes like other TM4SF molecules.

Intracellular lysosomal/endosomal/ granule protein in Weibel-Palade bodies of vascular endothelium.

Upon activation of platelets, endothelial cells and granulocytes, CD63 is rapidly translocated to the cell surface.

Detectable in exosomes secreted by a variety of cells, which appear to be capable of delivering antigens and other molecules to target cells. CD63 may function as an adhesion molecule in this system.

Antigen thought to be associated with early stages of melanoma tumour progression. Appears to regulate melanoma cell motility and adhesion to ligands of β1 integrins in extracellular matrix.

Expression

Activated platelets, activated endothelium, degranulated granulocytes, monocytes, macrophages, all T cells, low level on subset of B cells including CLL and neonatal B cells.

Also found on fibroblasts, osteoclasts, smooth muscle, white matter of brain and peripheral nerves, and synovial lining cells.

Applications

Marker of platelet activation, late endosomes and primary melanoma.

Gene Name   Entrez Gene#

CD63   967

Selected Monoclonal Antibodies

RUU-SP2.28 (Nieuwenhuis; Utrecht); CLB-gran/12 (Fijnheer; Amsterdam).

CD64

Other Names

FcgR1, FcγR1.

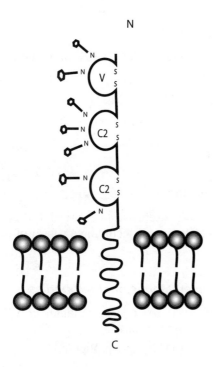

Molecular Structure

A type I transmembrane glycoprotein with three IgC-like domains in the extracellular region.

Extensively glycosylated.

Functional protein is encoded by the FcgRIA gene although there are two other genes FcgRIB and FcgRIC that possibly encode soluble FcgR, but no function has been assigned to these molecules.

Forms a multi-subunit receptor that requires association with the common FcR γ signaling chain for stable surface expression and to mediate phagocytosis.

Like other Fcγ receptors, CD64 has a unique cytoplasmic tail, which is suspected to have signaling properties, but no signaling motif has yet been identified.

Mol Wt: 72 kDa.

Function

Receptor for Fc segment of IgG, mediating phagocytosis of immune complexes, antibody-dependent cellular cytotoxicity, antigen capture for presentation to T cells, and release of cytokines and reactive oxygen intermediates.

CD64 deficiency has been described in four individuals. All are healthy which suggests other molecules can compensate for the lack of CD64.

Ligands

High affinity binding to IgG.

Expression

Constitutively expressed on monocytes, macrophages, and a subset of blood and germinal center dendritic cells.

Early myeloid lineage cells and granulocytes activated by IFNγ or G-CSF.

Applications

Potential marker for AML subsets: AML MO-M2 variable; M3 usually; M4, M5. Not present on AML M7.

Gene Name	Entrez Gene#
FCGR1A	2209

Selected Monoclonal Antibodies

32.2 (Guyre; Hannover); 22 (Guyre; Hannover).

CD65, CD65s

Other Names

Ceramide dodecasaccharide 4c.
CD65s: VIM2, Sialylated-CD65.

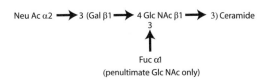

Molecular Structure

CD65s is a fucoganglioside with four lactosamine repeats, one fucose bound to the penultimate N-acetylglucosamine, and one terminal α2,3 linked N-acetyl-neuraminic acid (NeuAc-Gal-GlcNAc-Gal-GlcNAc (Fuc)-Gal-GlcNAc-Gal-GlcNAc-Gal-Glc-Cer).

CD65 is the same oligosaccharide without the terminal sialic acid.

The epitopes are carried by various glycolipids and glycoproteins.

Function

One study has implicated CD65 as a critical adhesion molecule for extravascular AML infiltration.

CD65s appears when CD34 disappears during myeloid differentiation.

Ligands

Potential ligand for CD62E and CD62L.

Expression

Granulocytes, monocytes (both forms); AML blasts and some ALL blasts express CD65s.

Applications

CD65s is useful as a marker for acute leukemia typing, including a subset of pre-preB ALL.

Selected Monoclonal Antibodies

CD65: HE10 (Tursz; Villejuif); VIM8 (Knapp; Vienna).
CD65s: VIM2 (Knapp; Vienna).

CD66a

Other Names

Biliary glycoprotein (BGP), NCA-160.

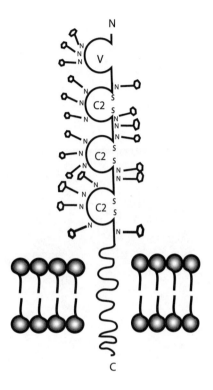

Molecular Structure

A member of the carcinoembryonic antigen (CEA) family of the Ig superfamily.

Thirteen splice variants have been identified (BGPa-z).

The structure consists of an N-terminal IgV-like domain and three Ig C2 domains.

Heavily N-glycosylated molecule with 20 potential glycosylation sites.

BGPa is the longest variant with a leader sequence of 34 amino acids, 382 amino acid extracellular domain, 43 amino acid transmembrane region, and 67 amino acid, cytoplasmic domain.

Short cytoplasmic tail with two YXXL motifs and two potential tyrosine phosphorylation sites.

Mol Wt: Reduced, 140–180 kDa.

Function

Cell adhesion molecule capable of homophilic and heterophilic adhesion with CD66c and CD66e probably via their protein core.

Carbohydrate groups of CD66a bind E-selectin (CD62E).

Capable of transmembrane signaling leading to the activation of neutrophils.

Binds type 1 fimbriae and is a receptor for *N. meningitis* and *N. gonorrhoeae*.

Displays mannose-sensitive binding to intestinal bacteria.

CD66 expression is dramatically down-regulated in malignancies, which suggests a possible role in tumor suppression.

May act as a regulator of bile transport in bile cannaliculi.

Ligands

CD62E, mannose-sensitive adhesin of gut bacteria, CD66a, CD66c, and CD66e.

Opa proteins of pathogenic *Neisseria* sp.

Expression

Primarily expressed on granulocytes and epithelial cells, but also found on NK cells, LAK and activated T cells, prostate glands and ducts, and bile canaliculi between liver cells.

Detectable on low grade prostatic carcinoma.

Gene Name	Entrez Gene#
CEACAM1	634

Selected Monoclonal Antibodies

Several antibodies recognize CD66a together with other CD66 family members: KAT4c (Turley; Oxford); 12-140-5 (Bormer; Oslo); (CD66a,b,c,e); YTH71.3 (Hale; Durham) (CD66a,c,d); CLB-gran/1 (van der Schoot; Amsterdam); HEA81 (Möller, Heidelberg);(CDa,c,d,e); F36-54 (Matsuoka; Saitama), 4/3/17 (Grunert; Freiburg) (CD66a,c,e); COL-4 (Schlom; Boston) (CD66a,d,e); 12-140-4 (Bormer; Oslo) (CD66a,e).

CD66b

Other Names

CGM6, NCA-95, previously CD67.

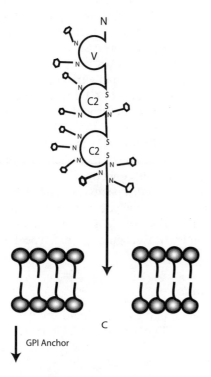

GPI Anchor

Molecular Structure

A member of the carcinoembryonic antigen (CEA) family of the Ig super-family.

This glycoprotein has a 34 amino acid leader sequence and an extracellular domain of 284 amino acid that is anchored to the membrane via GPI.

The structure is predicted to have an N-terminal IgV-like domain and two Ig C2 domains.

Heavily N-glycosylated with 11 potential N-glycosylation sites.

No splice variants have been described.

Mol Wt: Reduced, 95–100 kDa.

Function

Capable of heterophilic adhesion by binding the protein core of CD66c.

Associates with some Src family kinases in neutrophils and is involved in transmembrane signaling, which results in activation of neutrophils possibly by regulating activity of CD11/CD18.

Upon activation of neutrophils, CD66b is shed; however, no function has as yet been attributed to the soluble protein.

Ligands

CD66b binds CD66c.

Expression

Granulocytes.

Applications

Potential application in detecting sites of infection and inflammation.

Gene Name   Entrez Gene#

CEACAM8   1088

Selected Monoclonal Antibodies

B13.9 (van der Schoot; Amsterdam); 80H3 (Grunert; Freiburg); B4-EA4 (Micheel; Freiburg) recognizes CD66b, e.

CD66c

Other Names

NCA, nonspecific cross-reacting antigen, NCA-50/90.

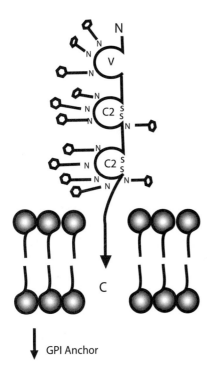

GPI Anchor

Molecular Structure

A glycophospatidylinositol (GPI)-anchored glycoprotein. Member of the carcinoembryonic antigen (CEA) gene family within the Ig superfamily.

The molecule has a 34 amino acid leader sequence followed by a 286 amino acid extracellular domain consisting of one IgV-like and two IgC-like domains linked to a GPI anchor.

Heavily and variably glycosylated with 12 potential N-glycosylation sites.

No splice variants have been found; however, NCA50 and NCA90 (formerly called TEX) are two gycosylation variants.

Mol Wt: 90 kDa.

Function

Capable of homophilic adhesion and heterophilic binding to CD66a–e, CD62E, and galectins.

Associates with some Src family kinases in neutrophils and is involved in transmembrane signaling, which results in activation of neutrophils possibly by regulating activity of CD11/CD18.

Evidence from an in vitro study suggests heterodimerization of CD66a–c molecules on the surface of neutrophils leads to concomitant clustering of the CD11b subunit of CD11b/CD18 (CR3) and activation of the integrin leading to increased adherence of the cells to fibronectin.

Interacts with opacity-associated (Opa) proteins of pathogenic *Neisseria* sp., acting as a receptor for *N. gonorrhoea* and *N. meningitidis*. Recognizes some type 1 fimbriae of *E. coli*.

Ligands

E-selectin and galectins bind the carbohydrate of CD66b, whereas CD66a, CD66b, CD66c, and CD66e bind the protein core of CD66c.

Opa proteins of pathogenic *Neisseria* sp.

Expression

Granulocytes and epithelial cells.

Applications

Has potential applications in the detection of sites of infection and inflammation.

Gene Name	Entrez Gene#
CEACAM6	4680

Selected Monoclonal Antibodies

F106-88 (Matsuoka; Saitama); 12G7 (Grunert; Freiburg); 4H12 (Grunert, Freiburg); By114 (Pulford; Oxford) recognizes CD66c, e.

CD66d

Other Names

CGM1.

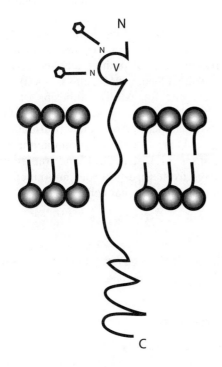

Molecular Structure

A member of the carcinoembryonic antigen (CEA) gene family within the Ig superfamily.

The protein has a 34 amino acid leader peptide, a 108 amino acid N terminal extracellular region consisting of one IgV-like domain, a 39 amino acid transmembrane domain, and a 71 amino acid cytoplasmic region that contains two YXXL motifs.

In contrast to some other members of the CEA family, which are glycophosphatidylinositol (GPI)-anchored, the CD66d molecule is a transmembrane glycoprotein. Alternative splicing results in three variants, one of which lacks the YXXL motifs due to a reading frame shift.

Binding site for opacity-associated (Opa) proteins of pathogenic *Neisseria* sp. occurs at the non-glycosylated face of the extracellular domain and requires Tyr-34 and Ile-91. Binding efficiency and specificity for particular Opa proteins is enhanced by other nonadjacent amino acids, which are found in close proximity to Tyr-34 and Ile-91 in the 3D-structure.

Mol Wt: Reduced, 35 kDa.

Function

May be involved in signaling and adhesion.

Capable of activating neutrophils and functions as a receptor for *Neisseria gonorrhoea* and *N. meningitidis*.

Its interaction with opacity-associated (Opa) proteins of pathogenic *Neisseria* sp results in signaling via Src family kinases and efficient uptake of the organism. Less-efficient CD66d-mediated uptake of *N. gonorrhoea* has also been observed in the absence of tyrosine phosphorylation.

Ligands

Opa proteins of pathogenic *Neisseria* sp.

Expression

CD66d is expressed by granulocytes.

Gene Name	*Entrez Gene#*
CEACAM3	1084

Selected Monoclonal Antibodies

COL-1 (Schlom; Boston) reacts with CD66d,e.

CD66e

Other Names

CEA, carcinoembryonic antigen, CEA-CAM5, meconium antigen100.

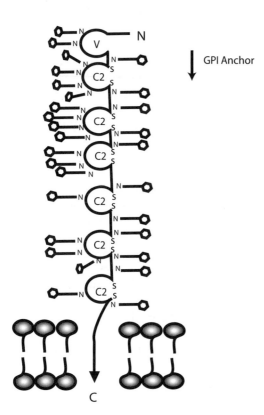

Molecular Structure

A member of the carcinoembryonic antigen (CEA) gene family within the Ig superfamily.

The protein structure consists of a leader peptide of 34 amino acids and a 642 amino acid extracellular region containing 1 IgV-like and 6 IgC-like domains and is glycophosphatidylinositol (GPI)-anchored to the membrane.

Heavily and variably N-glycosylated with 29 potential N-glycosylation sites.

No splice variants have been identified.

Mol Wt: Reduced, 100–200 kDa.

Function

Capable of homophilic and heterophilic adhesion to protein cores of CD66a and CD66c.

Is secreted by intestinal epithelial cells and is detectable in feces and pancreatico-biliary secretions.

May be involved in tumor metastasis.

Receptor for the opacity-associated (Opa) proteins of pathogenic *Neisseria* sp (see also CD66a, CD66c, and CD66d).

Receptor for Afa/Dr adhesins of diffusely adhering *E. coli*, which upon binding leads to activation of signal transduction pathways that result in proinflammatory responses and structural and functional damage to the brush border and junctions of intestinal epithelial cells.

Ligands

CD66a, CD66c, CD66e, Opa proteins of pathogenic *Neisseria* sp.

Expression

Epithelial cells.

Applications

Serum CEA is used as a clinical marker of tumor burden.

Potential target for tumor imaging and drug targeting.

CD66e promoter may have potential for use in tumor selective expression of pro-drugs.

Gene Name	Entrez Gene#
CEACAM5	1048

Selected Monoclonal Antibodies

T84.66 (Hefta; Duarte); 26/3/13 (Grunert; Freiburg); 26/5/1 (Grunert; Freiburg).

CD66f

Other Names

PSG, pregnancy-specific glycoprotein; Sp-1, pregnancy specific (b1) glycoprotein.

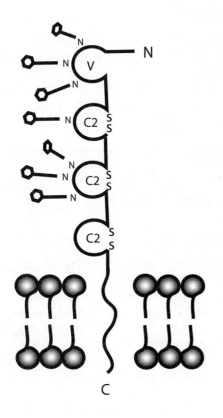

Molecular Structure

A member of the carcinoembryonic antigen (CEA) gene family within the Ig superfamily.

A glycoprotein has 34 amino acid leader sequence, 286 or 378 amino acid extracellular domain with 2 or 3 Ig C2 domains, and 1 IgG-V like domain followed by short hydrophilic sequences of 2–13 amino acids.

Many splice variants occur.

Heavily and variably glycosylated with between four and eight potential N-glycosylation sites.

Soluble protein.

Mol Wt: Reduced, 54–72 kDa.

Function

Essential for successful pregnancy.

May protect fetus from maternal immune system.

Expression

Produced by placental syncytiotrophoblasts and detectable in maternal serum, fetal liver, and myeloid cell lines.

Applications

Low levels in maternal blood predict spontaneous abortion.

Gene Name	Entrez Gene#
PSG1	5669

Selected Monoclonal Antibodies

G3, 11D10 (Chou; Bethesda).

CD68

Other Names

gp110, macrosialin (mouse).

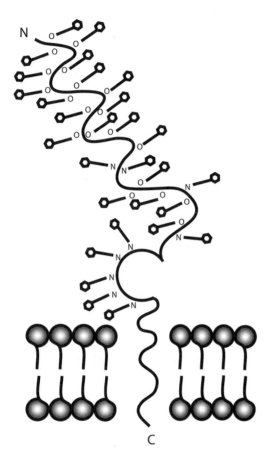

Molecular Structure

A type I transmembrane glycoprotein.

Mucin-like molecule (other members: CD34, CD43, CD164, and GlyCAM-1) and lysosomal/plasma membrane shuttling protein (see CD107a, and CD107b).

A 354 amino acid protein with a 298 amino acid extracellular region containing two domains linked by a proline-rich hinge.

N-terminal mucin-like domain that has short peptide repeats and several serine and threonine residues that are potentially O-glycosylated.

The membrane-proximal domain bears homology to the lysosomal/plasma membrane shuttling proteins (LGPs).

Mol Wt: Unreduced, 110 kDa.

Function

Scavenger receptor, which binds and internalizes oxidized low density lipoprotein (LDL).

One of several scavenger receptors of macrophages that contribute to foam cell formation in atherosclerosis.

Ligands

Oxidatively modified low density lipoprotein (LDL).

Expression

Mainly expressed in cytoplasmic granules, but also on the surface of monocytes and macrophages, dendritic cells, neutrophils, basophils, eosinophils, mast cells, subset of CD34+ hemopoietic bone marrow progenitors, and activated T cells.

Cytoplasmic expression in non-hemopoietic cells particularly in the liver, glomeruli, and renal tubules.

Soluble forms have been detected in serum and urine.

Applications

Probably the best macrophage marker in immunohistochemistry.

Gene Name	Entrez Gene#
CD68	968

Selected Monoclonal Antibodies

Y2/131 (Mason; Oxford); EBM11 (Johansson; Glostrup); Ki-M7 (Radzun; Kiel).

CD69

Other Names

AIM, activation-induced molecule, MLR3, EA1, VEA.

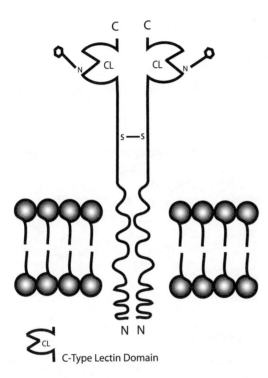

C-Type Lectin Domain

Molecular Structure

Member of the Ca^{++}-dependent (C-type) lectin superfamily of type II transmembrane receptors (see CD23, CD72, CD94, and CD161).

Disulphide-linked, homodimeric phosphorylated glycoprotein.

Core protein is 199 amino acids and is constitutively Ser and Thr phosphorylated.

One potential N-glycosylation site at position 166.

Mol Wt: Unreduced, 60 kDa. Although the protein cores are identical, the two chains of the homodimer are differentially glycosylated, leading to two bands at 22 and 33 kDa after reduction.

Function

Function has not been clearly demonstrated, and the results of *in vitro* studies appear to conflict with observations of CD69-deficient mice.

In vitro: Appears to have signaling functions and is involved in the early stages of activation of lymphocytes, monocytes, and platelets.

Induces Ca^{++} influx, synthesis of cytokines and their receptors, and expression of proto-oncogenes c-myc and c-fos during T-cell activation.

In platelets: Induces Ca^{++} influx, hydrolysis of arachidonic acid, and aggregation.

CD69 cross-linking induces cytotoxicity and cytokine release in NK cells.

CD69-deficient mice demonstrate an essential role for the molecule in downregulating the immune response by inducing production of pleiotropic cytokine transforming growth factor (TGF-β).

Overwhelming majority of T cells in inflammatory infiltrates of several diseases, including rheumatoid arthritis, viral hepatitis, and autoimmune thyroid disorders, are CD69[+].

Expression

Activtated leukocytes: T cells, thymocytes, B cells, NK cells, neutrophils, eosinophils.

Applications

Marker of early T-cell activation.

Gene Name	Entrez Gene#
CD69	969

Selected Monoclonal Antibodies

L78 (Buck; Mountain View); MLR3 (Cosulich; Genova); Bl-Ac/p26 (Fiebig; Leipzig).

CD70

Other Names

CD27 ligand, KI-24 antigen.

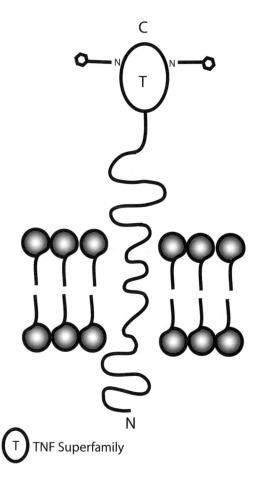

T TNF Superfamily

Molecular Structure

Type II transmembrane glycoprotein, member of the tumor necrosis factor (TNF) superfamily (see also CD153, CD154, CD95L).

A 193 amino acid protein has 155 amino acid C-terminal extracellular domain with two potential N-glycosylation sites, 18 amino acid transmembrane domain and a 20 amino acid cytoplasmic domain.

Forms trimeric structure.

Mol Wt: 50 kDa.

Function

Plays a role in T-cell activation, inducing proliferation of costimulated T cells and enhancing the generation of cytolytic T cells.

Involved in the generation and long-term maintenance of T-cell memory, particularly in CD8$^+$ cells.

Plays a role in expansion and differentiation of B cells and plasma cell differentation.

Ligands

Binds to CD27.

Expression

Transiently expressed on activated T and B lymphocytes and activated NK cells.

Constitutively expressed on B-cell chronic lymphocytic leukemias and large B-cell lymphomas.

Gene Name	Entrez Gene#
TNFSF7	970

Selected Monoclonal Antibodies

Ki-24 (Stein; Berlin); BU69 (Hardie; Birmingham).

CD71

Other Names

Transferrin receptor.

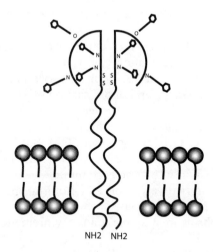

Molecular Structure

Disulfide-bonded homodimeric type II transmembrane molecule of 760 amino acids.

The protein has a 671 amino acid extracellular C-terminal domain that contains the transferrin-binding site, a 28 amino acid transmembrane domain, and a 61 amino acid N-terminal cytoplasmic tail that contains the conserved sequence YTRF essential for mediating rapid endocytosis and recycling.

Three N- and one O-glycosylation sites.

Cysteine residue in the transmembrane region proximal to the cytoplasmic domain is acylated.

Cytoplasmic domain is Ser and Thr phosphorylated.

Mol Wt: Reduced, 95 kDa; unreduced, 190 kDa.

Function

Mediates cellular iron uptake via internalization and recycling of transferrin.

N-terminal cytoplasmic domain mediates rapid endocytosis and recycling.

In addition to its role in delivering iron, the transferrin receptor may have further functions in the regulation of cell growth. (See CD178.)

Several CD71 antibodies block transferrin binding and lead to an arrest in cell division and an accumulation of cells in S-phase.

Can bind IgA complexes and is implicated in IgA nephropathy by mediating IgA1-complex deposition in glomerular mesangia.

Ligands

Transferrin, IgA

Expression

All proliferating cells.

Erythropoietic cells that use iron for heme synthesis and differentiation rather than proliferation.

Overexpressed in certain tumors such as glioma and colon cancer.

Applications

Marker of proliferation.

Target for monoclonal antibodies that inhibit proliferation.

Has been used to target cytotoxic molecules to proliferating cells.

Transfection of DNA into cells (transferrinfection).

Gene Name   *Entrez Gene#*

TFRC   7037

Selected Monoclonal Antibodies

T9 (Schlossman; Boston); 42.6.3 (Trowbridge; LaJolla); VIP1 (Knapp; Vienna).

CD72

Other Names

Lyb-2 (mouse homologue), Ly-19.2, Ly32.2.

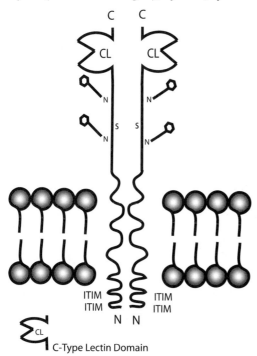

C-Type Lectin Domain

Molecular Structure

A type II transmembrane protein and a member of the Ca^{++}-dependent (C-type) lectin superfamily (see CD23, CD69, CD94, and CD161).

A 359 amino acid protein with extracellular, C-terminal lectin domain followed by an α-helical coiled coil that forms a 15-nm stalk and spacer between the lectin domain and the membrane.

Glycosylation sites are present within the stalk region.

Cytoplasmic tail has two immunoreceptor tyrosine-based inhibitory motifs (ITIMs).

Forms disulphide-linked homodimers.

Alternatively spliced isoform displays polymorphism.

Mol Wt: 45 kDa.

Function

Putative ligand for CD100 and for CD5.

Plays a role in B-cell proliferation and differentiation.

Downregulates signaling by B-cell receptor (BCR) containing either IgM or IgG.

CD100 (Sem4D) appears to prevent negative regulation by CD72 as upon binding to CD72, dephosphorylation of ITIMs occurs and disassociation of SHP-1.

Some evidence to suggest that positive signaling may occur through the recruitment of Grb2 to the other ITIM. B cells of CD72-deficient mice are hyperproliferative in response to various stimuli.

Alternatively spliced isoform polymorphism associated with presence of nephritis in systemic lupus erythrematosis (SLE).

Interaction with FcγR2B modifies susceptibility to SLE.

Ligands

CD72 binds CD100.

CD5 is a putative ligand.

Expression

All B lymphocytes from early progenitors through to mature cells, but expression is downregulated during differentiation into plasma cells.

Expressed on macrophages and dendritic cells.

Gene Name   Entrez Gene#

CD72   971

Selected Monoclonal Antibodies

S-HCL2 (Schwarting; Berlin); BU-40 (Hardie; Birmingham); J3-109 (Pesando; Seattle).

CD73

Other Names

Ecto-5′-nucleotidase.

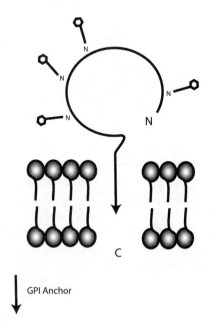

GPI Anchor

Molecular Structure

A glycophosphatidylinositol (GPI)-linked 5′-nucleotidase.

Mature protein predicted to be 548 amino acids.

C-terminus has a stretch of uncharged and hydrophobic amino acids, which are substituted for a GPI anchor bound to Ser-523.

Molecule is N-glycosylated in a tissue-specific manner.

CD73 does not appear to be O-glycosylated but is sialylated.

Mol Wt: 69–72 kDa.

Function

Catalyses the dephosphorylation of purine and pyrimidine ribo- and deoxyiribonucleoside monophosphates to the nucleoside.

Putative role in regulating the availability of adenosine for interaction with cell surface adenosine receptor.

Can mediate costimulatory signals in T-cell activation and can do so in the absence of the GPI anchor or its 5′-nucleoside activity. May contribute to lymphocyte adhesion to the endothelium.

Implicated in B-cell–follicular dendritic cell interactions although no ligand has been identified.

Monoclonal antibody triggering of CD73 results in rapid shedding of CD73 and protein phosphorylation in lymphocytes, but the same does not occur in endothelial cells, suggesting control of CD73 expression differs between the two cell types.

Expression

Expression increases during development of T and B lymphocytes.

25% CD3$^+$, 10% CD4$^+$, and 50% CD8$^+$ peripheral blood T cells and expression is restricted to a CD28$^+$ subset of T cells.

75% adult peripheral blood B cells.

Various lymphomas and leukemias.

Expressed on follicular dendritic cells and epithelial and endothelial cells.

Applications

High CD73 expression in leukemia or lymphoma is a poor prognostic indicator.

Low CD73 expression found in some immunodeficiency diseases.

Gene Name	Entrez Gene#
NT5E	4907

Selected Monoclonal Antibodies

1E9.28.1 (Thompson; La Jolla); AD2 (Gwin/Cooper; Birmingham); FG2.2.11 (Thompson; La Jolla).

CD74

Other Names

MHC class II associated invariant chain (Ii), class II-specific chaperone.

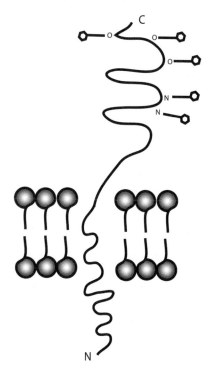

Molecular Structure

A type II membrane protein.

CD74 gene consists of nine exons, and four major isoforms are generated by variable splicing and alternative usage of two in-phase initiation codons.

Isoforms Ii33 and Ii35 are both encoded by 8 exons but differ by 16 N-terminal amino acids due to alternative translation initiation.

Ii41 is encoded by nine exons and is derived by alternative splicing of a pre-mRNA.

Addition of exon 6b in Ii41 and Ii43 results in a cysteine-rich stretch of 64 residues near the C-terminus with significant homology to a repetitive sequence of thyroglobulin.

Isoform Ii35 has an ER retention signal and a sorting signal close to the N-terminus.

Residues 81–104 form the class II binding site, and this sequence is referred to as the class II associated invariant chain peptide (CLIP).

Residues 91–99 within CLIP occupy the groove of class II heterodimers during intracellular transport.

Residues 163–183 form the site where emergent CD74 molecules trimerise.

Ii 33 protein has a 160 amino acid extracellular domain, 26 amino acid transmembrane domain, and 33 amino acid cytoplasmic domain.

Two or four N-glycosylation sites as well as two O-glycoslation sites and minor subfractions are palmitylated, sulfated, and phosphorylated or contain glycosaminoglycan side chains.

Soluble forms detectable in plasma.

Mol Wt: 33, 35, 41 (43), 43 (45) kDa.

Function

Regulates loading of exogenous-derived peptides onto MHC class II heterodimers.

CD74 homotrimers associate in the endoplasmic reticulum (ER) with three MHC class II α/β dimers, thus preventing binding of endogenous peptides. Following targeting to the trans-Golgi network and then into endosomal/lysosomal compartments, CD74 is proteolytically degraded leaving only the CLIP fragment occupying the peptide-binding groove of the α/β dimers until this complex associates with HLA-DM. CLIP is then released, and the class II molecules can bind exogenous peptide.

Required for normal positive selection of CD4[+] T cells.

May be required for endocytosis of MHC class II molecules as cell surface MHC class II–CD74 complexes are rapidly internalized to endosomes.

Cell surface form of CD74 binds macrophage migration inhibitory factor (MIF) with high affinity, and this interaction leads to activation of the extracellular signal-regulated kinase (ERK)-1/2 MAP kinase signal cascade, PGE2 production, and cell proliferation. In certain cell types, CD44 recruitment into the CD74–MIF complex may be necessary for MIF signal transduction to occur.

In vitro, chondroitin sulphated CD74 (Ii-CS) can act as an accessory molecule enhancing activation of primary T-cell responses through interaction with CD44 on CD44$^+$ T cells.

Knockout mice have deficient MHC class II assembly and transport, decreased surface expression of class II molecules, altered antigen presentation, and inefficient positive selection of CD4$^+$ T cells. Those CD4$^+$ cells that do mature display aberrant peripheral activation.

Ligands

HLA-DR heterodimers, macrophage migration inhibitory factor (MIF), and CD44.

Expression

MHC class II positive cells, including B cells and other antigen presenting cells and activated T cells, and activated endothelial and epithelial cells.

Applications

Useful in the study of antigen presentation and processing and analysis of subcellular compartments.

Phenotyping of leukemias and lymphomas.

Potential therapeutic target for treatment of malignancies and immunologic diseases due to its restricted expression in normal tissues and rapid internalization.

Gene Name	Entrez Gene#
CD74	972

Selected Monoclonal Antibodies

LN2 (Epstein; Frankfurt); BU-43 (Hardie; Birmingham); BU-45 (Hardie; Birmingham).

CD75, CD75s, CDw76

Other Names

CD75 indicates lactosamines; CD75s indicates sialylated lactosamines; CDw76.

Neu Ac α2 ⟶ 6 (Gal β1 ⟶ 4GlcNAcβ1 ⟶ 3) n-R

Molecular Structure

CD75 comprises lactosamine structures, whereas CD75s describes sialylated lactosamines (CD75s).

The carbohydrate epitopes are expressed in association with a variety of glycoproteins and glycolipids.

Different antibodies show somewhat different reactivities, and CDw76, previously regarded as a different entity, is now subsumed in CD75 and CD75s.

The expression of the sialylated form is dependent on the activity of the β-galactose α2,6 sialyltransferase.

Mol Wt: Immunoprecipitation reveals proteins at 67 and 85 kDa.

Expression

CD75: Germinal center B cells, with lower levels on other mature B cells but down-regulated on differentiation to plasma cells.

CD75s: Mature B cells in blood and lymphoid tissue, lost on germinal center and plasma cell differentiation.

T-cell subsets ($CD8^+$ cells more than $CD4^+$ cells).

Mature B-cell leukemias but not B-ALL.

Subsets of endothelial and epithelial cells.

Applications

Differentiates between malignant B-cell types.

Selected Monoclonal Antibodies

CD75: OKB4 (Goldstein; Raritan).

CD75s: HH2 (Funderud; Oslo); EBU-141 (Gramatzki; Erlangen).

Classified as CDw76: HD66 (Dörken; Berlin); CRIS-4 (Vilella; Barcelona).

CD77

Other Names

Globotriaosylceramide (Gb3); Pk blood group antigen; Burkitt's lymphoma associated antigen (BLA), ceramide trihexoside (CTH).

Gal α1 ➤ 4 Gal β1 ➤ 4 Glc β1 - Ceramide

Molecular Structure

Neutral glycosphingolipid of the globoside series (Gal-α1-4 Gal-β1-4 Glc-β1-Cer) and is the rare Pk blood group antigen.

Consists of three carbohydrate molecules linked to a lipid moiety in the cell membrane.

Exposure of CD77 depends on the length and extent of unsaturation of the fatty acid chain.

Mol Wt: 1 kDa.

Function

Receptor for Shiga toxin and Verotoxin, which cause dysentery and hemolytic uremic syndrome.

Physiological function not known but may bind CD19.

Function has not been clearly demonstrated, but there is evidence to suggest CD77 is involved in elimination of germinal center B cells that fail to produce high affinity antibody.

CD77 expression is lost from cells that are rescued from death by binding antigens on follicular dendritic cells. CD77 antibodies and Verotoxin (VT-B) induce apoptosis of Burkitt's lymphoma cells.

Ligands

Shiga toxin of *Shigella dysenteriae* type 1 and verotoxin 1 of enterohemorrhagic *Escherichia coli*.

Possibly binds CD19 due to its similarity to the binding subunit of verotoxin.

Expression

Germinal center B cells, more strongly on centroblasts, but can be induced on extrafollicular B cells.

Strongly expressed on Burkitt's lymphoma cells.

Endothelia and epithelia.

Applications

Used as a centroblast marker.

Potential use as a target for cancer therapy particularly hematological malignancies such as follicular lymphoma, multiple myeloma, and chronic lymphocytic leukemia.

Selected Monoclonal Antibodies

38.13 (BLA) (Wiels/Tursz; Villejuif); 424/4A11 (Brodin; Lund); 424/3D9 (Brodin; Lund).

CDw78

Other Names

Ba.

Molecular Structure

CDw78 antibodies turn out to be against MHC class II, and CDw78 has therefore been deleted from CD classification. The epitope detected by CDw78 antibodies is present on a restricted subset of MHC class II molecules.

CD79a

Other Names

mb-1, IGA, Ig-alpha.

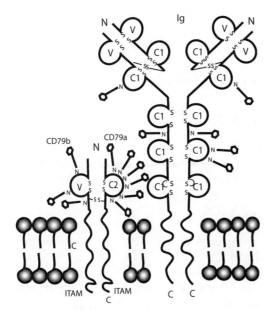

Molecular Structure

A type I integral membrane protein and a member of the Ig superfamily.

The 109 amino acid extracellular region consists of 1 IgC-like domain followed by a 22 amino acid transmembrane region and the 61 amino acid cytoplasmic domain that contains a cytoplasmic immunoreceptor tyrosine-based activation motif (ITAM).

Six potential N-glycosylation sites.

Forms a disulphide-linked heterodimer with CD79b.

The Cys reside found in the Ser-Cys-Gly-Thr sequence present in both CD79a and b is considered to be the site where the disulphide bond occurs.

Mol Wt: 32–33 kDa.

Function

CD79a (Igα) associates with CD79b (Igβ) creating a heterodimer that then interacts with membrane Ig (mIgM) to form the B-cell antigen receptor (BCR).

The CD79 heterodimer is necessary to escort the receptor complex to the cell membrane. When mIgM binds antigen, the CD79 heterodimer transduces the signal and promotes endocytosis of bound antigen for intracellular degradation and presentation to T helper cells.

CD79 heterodimer has been shown to function synergistically to induce apoptosis via the BCR.

Expression

Present early in B-cell maturation with marginal zone and follicular mantle B cells having stronger expression than germinal center.

Found intracellularly in plasma cells.

Applications

Useful in differential diagnosis of B-cell neoplasms from T-cell or myeloid neoplasms.

Useful marker of precursor B acute lymphoblastic leukemia (pre-B-ALL).

Gene Name   Entrez Gene#

CD79A   973

Selected Monoclonal Antibodies

HM47 (Cordell; Oxford).

CD79b

Other Names

B29; IGB, Ig-beta.

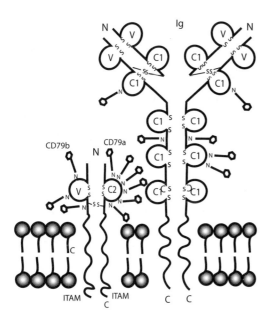

Molecular Structure

A type I integral membrane protein encoded by the B29 gene.

A member of the Ig superfamily.

The 131 amino acid extracellular region consists of 1 IgV-like domain followed by a 21 amino acid transmembrane region and a 49 amino acid cytoplasmic domain containing a cytoplasmic immunoreceptor tyrosine-based activation motif (ITAM).

Three potential N-glycosylation sites.

A truncated variant form of CD79b of only 125 amino acids also occurs in human B cells and B-cell lines.

Forms disulfide linked heterodimer with CD79a (see CD79a).

Mol Wt: 37–39 kDa.

Function

See CD79a.

The progression of pro B cells to pre B cells is blocked in CD79b deficient mice.

Expression

Expression of truncated CD79b is upregulated in B-CLL.

Present early in B-cell maturation with marginal zone and follicular mantle B cells having stronger expression than germinal center.

Found intracellularly in plasma cells.

Gene Name   Entrez Gene#

CD79B   974

Selected Monoclonal Antibodies

SN8 (Seon; Buffalo).

CD80

Other Names

B7-1; BB1.

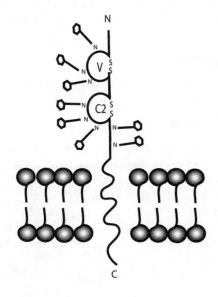

Molecular Structure

A type I integral membrane protein related to CD86.

A member of the Ig superfamily.

The extracellular region consists of one IgV-like and one IgC-like domain, both of which are highly glycosylated.

Single transmembrane domain and variable cytoplasmic domain ranging from 16 to 31 amino acids depending on species and splice variant.

Alternative splicing of two exons encoding cytoplasmic domain.

Eight N-linked glycosylation sites.

Mol Wt: Unreduced, 60 kDa (immunoprecipitation).

Function

Costimulation of T cells through ligation of CD28 and CTLA-4 (CD152).

Coregulator of T-cell activation with CD86.

Binding to CD28 results in T-cell activation, whereas CD80 binding to CD152 provides inhibitory signals to T cells.

Putative susceptibility gene for rheumatoid arthritis.

Ligands

CD80 binds CD28 and CD152 (CTLA-4).

Expression

Activated B cells, activated T cells, macrophages, and dendritic cells.

Applications

CD28–CD80 complex is a potential therapeutic target in the treatment of rheumatoid arthritis.

Gene Name	Entrez Gene#
CD80	941

Selected Monoclonal Antibodies

BB1 (Clark; Seattle); L307 (Warner; San José).

CD81

Other Names

Target of an antiproliferative antibody (TAPA-1); M38.

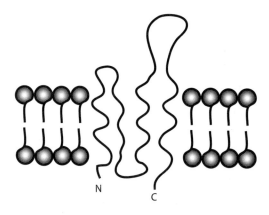

Molecular Structure

A member of the TM4SF tetraspanin family (see CD9).

Two extracellular domains of unequal size and four transmembrane domains.

The NH2- and COOH- termini are both intracellular.

No N-glycosylation.

Mol Wt: 26 kDa.

Function

Involved in a signal transduction complex with CD19, CD21, and Leu13 that regulates the threshold response to antigen.

Surface expression of CD81 is downregulated on lymphocytes during infections.

Receptor for hepatitis C virus and is required for hepatic infection by malarial parasites.

Knockout mice show subtle defects in B-cell maturation and antibody production.

Ligands

Envelope (E) 2 protein of hepatitis C virus.

Expression

Widely expressed among leukocytes with greatest expression in T cells followed by monocytes and then B cells. Expression increases after activation.

Lowest expression in granulocytes; however, the small subgroup of CD81+ granulocytes has high intensity levels per cell.

Also found on endothelia.

Gene Name	Entrez Gene#
CD81	975

Selected Monoclonal Antibodies

1D6 (Levy; Stanford); 4TM-1 (Tedder; Boston); JS64 (Pesando; Seattle).

CD82

Other Names

R2; 4F9; C33; IA4.

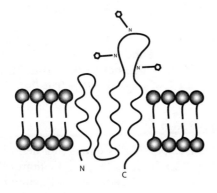

Molecular Structure

CD82 is a member of the tetraspan family (see CD9).

The protein has four putative trans-membrane domains (each at least 23 amino acids) with two unequal extracellular loops.

The NH2- and COOH- termini are short (9,15 amino acids) cytoplasmic sequences.

There are three putative N-glycosylation sites in the large extracellular loop.

Mol Wt: 45–90 kDa depending on the cell type and state of cell activation.

Function

CD82 plays a role in signal transduction. It forms a complex with other members of this family (CD37, CD53, and CD81), as well as integrins and MHC molecules.

CD82 cross-linking promotes activation of human monocytic cell lines.

Immobilized anti-CD82 antibody induces T-cell spreading, pseudopod formation, and modulation of T-cell proliferation and provides costimulatory signals for cytokine production.

May play a role in regulating tumor metastasis as loss of or reduced CD82 expression correlates with increased motility of prostate tumor cells as well as lung, pancreas, and colorectal cancers.

Expression

CD82 is expressed in polymorphonuclear cells and monocytes and has a weaker expression in T cells and B cells.

Expression of CD82 appears to be downregulated in all peripheral blood leukocytes during infections.

Epithelial cells, endothelial cells, and fibroblasts express CD82.

Applications

CD82 is a prognostic marker of metastatic potential in prostate, lung, breast, pancreas, and colon carcinomas and hepatoma.

Gene Name	Entrez Gene#
KAI1	3732

Selected Monoclonal Antibodies

4F9 (Morimoto; Boston); IA4 (Fradeliz; Villejuif).

CD83

Other Names

HB15.

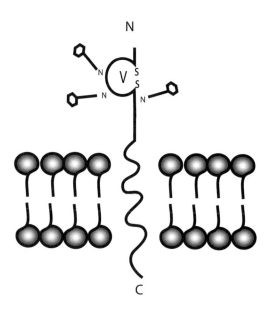

Molecular Structure

CD83 is a type I transmembrane protein and a member of the Ig superfamily.

The extracellular region has one IgV-like domain and is heavily glycosylated.

The protein has one transmembrane domain and a short cytoplasmic domain of 39 amino acids.

Alternative splicing of exons 3 and 4 generates three isoforms CD83a, b, and c.

Apart from the full-length membrane-bound molecule, only one variant, CD83c, has thus far been found to be a functional soluble isoform detectable in serum.

Mol Wt: 40–45 kDa.

Function

Function unknown but may be involved in activating immune effector cells.

CD83c levels are increased in serum of leukemia patients.

Knockout mice have arrested development of CD4$^+$ single-positive T cells.

Expression

CD83 is expressed by circulating dendritic cells (DCs), interdigitating reticulum cells present in the T-cell areas of lymphoid organs, Langerhans cells, and thymic DC and polymorphonuclear cells.

It is expressed on some EBV-transformed lymphoblastoid cell lines, Hodgkin cells, and with some germinal center B cells in vivo.

Applications

Dendritic cell marker.

Gene Name	Entrez Gene#
CD83	9308

Selected Monoclonal Antibodies

HB15a (Tedder; Boston); HB15b (Tedder; Boston).

CD84

Other Names

p75, GR6, SLAMF5, Hly9-β.

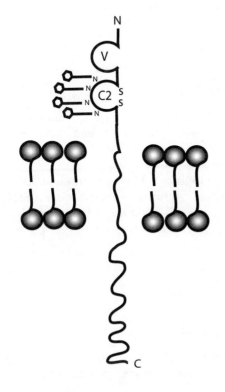

Molecular Structure

CD84 is a type I integral membrane glycoprotein and a member of the CD2 family of the Ig gene superfamily.

The extracellular domain has two Ig-like domains and is highly N-glycosylated.

The NH2-terminal domain is an IgV-type domain that lacks the disulphide bond between the β sheets.

The second domain is a C2-type Ig-like domain with two putative disulphide bonds.

The 83 residue cytoplasmic domain contains 5 tyrosines and Src homology 2 (SH2) domain binding motifs (TxYxxV/I) common to the cytoplasmic domains of CD2 family members.

Mol Wt: 64–82 kDa.

Function

Not known, but structural similarties to other adhesion molecules such as CD2 and CD48 suggest a function in intercellular interaction and signaling.

Putative function as a homotypic adhesion molecule and as a lymphocyte costimulatory molecule.

Ligation of CD84 by mAb enhances proliferation of anti-CD3 mAb stimulated human T cells and enhances IFN-γ secretion by lymphocytes.

CD84 associates with cytoplasmic, SH2 domain-containing peptides SAP and EAT-2.

Ligands

Homotypic adhesion.

Expression

Predominantly expressed on mature B cells and monocytes. CD45RO⁺ T cells, NK cells, and at low levels on polymorphs and platelets.

Strongly expressed on tissue macrophages.

Gene Name	Entrez Gene#
CD84	8832

Selected Monoclonal Antibodies

152-1D5 (Vilella; Barcelona); 2G7 (Tedder; Boston).

CD85a

Other Names

LIR-3 (leukocyte immunoglobulin-like receptor-3); ILT-5 (immunoglobulin-like transcript-2); HL9.

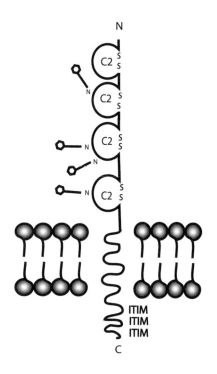

Molecular Structure

CD85a is a transmembrane glycoprotein and a member of the ILT/LIR family within the Ig gene superfamily.

CD85a has four extracellular C2-like Ig domains and a long cytoplasmic tail con-taining three immunoreceptor tyrosine-based inhibitor motif (ITIM) sequences.

Predicted to have a 608 amino acid extracellular domain, 21 amino acid trans-membrane region, and 167 amino acid cyto-plasmic domain.

Four potential N-glycosylation sites.

Mol Wt: 110 kDa.

Function

CD85a is involved in the activation of NK-mediated cytotoxicity and acts as an inhibitory receptor for MHC class I mole-cules.

Cytoplasmic ITIMs recruit and activate protein tyrosine phosphatases SHP-1 and/or SHP-2 that act as inhibitory signal-ing effector molecules.

Ligands

MHC class I.

Expression

CD85a is expressed on NK cells, mono-cytes, macrophages, granulocytes, and a subset of T cells.

Gene Name	Entrez Gene#
LILRB3	11025

Selected Monoclonal Antibodies

7H5 (van Agthoven, Marseille).

CD85d

Other Names

LIR-2 (leukocyte immunoglobulin-like receptor-2); ILT-4 (immunoglobulin-like transcript-4); MIR10.

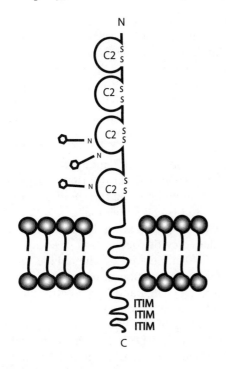

Molecular Structure

CD85d is a transmembrane glycoprotein and a member of the ILT/LIR family within the Ig gene superfamily.

CD85d is predicted to have a 440 amino acid extracellular region containing 4 C2-like Ig domains, a 21 amino acid transmembrane region, and a 116-residue cytoplasmic tail containing 3 immunoreceptor tyrosine-based inhibitor motif (ITIM) sequences.

Mol Wt: 110 kDa.

Function

CD85d is involved in the suppression of NK cell-mediated cytotoxicity.

Inhibitory receptor for MHC class I.

Cytoplasmic ITIMs recruit and activate protein tyrosine phosphatases SHP-1 and/or SHP-2 that act as inhibitory signaling effector molecules.

Antigen presenting cells expressing CD85k and CD85d appear to be crucial to the generation of $CD8^+$ suppressor T cells and $CD4^+$ regulatory T cells.

CD40-stimulated chemokine and cytokine production in monocytes is modulated by CD85j and CD85d after engagement by class I molecules.

The trophoblast-specific HLA-G1 protein binds CD85j and CD85d. This interaction possibly contributes to maternal tolerance of the fetus by inhibiting maternal leukocytes.

Ligands

CD85d binds HLA class I molecules and the trophoblast-specific, nonclassic class I molecule HLA-G1.

Expression

NK cells, monocytes, and macrophages; granulocytes (weakly); some DC (but not fresh blood DC).

Gene Name	*Entrez Gene#*
LILRB2	10288

Selected Monoclonal Antibodies

42D1 (van Agthoven; Marseille).

CD85j

Other Names

LIR-1 (leukocyte immunoglobulin-like receptor-1); ILT-2 (immunoglobulin-like transcript-2); MIR7.

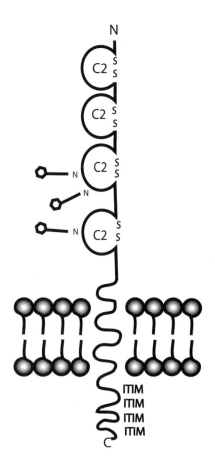

Molecular Structure

CD85j is a transmembrane glycoprotein and a member of the ILT/LIR family within the Ig gene superfamily.

CD85j is predicted to have an extracellular region of 438 amino acids containing four C2-type Ig domains, a 21 amino acid transmembrane region, and a long cytoplasmic tail of 168 amino acids containing four immunoreceptor tyrosine-based inhibitor motif (ITIM) sequences.

Mol Wt: 110 kDa.

Function

Inhibitory receptor for MHC class I.

Ligation of CD85j produces an inhibitory signal mediated by SHP-1 phosphatase.

CD85j has been shown to downregulate antigen-specific cytolytic activity of CD8$^+$ T cells and inhibits responses to recall antigens by CD4$^+$ T cells.

Co-engagement of CD85j with the B-cell receptor (BCR) inhibits Ca2$^+$ mobilization triggered via the BCR, suggesting CD85j modulates the threshold of antigen-mediated B-cell activation.

CD85j mediates inhibition of NK-cell-mediated cytotoxicity.

CD40-stimulated chemokine and cytokine production in monocytes is modulated by CD85j and CD85d after engagement by class I molecules.

Binding of the human cytomegalovirus (HCMV) to CD85j has the potential to block leukocyte activation and prevent an anti-viral response. The trophoblast-specific HLA-G1 protein binds CD85j and CD85d. This interaction possibly contributes to maternal tolerance of the fetus by inhibiting maternal leukocytes.

Ligands

CD85j binds a broad range of HLA-A and -B molecules, some HLA-C molecules, the trophoblast-specific, nonclassic class I molecule HLA-G1, and the human cytomegalovirus UL18 protein.

Expression

CD85j is expressed on NK cells, dendritic cells, monocytes, the majority of T cells, plasma cells, and at lower levels on B cells.

Gene Name   **Entrez Gene#**

LILRB1   10859

Selected Monoclonal Antibodies

VMP-55 (Pulford; Oxford); GH1/75 (Pulford; Oxford), HP-F1 (van Agthoven; Marseille).

CD85k

Other Names

LIR-5 (leukocyte immunoglobulin-like receptor-5); ILT-3 (immunoglobulin-like transcript-3); HM18.

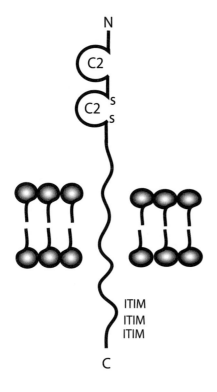

Molecular Structure

CD85k is a transmembrane glycoprotein and a member of the ILT/LIR family within the Ig gene superfamily.

The CD85k protein is predicted to have a 608 amino acid extracellular region containing two C2-type Ig domains, a 21 amino acid transmembrane region and a long cytoplasmic tail comprised of 168 amino acids and containing three immunoreceptor tyrosine-based inhibitor motif (ITIM) sequences.

Mol Wt: 60 kDa.

Function

Putative inhibitory receptor with unknown ligand.

Cytoplasmic ITIMs recruit and activate protein tyrosine phosphatases SHP-1 and/or SHP-2, which act as inhibitory signaling effector molecules.

Antigen presenting cells expressing CD85k and CD85d appear to be crucial to the generation of CD8$^+$ suppressor T cells and CD4$^+$ regulatory T cells.

Expression

CD85k is expressed by monocytes, macrophages, and dendritic cells.

Expression of CD85k by endothelial cells has been induced in vitro.

Applications

Useful marker for the purification of plasmacytoid monocytes.

Gene Name   Entrez Gene#

LILRB4   11006

Selected Monoclonal Antibodies

ZM3.8 (van Agthoven; Marseille).

CD86

Other Names

B7-2; B70.

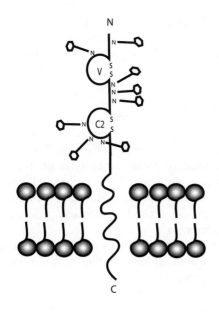

Molecular Structure

CD86 is a type I transmembrane glycoprotein and a member of the Ig gene superfamily.

CD86 is predicted to have 224 amino acids in the extracellular region, 21 amino acids in the transmembrane domain, and 61 amino acids in the cytoplasmic tail.

The extracellular region consists of one IgV-like and one IgC-like domain and has eight N-glycosylation sites.

The cytoplasmic tail has three potential sites for protein kinase C phosphorylation.

CD86 is structurally related to the CD80 molecule and functions as a counter-receptor for the T-cell accessory molecules CD28 and CD152.

Mol Wt: 80 kDa.

Function

CD86 acts a ligand for costimulatory molecule CD28 of T cells.

CD86 also binds CD152 with 20- to 100-fold higher affinity than to CD28. CD152 (CTLA4) on T cells plays a critical role in inhibiting T-cell activation.

The level of IgG1 produced by B cells is increased after CD86 and β-2-adrenergic receptor stimulation.

CD86 knockout mice have deficient antibody responses.

Ligands

CD86 binds CD28 and CD152 (CTLA4).

Expression

CD86 is constitutively expressed by interdigitating dendritic cells in T-cell zones of secondary lymphoid organs.

Lower level expression by Langerhans cells and peripheral blood dendritic cells (DC), memory B cells, and germinal center B cells.

Low level expression by monocytes can be increased in the presence of IFN-γ.

Gene Name	Entrez Gene#
CD86	942

Selected Monoclonal Antibodies

BU63 (Hardie; Birmingham); FUN-1 (Nozawa; Fukushima).

CD87

Other Names

Urokinase plasminogen activator-receptor (uPA-R).

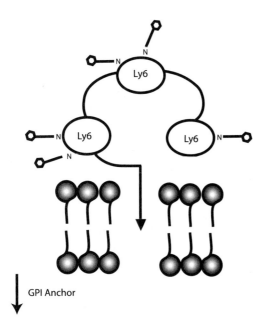

GPI Anchor

Molecular Structure

CD87 is a single-chain, glycophosphotidylinositol (GPI)-anchored glycoprotein and a member of the Ly-6 superfamily (see CD59).

The extracellular region consists of three homologous domains, DI, DII, and DIII, and five N-glycosylation sites.

Each domain consists of approximately 90 residues with three to four disulphide bonds and adopts a three-finger fold with three adjacent loops rich in β-pleated sheets and a small C-terminal loop.

Domains DI and DII have a folding topology similar to an α-neurotoxin, whereas DIII resembles CD59.

DI, DII, and DIII are arranged in an almost circular fashion, which generates a

deep central cavity where urokinase plasminogen activator (uPA) can bind.

Binding of uPA does not interfere with binding of ligands to the external receptor surface of CD87, enabling CD87 to be a multimeric receptor.

Alternative splicing generates truncated, soluble forms of CD87.

Mol Wt: Reduced, 32–66 kDa; unreduced, 35–68 kDa.

Function

CD87 can act as a multimeric receptor, capable of orchestrating complex events required to focus proteolysis on the cell surface and assist in controlled extracellular matrix degradation followed by intravasation and metastasis in various carcinomas.

CD87-bound uPA converts plasminogen to plasmin, which then binds other adjacent cell-surface receptors.

Expression of CD87 is localized at the leading edge of migrating leukocytes during inflammatory responses and of metastatic tumor cells enabling plasmin-mediated hydrolysis of extracellular matrix in the path of cellular invasion.

Binding of CD87 to β2 integrins may contribute to adherence and chemotaxis.

In tumor cells and smooth muscle cells, CD87 associates with CD130 and activates CD130 associated signaling components JAK1 and STAT1.

C87 associates with G-protein coupled chemotactic receptor FPRL1/LXA4R.

Patients with LAD (lacking β2 integrin function) show CD87 signaling deficits.

Knockout mice show a defect in uPA-mediated plasminogen activation.

Ligands

CD87 binds urokinase plasminogen activator, vitronectin, β1 and β2 integrins, and kininogen.

Expression

CD87 is expressed by monocytes, poly-morphs, dendritic cells, activated T cells, NK cells, fibroblasts, endothelial cells, smooth muscle cells, keratinocytes, placental trophoblasts, hepatocytes, and several tumors, including breast, colon, and prostate carcinoma and melanoma.

Leukocyte expression of CD87 is weak but is upregulated when the cells become activated.

Applications

Elevated expression of CD87 correlates with a poor prognosis in several tumors.

Gene Name	Entrez Gene#
PLAUR	5329

Selected Monoclonal Antibodies

3B10 (Todd; Ann Arbor); VIM5 (Knapp; Vienna).

CD88

Other Names

C5a-receptor, C5aR.

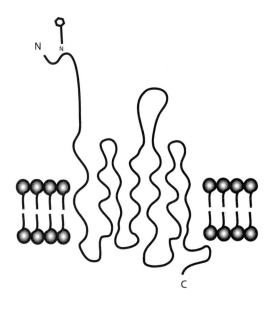

Molecular Structure

A member of the rhodopsin superfamily that contains seven transmembrane domains and couples to GTP-binding proteins.

CD88 is related to the CD128 molecule and the N-fomyl peptide receptor.

350 amino acids, glycosylated protein.

Mol Wt: 43 kDa.

Function

CD88 is a G-protein-coupled receptor, involved in C5a-mediated inflammation and activation of granulocytes.

Ligands

CD88 binds C5a/5a(desArg) and anaphyla-toxin.

Expression

CD88 is expressed on granulocytes, monocytes, dendritic cells, astrocytes, and microglia.

Gene Name	Entrez Gene#
C5R1	728

Selected Monoclonal Antibodies

S5/1 (Opperman; Durham); W17/1 (Opperman; Durham).

CD89

Other Names

Fc-α-receptor, IgA-receptor.

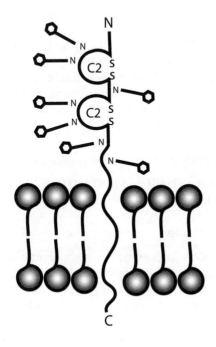

Molecular Structure

A type I transmembrane glycoprotein of 266 amino acids.

A member of the Ig gene superfamily.

CD89 has two extracellular Ig-like (C2 type) domains, a 19 amino acid single transmembrane segment containing a charged Arg residue, and a 41 amino acid cytoplasmic tail.

The cytoplasmic tail is devoid of known signaling motifs and requires interaction with FcR γ-chain homodimers for CD89-mediated signal transduction. The charged arginine (Arg209) is essential for this association.

The IgA binding site of CD89 is located in the extracellular domain 1.

Soluble CD89 is detectable in serum and retains its IgA binding capacity.

Mol Wt: 45–100 kDa. There is a wide variation in molecular weight between and within cell types.

Function

CD89 is a low affinity, myeloid receptor for monomeric, secretory IgA and polymeric IgA.

Binding of IgA to CD89 initiates several immune effector functions including phagocytosis, cytotoxicity, degranulation, the release of inflammatory cytokines, respiratory burst, and killing of microorganisms. CD89 associates with the common Fc receptor γ chain that acts as a signal transduction molecule.

The association of β2-integrin Mac-1 (CD11b/CD18) with CD89 is required for binding of sIgA to CD89 on phagocytes.

Ligands

CD89 binds IgA1 and IgA2.

Expression

CD89 is expressed on granulocytes, monocytes, macrophages, dendritic cells, activated eosinophils, and myeloid cell lines.

Expression of CD89 is upregulated in the presence of IgA-immune complexes, TNF-α, IL1-β, GM-CSF, and stimulators such as LPS and PMA.

CD89 expression is downregulated in the presence of TGF-β and suramin.

Applications

CD89 is a potential target for immunotherapy of infectious disease and malignancies.

Gene Name	Entrez Gene#
FCAR	2204

Selected Monoclonal Antibodies

A3 (Cooper; Birmingham); A59 (Cooper; Birmingham); A62 (Cooper; Birmingham).

CD90

Other Names

Thy-1.

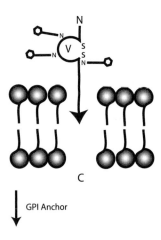

GPI Anchor

Molecular Structure

A glycophosphatidylinositol (GPI)-anchored protein.

A member of the Ig gene superfamily.

The 112 amino acid, extracellular region consists of a single IgV-like domain with three N glycosylation sites.

The complex carbohydrate side chains vary in composition between tissues and species.

Mol Wt: Reduced, 25–29 kDa; unreduced, 25–35 kDa.

Function

In the mouse, CD90 associates with CD45 and has a costimulatory role in activation of lymphocytes.

Murine CD90 acts as an adhesion molecule mediating $Ca2^+$-independent cell contact between thymocytes and thymic epithelial cells.

CD90 may contribute to inhibition of proliferation and differentiation of hemopoietic stem cells and neuron memory formation in the central nervous system.

CD90 antibodies inhibit proliferation of CD90$^+$/CD34$^+$ cord blood cells.

CD90 has been demonstrated to be an activation associated cell adhesion molecule on human dermal microvascular endothelial cells.

CD90 expressed on the surface of activated endothelial cells specifically interacts with Mac-1 (CD11b/CD18) on the surface of myeloid cells, mediating cell-to-cell adhesion and subsequent transendothelial migration, thereby contributing to leukocyte recruitment to sites of inflammation, tissue injury, and infection.

Ligands

CD90 binds Mac-1 (CD11b/CD18 complex).

Expression

CD90 is expressed on hemopoietic stem cells, neurons, few fetal thymocytes, 10–40% CD34 positive cells in bone marrow, and less than 1% of CD3$^+$ CD4$^+$ peripheral blood lymphocytes.

The endothelium of high endothelial venules of human lymph and dermal microvascular endothelial cells expresses CD90 when activated by inflammatory mediators.

CD90 is expressed by some lymphoblastoid and leukemic cell lines.

Applications

Marker for hemopoietic stem cells, when coexpressed with CD34.

CD34$^+$ CD90$^+$ hemopoietic stem cells serve as autologous grafts to replace bone marrow in patients with malignancies.

Gene Name	Entrez Gene#
THY1	7070

Selected Monoclonal Antibodies

5E10 (Landsdorp; Vancouver).

CD91

Other Names

α2-macroglobulin receptor (α2M-R); low density lipoprotein receptor-related protein (LRP).

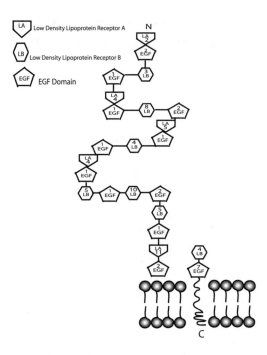

Molecular Structure

A glycoprotein that is cleaved in the Golgi into the 85-kDa transmembrane β-chain and the extracellular 515-kDa α-chain that is noncovalently bound by the β-chain.

The α-chain contains four clusters of cysteine-rich LDL receptor class A repeats, each flanked by epidermal growth factor (EGF) motifs.

The spacing regions between the cysteine-rich repeats consist of EGF and YWTD repeats.

CD91 ligands interact in part or entirely with the second and fourth cysteine-rich domains.

The β-chain has a single transmembrane region and a short cytoplasmic tail that contains signals for endocytosis.

Mol Wt: 515 kDa (α chain) and 85 kDa (β chain).

Function

The role of CD91 is to mediate the uptake and elimination of ligands. The affinity of CD91 for heat-shock protein gp96 allows antigen-presenting cells to take up peptides chaperoned by gp96, for subsequent presentation to T cells.

A 40-kDa intracellular protein called receptor-associated protein (RAP) can inhibit the ligand binding involved in the regulation of extracellular proteolytic activity and lipoprotein levels and provision of nutrients for the cell.

High level expression of CD91 is detectable in Alzheimer plaques and in atherosclerotic lesions.

CD91 is upregulated on monocytes of patients with slow progression of advanced melanoma. This observation may be related to CD91-mediated internalization and cross-presentation via MHC class I pathway of tumor antigens that may maintain anti-tumor CD8[+] cytotoxic T-cell responses and slow tumor progression.

Similarly, increased surface expression of CD91 on CD14[+] monocytes of human immunodeficiency virus type 1 (HIV-1)-infected but seronegative patients correlates with apparent resistance to HIV-1.

Binding of calreticulin to CD91 complexed with surfactant proteins (SP-A and SP-D) associated with foreign debris can initiate phagocytosis and a pro-inflammatory response in the lungs.

Deletion of the CD91 gene in mice is fatal.

Ligands

CD91 is the receptor for a variety of ligands including α2–macroglobulin–proteinase complex, plasminogen activators (urokinase and tissue) in complex with type-1 inhibitors, chylomicron remnants, lipoprotein lipase, *Pseudomonas* exotoxin A, and various heat shock proteins including gp96/GRP94, calreticulin, and HSP90.

Expression

CD91 is expressed by many cell types including hepatocytes, neurons, fibroblasts, and syncytiotrophoblasts.

Hemopoietic cells of monocytic lineage and erythroblasts/reticulocytes express CD91.

Gene Name	Entrez Gene#
LRP1	4035

Selected Monoclonal Antibodies

α2MRa-1 (Moestrup; Aarhus); α2MRa-2 (Moestrup; Λarhus).

CD92

Other Names

p70, CHTL1.

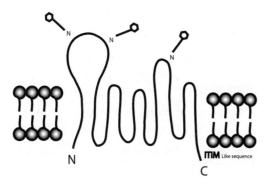

Molecular Structure

A member of the choline transporter-like family characterized by multi-transmembrane surface proteins.

CD92 is predicted to have 10 transmembrane domains, 3 potential N-linked glycosylation sites, and an immunoreceptor tyrosine-based inhibitory motif (ITIM)-like sequence in the cytoplasmic C-terminal region.

Mol Wt: 70 kDa.

Function

Potentially a ligand transporter, based on structural similarity to the choline transporter family.

Transports choline for membrane phospholipid synthesis by immune cells but may also be involved in specific regulation of immune function via negative signaling pathways; however, signaling via the ITIM-like region has yet to be demonstrated.

Ligands

CD92 binds choline.

Expression

CD92 is preferentially expressed on human peripheral blood monocytes and neutrophils as well as several myeloid and T-cell lines.

Expression of CD92 is detectable on mast cells but not eosinophils and is weakly expressed on peripheral blood lymphocytes, fibroblasts, epithelial cells, and endothelial cells.

Gene Name	Entrez Gene#
SLC44A1	23446

Selected Monoclonal Antibodies

VIM15 (Knapp; Vienna); VIM15b (Knapp; Vienna).

CD93

Other Names

GR11, C1qR1, C1qRP (C1q receptor precursor).

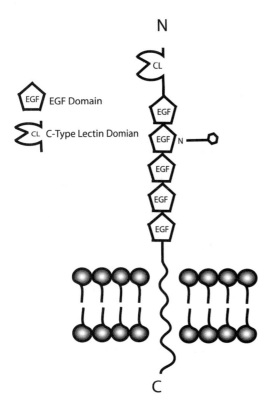

Molecular Structure

A 110-kDa O-sialoglycoprotein.
  Sequence predicts a 652-residue protein with an N-terminal C-type lectin domain followed by five EGF-like domains. The three membrane-proximal EGF-like domains potentially bind Ca2+. A 22-residue membrane-spanning sequence is followed by a 46-residue cytoplasmic region.

Mol Wt: Reduced, 126 kDa; unreduced, 110 kDa.

Function

C1q receptor. Postulated to assist phagocytosis of micro-organisms coated with complement. However, evidence for this role is contradictory.

Ligands

Complement component C1q.

Expression

CD93 is expressed on NK cells, monocytes, granulocytes AML blasts, myeloid cell lines, platelets, and endothelial cells.

Gene Name	Entrez Gene#
CD93	22918

Selected Monoclonal Antibodies

VIMD2 (Knapp; Vienna); x2 (Peters; Göttingen); WDS4.B4 (De Smet; Brüssel).

CD94

Other Names

Kp43.

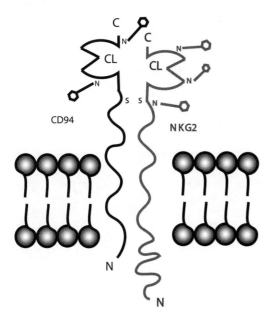

Molecular Structure

A type II transmembrane glycoprotein.

Member of the Ca^{++}-dependent (C-type) lectin superfamily (see CD23, CD69, CD72, and CD161).

CD94 is an approximately 180 amino acid protein with a 148 amino acid extracellular region containing one C-type lectin domain and two potential N-linked glycosylation sites.

The 10 amino acid cytoplasmic tail does not contain any known signaling motifs.

The CD94 molecule forms a disulfide-linked heterodimer with two other members of the C-type lectin superfamily, NKG2A (43 kDa subunit) and NKG2C (39-kDa subunit).

Mol Wt: 30 kDa.

Function

CD94 covalently associates with NKG2A, C, and E to form receptors for HLA class I molecules.

The CD94/NKG2A complex is the predominant form and functions as an inhibitory receptor.

Cross-linking of CD94/NKG2 dimers by HLA-E-bearing target cells results in the phosphorylation of two immunoreceptor tyrosine-based inhibition motifs (ITIMs) present in the cytoplasmic domain of NKG2A. The subsequent binding of Src homology 2 domain-bearing tyrosine phosphatases SHP-1 and SHP-2 to the phosphorylated ITIMs leads to their activation and results in suppression of NK cytotoxicity.

Expression of CD94/NKG2A complexes on the cell surface of a large subset of NK cells appears to be constant via rapid recycling of internalized receptors, thus ensuring that interaction with ligand-bearing normal cells does not result in an autoimmune response. In contrast, CD94/NKG2C and CD94/NKG2E complexes seem to be expressed at lower levels on the NK cell surface and act as activatory receptors. Both NKG2C and NKG2E lack cytoplasmic signaling motifs, but the CD94/NKG2C and CD94/NKG2E complexes associate with the signal transducing protein DAP12.

CD94 antibodies modulate NK cell function, triggering or inhibiting cytotoxicity and tumor necrosis factor production.

Ligands

The CD94/NKG2a, CD94/NKG2C, and CD94/NKG2E complexes bind the non-classic, class I molecule HLA-E but can also bind peptides derived from other MHC class I molecules (HLA-A, HLA-B, HLA-C and HLA-G, H-2D, and H-2K).

Expression

CD94/NKG2 complexes are expressed on NK cells and subsets of α/β and γ/δ T cells.

In mice, CD8$^+$ cytotoxic T cells can upregulate CD94/NKG2 expression, thus reducing their cytotoxic activity.

Gene Name	Entrez Gene#
KLRD1	3824

Selected Monoclonal Antibodies

HP-3B1 (Lopez-Botet; Madrid); XA185 (Moretta; Genova).

CD95

Other Names

APO-1, Fas, TNFRSF6, APT1, apoptosis antigen 1.

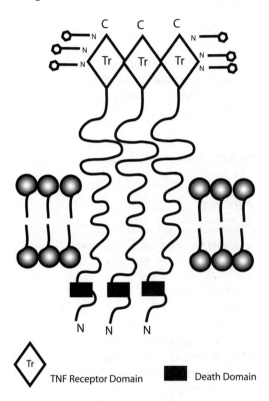

| Tr | TNF Receptor Domain | ▇ Death Domain |

Molecular Structure

A type I integral membrane protein with 320 amino acids.

CD95 is a member of the tumor necrosis factor (TNF)/nerve growth factor (NGF) receptor family (see CD27, CD30, CD40, CD120a, CD120b, CD134, and CD137).

The 157 amino acid extracellular domain consists of three cysteine-rich repeats and contains two O-glycosylation sites.

The cytoplasmic region has a "death domain" sequence between amino acids 214 and 295.

Alternative splicing yields soluble forms.

CD95 molecules form trimers and upon ligation trimers can form dimers and oligomers.

Mol Wt: Reduced, 45 kDa; unreduced, 45, 90 > 200 kDa.

Function

The binding of CD95L to CD95 trimers results in dimerization of the two trimers and higher levels of oligomerization. Once activated, the FADD protein binds to the CD95 cytoplasmic death domain to form the death inducing signal complex (DISC). This complex triggers a caspase-dependent cascade that ultimately results in cell death.

CD95 antibodies induce apoptosis.

Ipr/Ipr mice do not express CD95 and develop lymphadenopathy.

Ligands

CD95 (Fas) binds CD178 (CD95L, Fas ligand).

Expression

CD95 is expressed at high levels on activated T and B cells.

Applications

Marker of apoptotic cells.

Gene Name	*Entrez Gene#*
TNFRSF6	355

Selected Monoclonal Antibodies

APO-1 (Krammer; Heidelberg); ANTI-FAS (Yonehara; Yokohama).

CD96

Other Names

TACTILE (T-cell activation increased late expression).

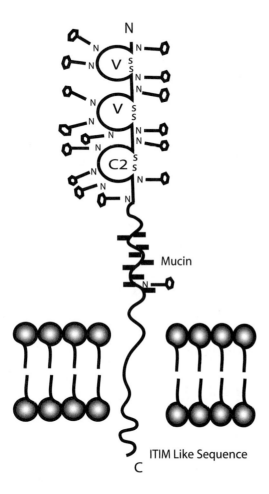

Molecular Structure

A type I integral membrane protein and member of the Ig gene superfamily.

The extracellular region consists of two IgV-like domains, one C2-type Ig-like domain, and one mucin-like domain, and it is extensively N- and O-glycosylated and can be sialylated and sulfated.

CD96 has a 45 amino acid, proline-rich cytoplasmic domain with ITIM-like sequences; however, no inhibitory signaling function has been attributed to these sequences.

CD96 can form disulphide-linked homodimers.

Alternative splicing results in several transcripts including one, which encodes a soluble molecule consisting of the three Ig-like domains only.

Mol Wt: Reduced, 160 kDa; unreduced, 160 kDa, 180 kDa, 240 kDa.

Function

CD96 is thought to be involved in the adhesive interactions of T cells and NK cells during the late phase of the immune response.

CD96 promotes T lymphocyte and NK-cell adhesion to target cells expressing poliovirus receptor (PVR).

Strong adhesion between CD96 and PVR stimulates cytotoxicity of activated NK cells and promotes transfer of PVR from the target cell to the NK cell.

PVR is expressed at high levels in many tumors, and it has been suggested that recognition of PVR via binding to CD96 may be important for NK-cell recognition of tumors.

Ligands

CD96 binds the poliovirus receptor (PVR, CD155).

Expression

Expressed at low levels on resting T and NK cells, but expression is strongly up-regulated when these cells become activated.

Expression of CD96 is found on 78% of T-cell leukemias and 29% of acute myeloid leukemias.

Applications

Useful marker for immunophenotyping of T-cell acute lymphoblastic leukemias as well as a subgroup of acute myeloid leukemias.

Gene Name	Entrez Gene#
CD96	10225

Selected Monoclonal Antibodies

TH-111 (Gramatzki; Erlangen); G8.5 (Wang; Manchester).

CD97

Other Names

BL-KDD/F12.

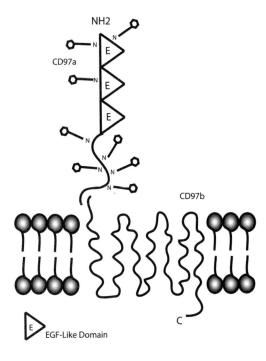

EGF-Like Domain

Molecular Structure

CD97 is a seven-span transmembrane protein belonging to the secretin receptor superfamily, the G protein-coupled receptor superfamily, and the EGF-TM7 family of class II seven span transmembrane molecules.

CD97 is translated as a single polypeptide that is then cleaved into two subunits (a and b) within the endoplasmic reticulum. The two subunits associate noncovalently on the cell surface.

CD97a is the extracellular subunit that consists of between three to five tandem EGF-like domains, an RGD motif, and eight potential N-glycosylation sites. Two EGF-like domains have Ca^{2+} binding sites.

Three isoforms that arise from three alternatively spliced transcripts, have extra-cellular regions with three (EGF1,2,5), four (EGF1,2,3,5), or five (EGF1,2,3,4,5) EGF domains, respectively.

CD55 can bind all isoforms but with differing affinity, having the highest affinity for the three EGF domain-containing isoform and the lowest affinity for the five EGF domain-containing isoform.

The EGF4 domain has the binding site for chondroitin sulphate (CS); therefore, only the largest isoform binds CS.

CD97b is the seven-span transmembrane segment (7TM) of 243 amino acids and has an intracellular region of 46 amino acids.

The two subunits are associated via a mucin-like spacer.

Mol Wt: CD97a: Reduced, 75–85 kDa; unreduced, 74–78 kDa, 80–82 kDa, 86–89 kDa.

Mol Wt: CD97b: 28 kDa.

Function

Acts as a receptor involved in adhesion and signaling processes early after leukocyte activation.

There is some evidence from in vivo studies that CD97 plays an important role in the migration of neutrophils as pre-incubation of neutrophils with anti-CD97 mAb delayed migration of these cells to sites of inflammation in experimental colitis.

Similarly, the presence of CD97 mAb impaired granulocyte recruitment to the lungs and reduced bacterial clearance in a model of pneumococcal pneumonia.

CD97 can coengage chondroitin sulphate (CS) and α5/β1 integrin to synergistically initiate endothelial cell invasion and may stimulate angiogenesis.

CD97 on activated T cells, dendritic cells, and macrophages can bind CS expressed on B cells, but this interaction has not been shown to stimulate B-cell proliferation, Ig synthesis, or class switching.

CD97 has been implicated as having an important role in tumor cell migration and invasion as the level of expression of CD97 is proportional to the aggressiveness and lymph node involvement in thyroid carcinomas. Similarly, in colorectal carcinoma, strong expression of CD97 in scattered tumor cells at the invasion front correlates with an increased likelihood of lymph node involvement and poor prognosis.

Ligands

CD97 binds CD55 and chondroitin sulphate.

Expression

Expressed on activated T cells and B cells and constituitively by monocytes, macrophages, dendritic cells, and granulocytes.

Expression of CD97 is also found on smooth muscle cells and on a subset of thyroid and gastrointestinal tract carcinoma cells.

Applications

Prognostic marker and a marker of dedifferentiation for thyroid carcinomas and gastrointestinal tract carcinomas.

Gene Name	Entrez Gene#
CD97	976

Selected Monoclonal Antibodies

VIM3 (Knapp; Vienna); VIM3b (Knapp; Vienna); VIM3c (Knapp; Vienna); MEM180 (Horejsi; Prague).

CD98

Other Names

4F2, FRP-1.

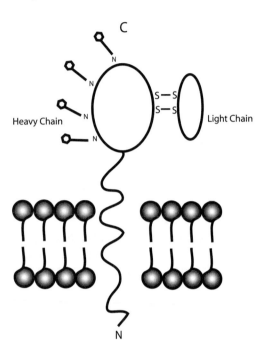

Molecular Structure

CD98 is a disulphide-linked heterodimer.

The CD98 heavy chain (CD98hc) is a glycosylated, type II transmembrane glycoprotein that forms disulphide bonds with at least six different light chains (LAT1, LAT2, y⁺LAT1, y⁺LAT2, Asc-1, xCT) that act as amino acid transporters.

The CD98hc transmembrane domain and in particular the N-terminal five amino acids of this domain are required for interaction with β1 integrins.

Mol Wt: CD98hc: 80 kDa.

Function

CD98hc functions as a chaperone for amino acid transporters closely associated with actin.

CD98hc is implicated in the regulation of cell fusion and β1 integrin adhesive functions by associating either directly or indirectly with β1 integrins.

The interaction of CD98hc, basolateral amino acid transporters, and β1 integrins alters diverse cellular functions in polarized renal epithelial cells including amino acid transport, cell adhesion, migration, and branching morphogenesis.

Overexpression of CD98hc was demonstrated to result in anchorage-independent cell growth in 3T3 fibroblasts and activation of certain integrin-regulated signaling pathways that promote tumorigenesis.

A complex of CD98hc-amino acid transporter LAT1 can associate with CD147, monocarboxylate transporters, and a regulator of cell proliferation (epCAM) to form a potential supercomplex that regulates cellular energy metabolism.

Expression of CD98 is upregulated in the presence of IFN-γ.

CD98 antibodies inhibit lectin-induced T-cell proliferation, but not the mixed lymphocyte reaction, antibody-dependent cellular cytotoxicity, or T-cell-mediated cytotoxicity.

Ligands

β1 integrins.

Expression

Broadly expressed and not restricted to hemopoietic cells. High level expression is found on proliferating cells, particularly neoplastic cells.

Expression of CD98 may be upregulated in the presence of IFN-γ.

Gene Name	Entrez Gene#
SLC3A2	6520

Selected Monoclonal Antibodies

4F2 (Haynes; Durham); 2F3 (Ritz; Boston); BU53 (Hardie; Birmingham).

CD99

Other Names

MIC2, E2.

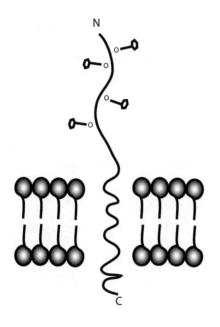

Molecular Structure

A type I transmembrane glycoprotein and is a mucin.

The 100 amino acid extracellular domain contains three EF hand motifs, a proline-rich region, and a collagen-like region (G-X-Y), and it is not predicted to have any α helices or β sheets.

The transmembrane region consists of 25 amino acids, and the cytoplasmic domain consists of 35 residues.

CD99 is heavily O-glycosylated but not N-glycosylated.

Two alternative splice forms have been described that appear to be differentially expressed in a cell-type specific manner. The CD99 type II molecule is a truncated form of CD99 type I and is expressed in varying lower levels than CD99 type I.

The MIC2 gene locus is in the pairing region of the human X and Y chromosomes and is the first pseudoautosomal gene to be described in humans.

Mol Wt: 32 kDa.

Function

Participates in the positive selection of thymocytes via its ability to act as an adhesin and its ability to induce apoptosis.

CD99 acts as an adhesion molecule and is involved in the transendothelial migration of leukocytes during inflammation.

The major isoform, CD99 type 1, may also indirectly mediate lymphocyte adhesion by postively regulating LFA-1 expression in lymphocytes, whereas the CD99 type II appears to inhibit adhesion via the LFA-1/ICAM-1 pathway.

Activation of a distinct domain of CD99 on T cells induces caspase-independent cell death and is a far more potent inducer of cell death than either CD95 or TRAIL.

CD99 mediates TCR/CD3-dependent activation of resting peripheral T cells and induces production of TNF-α and IFN-γ.

CD99 regulates the transport of MHC class I molecules from the Golgi complex to the cell surface and is responsible for the downregulation of MHC class I molecules on the surface of Hodgkin's and Reed–Sternberg cells.

Downregulation of CD99 expression is important for the generation of Hodgkin's and Reed–Sternberg cells.

CD99R antibodies do not induce the cellular responses seen with CD99 antibodies.

Ligands

No other ligand has been identified for CD99 other than itself.

Expression

CD99 isoforms are broadly expressed in most hematopoietic cells, Ewing tumor cells, endothelial cells, and many other cell types.

The name CD99R (restricted) was given to several antibodies that showed a more restricted expression pattern.

CD99R is expressed by myeloid cells, NK cells, and double positive thymocytes.

Applications

Useful marker in the differential diagnosis of Ewing's sarcoma from neuroblastoma.

Potential therapeutic target in the treatment of Ewing's tumors.

Gene Name	Entrez Gene#
CD99	4267

Selected Monoclonal Antibodies

O662 (Bernard; Nice); 12E7 (Levy; Stanford); MEM-131 (Horejsi; Praha).

Antibodies classified as CD99R: D44 (Boumsell; Paris); FMC29 (Zola; Adelaide).

CD100

Other Names

Semaphorin 4D (SEMA4D).

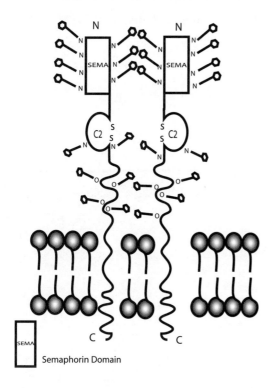

Semaphorin Domain

Molecular Structure

A type I integral membrane protein belonging to subclass 4 of the semaphorin family within the Ig gene superfamily and is the first semaphorin described in the immune system.

The extracellular region incorporates a semaphorin domain containing potential N-linked glycosylation sites and conserved cysteines followed by an Ig-like domain and a lysine-rich stretch.

Cys679 is essential for homodimerization and biological function of the molecule.

There are no catalytic domains in the cytoplasmic tail, but there are consensus sites for tyrosine and serine phosphorylation.

Soluble CD100 is generated from the transmembrane form via a proteolytic cascade initiated after activation of primary T and B cells.

Mol Wt: Reduced, 150 kDa; unreduced, 300 kDa (soluble form, 120 kDa).

Function

CD100 increases PMA, CD3, and CD2 induced T-cell proliferation.

CD100 mediates axon repulsion via its receptor plexin-B1 and may help guide developing neuronal cells.

In epithelial cells, the binding of CD100 to plexin-B1/Met (scatter factor 1) complex induces phosphorylation of the complex that is crucial for epithelial cell invasive growth.

Exogenous expression of CD100 or soluble CD100 (sCD100) promotes B-cell activation by inducing homotypic adhesion of B cells, downregulating expression of CD23, and modifying CD40-CD40L B cell signaling.

CD100 may exert its positive effects on B cells by binding to CD72 and dampening CD72-mediated negative signaling. Evidence for this comes from the observations that CD72 is constitutively tyrosine phosphorylated and associated with SHP-1 and that B cells are hyporesponsive in CD100-deficient mice.

Recombinant sCD100 has been shown to induce proinflammatory cytokine release by monocytes and inhibit spontaneous and MCP-3-induced migration of monocytes or a monocytic cell line.

CD100-deficient mice have both impaired antibody production and T-cell priming against specific antigens.

Ligands

Binds CD72 in the immune system and displays high affinity binding to plexin-B1 in non-hematopoietic tissues.

Expression

Detectable on most hemopoietic cells with the exception of immature bone marrow cells, erythrocytes, and platelets. It is strongly expressed on resting T cells but weakly on resting B cells and antigen presenting cells but is upregulated upon activation.

Expression is detectable on many non-hematopoetic tissues including embryonic and adult brain, kidney, and heart.

Gene Name	Entrez Gene#
SEMA4D	10507

Selected Monoclonal Antibodies

BD16 (Boumsell; Paris); 148-2D12 (Vilella; Barcelona).

CD101

Other Names

V7, P126.

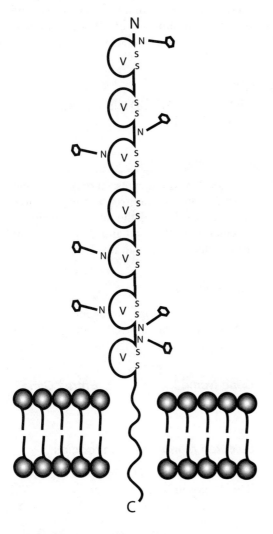

Molecular Structure

A type I transmembrane glycoprotein and member of the EWI family within Ig superfamily.

The protein forms homodimers.

The extracellular domain consists of seven IgV-like domains with seven potential N-linked glycosylation sites.

The transmembrane domain is predicted to consist of 25 amino acids, and the cytoplasmic domain consists of 42 amino acids and contains several phosphorylation consensus sites.

Mol Wt: Reduced, 120kDa; unreduced, 240kDa.

Function

The function of CD101 has not yet been clearly demonstrated.

MAbs against CD101 inhibit allogeneic T-cell responses and costimulate T-cell proliferation with suboptimal anti-CD3 activation.

Triggering of CD101 on cutaneous dendritic cells (DCs) was found to induce IL-10 secretion by the DCs, which inhibited T-cell proliferation in vitro.

CD101 is found on a subpopulation of T cells (CD101$^+$, CD8$^+$, and CD103$^+$) with a possible role in preventing fetal rejection and inflammatory bowel disease in the gut mucosa.

Expression

High level expression of CD101 is found on monocytes, granulocytes, dendritic cells, and activated T cells.

Gene Name	Entrez Gene#
IGSF2	9398

Selected Monoclonal Antibodies

BA27 (Boumsell; Paris); BB27 (Boumsell; Paris).

CD102

Other Names

Intercellular adhesion molecule-2 (ICAM-2).

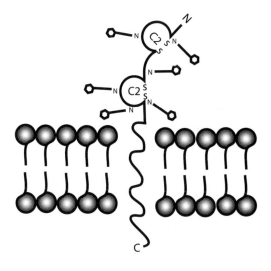

Molecular Structure

A type I transmembrane glycoprotein, member of the intercellular adhesion molecule (ICAM) family, with 34% homology to ICAM-1. Apparent Mol Wt 55–65 kDa. The extracellular region consists of two IgC-like domains and is N-glycosylated. The N-linked carbohydrate is involved in the conformation and function of CD102.

Function

CD102 is an intercellular adhesion molecule and is believed to be involved in lym-phocyte recirculation and homing to inflammatory sites. It also provides a cos-timulatory signal in the immune response, through interaction with integrins.

CD102 knockout mice show impaired recruitment of inflammatory cells and reduced numbers of bone marrow megakaryocyte precursors.

Ligands

LFA-1 (CD18/CD11a) and CR3 (CD18/CD11b).

Expression

In blood, lymphocytes, monocytes, and platelets, but not neutrophils, express low levels of CD102 on the surface. In tissue, vascular endothelium and follicular dendritic cells express high levels.

Applications

Potential pathology reagent, because CD102 levels are reportedly upregulated in lymph nodes with malignant infiltration.

Gene Name	Entrez Gene#
ICAM2	3384

Selected Monoclonal Antibodies

6D5 (Gahmberg; Helsinki); CBR-1C2/1 (De Fougerolles; Cambridge).

CD103

Other Names

Integrin αE-subunit, HML-1.

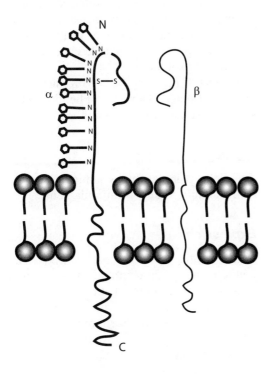

Molecular Structure

A type 1 transmembrane glycoprotein 1160 amino acid residues long. The extracellular domain has seven repeats characteristic of integrin α chains, including three EF-Hand cation-binding motifs. The extracellular region also contains a 193-residue integrin A domain and an unusual 55-residue domain, which contains a cleavage site. Enzymic cleavage at this site produces a 25-kDa N-terminal protein containing the first two (membrane-distal) repeats, which remains disulphide-linked to the 150-kDa chain.

The 30-residue intracytoplasmic sequence contains a GFKKR motif involved in ligand-induced conformation changes in integrins.

Function

CD103 associates with integrin β7 to form the human mucosal lymphocyte antigen, and the complex binds E-cadherin, which is a component of epithelial cell membranes. The interaction appears to be involved in lymphocyte homing to epithelia.

In vitro experiments using antibody suggest that CD103 is able to submit an activation signal, particularly in intraepithelial lymphocytes (IELs).

Knockout mice have reduced numbers of IELs, but this is strain-dependent, suggesting a redundancy in the major function of CD103.

Ligands

The integrin αEβ7 complex binds E-cadherin.

Expression

Expressed on most IELs and a smaller proportion of intestinal lamina propria T cells. Also expressed on T cells in other epithelial tissues, including bronchi, and inflamed tissues, including skin. Present on only 1–2% of circulating T cells and absent from most cells in secondary lymphoid tissue.

Expressed on lymphomas associated with IELs. Also expressed on hairy cell leukemia.

Applications

A marker for IELs and for lymphomas deriving from IELs, but must be interpreted conservatively, because CD103 can be induced on non-IELs by TGF β.

Gene Name	Entrez Gene#
ITGAE	3682

Selected Monoclonal Antibodies

HML-1 (Cerf-Bensussan; Paris); BER-ACT8 (Stein; Berlin).

CD104

Other Names

Integrin β4-subunit, TSP-1180.

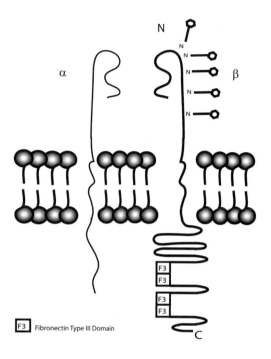

F3 Fibronectin Type III Domain

Molecular Structure

A type I transmembrane glycoprotein that associates with CD49f (integrin α6-chain) to form the integrin α6β4 and laminin receptor. The protein consists of 1822 residues and has an apparent Mol Wt of 205 kDa. The extracellular domain has the characteristics of an integrin β chain, whereas the large cytoplasmic region has four fibronectin type 3 domains and an intervening 142-residue segment that can be tyrosine phophorylated.

Function

The α6β4 complex is an adhesion receptor for laminins (especially laminin 5), which occur in basement membranes. The α6β4 complex interacts with keratin filaments, in the formation of hemidesmosomes, unlike other integrins, which interact with actin fibers to form focal adhesions. The cytoplasmic domain is necessary for hemidesmosome formation.

The complex also transduces signals through the interaction with laminin. It is expressed selectively in areas of proliferation and appears to be involved in cell activation and proliferation.

Knockout mice are born with blistering of gut and skin and absence of hemidesmosomes; they survive only hours.

Ligands

The α6β4 complex binds laminins (especially laminin 5) and keratin filaments.

Expression

Highly expressed in the basal cell layer of epithelia, including skin and the gastrointestinal tract. Expressed on endothelium undergoing angiogenesis and in myelinating nerve fibers. In the immune system, CD104 is expressed in double-negative pre-T thymocytes.

Applications

Mutation or loss of CD104 is associated with junctional epidermolysis bullosa with pyloric atresia (JEBPA). Increased CD104 expression is seen in squamous cell carcinomas and in thyroid, colorectal, gastric, and pancreatic carcinomas. Decreased levels are found in breast, bladder, and prostate tumors.

Gene Name	Entrez Gene#
ITGB4	3691

Selected Monoclonal Antibodies

UM-A9 (Carey; Ann Arbor); 439-9B (Kennel; Oak Ridge).

CD105

Other Names

Endoglin.

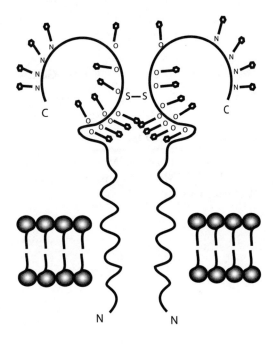

Molecular Structure

A type I transmembrane glycoprotein and a member of the transforming growth factor-β (TGF-β) type III receptor family.

CD105 disulphide-linked homodimers form part of the TGF-β receptor (TGF-β R) complex but can exist independently on the cell surface.

The 561 amino acid extracellular domain has five potential N-linked glycosylation sites, a region of potential O-linked glycosylation between residues 311 and 551, and an RGD motif in an exposed region. The presence of the RGD sequence suggests the protein may interact with integrins or integrin-like molecules although none have as yet been identified as ligands of CD105.

CD105 has a 25 amino acid transmembrane region and 47 amino acid cytoplasmic domain.

A short form of CD105 (sCD105) with a 14-residue cytoplasmic tail is also detectable by RT-PCR; however, it appears to be only weakly expressed on the cell surface.

TGF-β RI complexes with CD105 only when its kinase domain is active and binds a different region of the CD105 extracellular domain to TGF-β RII. TGF-β RII remains associated with CD105 whether it is active or inactive.

Mol Wt: Reduced, 90 kDa; unreduced, 180 kDa.

Function

Although not fully understood, there is evidence that suggests CD105 is involved in angiogenesis, in vascular development, and in maintaining vessel wall integrity. Evidence for a role in angiogenesis comes from the observation that CD105 gene mutations are associated with hereditary hemorrhagic telangiectasia and vascular and bleeding disorders in humans and mice. Furthermore, CD105 null mice have several vascular and cardiac defects resulting in death at an early embryonic stage.

Expression of CD105 is elevated in proliferating endothelial cells in vitro.

Expression of different extracellular matrix components such as fibronectin and collagen are regulated by CD105 levels suggesting a role for CD105 in cellular transmigration.

CD105 expression is induced by hypoxia, and in the absence of TGF-β1, CD105 displays anti-apoptotic effects in endothelial cells under hypoxic stress.

Only a small proportion of surface-expressed CD105 molecules bind TGF-β, but it appears to modulate the negative effects of TGF-β1 on cell proliferation, migration, and microvessel formation.

Ligands

CD105 in association with TGF-βRI or TGF-βRII binds TGF-β1 and TGF-β3 isoforms with high affinity.

Expression

Strongest expression of CD105 occurs in vascular endothelial cells, particularly microvascular endothelium and vascular endothelial cells in normal and neoplastic tissues undergoing angiogenesis.

CD105 is strongly expressed by syncytiotrophoblasts. Weaker expression is detectable in activated macrophages, tissue macrophages, follicular dendritic cells, pre-B cells in fetal marrow, erythroid precursors, fibroblasts, melanocytes, heart mesenchymal cells, and vascular smooth muscle and mesangial cells.

Applications

CD105 is a useful marker of angiogenesis and is a good target for tumor imaging.

It can be used as a prognostic marker for several types of cancer where increased intra-tumor expression of CD105 on microvasculature correlates with disease progression and metastasis. Serum CD105 levels may also be a prognostic indicator.

Recent studies have shown CD105 has potential as a therapeutic target in the treatment of breast cancer.

Gene Name	Entrez Gene#
ENG	2022

Selected Monoclonal Antibodies

1G2 (van Agthoven; Marseille); CLB-HEC-19 (van Mourik; Amsterdam); 44G4 (Letarte; Toronto).

CD106

Other Names

VCAM-1 (vascular cell adhesion molecule-1), INCAM-110.

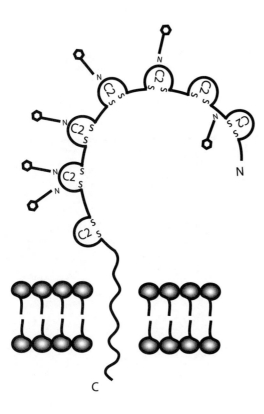

Molecular Structure

A type I transmembrane sialoglycoprotein and is a member of the Ig superfamily.

The extracellular region consists of seven IgC-like domains. Sequence similarity between domains 1 and 3 and domains 4 and 5 suggest an internal gene duplication event during evolution.

The regions spanning domains 1 and 2 and domains 4 and 5 are closely related to the two IgSF domains of MAdCAM-1 (which also binds the integrin α4β7) as well as domains 1 and 2 of the CD18

binding molecules CD50, CD54, and CD102.

Alternative splicing can give rise to an isoform with six IgC-like domains.

Mol Wt: 100–110 kDa.

Function

CD106 is involved in leukocyte adhesion, transmigration, and costimulation of T-cell proliferation.

Expression of CD106 on endothelial cells promotes extravasation of lymphocytes, monocytes, basophils, and eosinophils but not neutrophils, particularly at the sites of inflammation.

The CD106/VLA-4 interaction mediates both tethering and rolling of lymphocytes on endothelium as well as their subsequent firm adhesion.

In nonvascular tissue, CD106 has been implicated in the interaction of hematopoietic progenitors with bone marrow stromal cells, B cell binding to follicular dendritic cells, and costimulation of T cells and embryonic development.

CD106-knockout mice have severe organogenesis defects and die as embryos.

Ligands

CD106 binds the integrins α4β1 (CD49d/CD29, VLA-4) and α4β7. CD49d/CD29 is the dominant ligand in cells expressing both integrins.

Expression

Predominantly expressed on endothelial cells but is expressed by follicular dendritic and interfollicular dendritic cells, some macrophages, bone marrow stromal cells, and nonvascular cell populations within joints, kidney, muscle, heart, placenta, and brain. Activated vascular endothelium secretes a soluble form.

Gene Name   **Entrez Gene#**

VCAM1   7412

Selected Monoclonal Antibodies

HAE-2a   (Tedder;   Boston);   E1/6 (Bevilacqua; La Jolla).

CD107a and b

Other Names

Lysosomal associated membrane protein, LAMP-1 (CD107a) and LAMP-2 (CD107b).

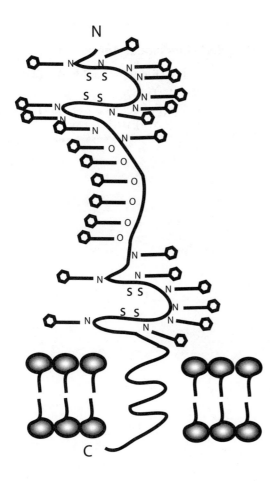

Molecular Structure

CD107a and b are type 1 transmembrane glycoproteins of 389 and 382 residues, respectively, with 37% homology. The extracellular domain of 350 residues is heavily glycosylated (19 and 16 N-glycosylation sites and 6 and 10 O-glycosylation sites for CD107a and b). Both proteins have membrane-spanning sequences of 24 residues followed by an 11 amino acid cytoplasmic sequence.

The carbohydrate constitutes about 60% of the 100–120-kDa apparent Mol Wt. The N-glycosylation sites cluster in two homologous domains, separated by a hinge-like structure enriched with proline and serine (CD107a) or proline and threonine (CD107b). The hinge region bears the O-linked carbohydrate. Each N-glycosylated domain contains two disulfide loops. Some N-linked oligosaccharides bear the sialyl Lewis X (LeX) Antigen (see CD15).

Function

CD107a and b line the external surface of lysosomes and are present in large amounts. However, enzymatic removal of the carbohydrate does not affect lysosomal integrity, and their specific function remains unclear. They bind macromolecules such as galectin-3 (a ligand for CD107a) and may act to bring such molecules into lysosomes for degradation.

On the cell surface, the carbohydrate groups borne by CD107, including Lewis X, are ligands for lectins such as the selectin family.

Knockout mice have normal lysosomal function, although in the absence of double knockouts, this may reflect a redundancy in their lysosomal function. CD107a knockout mice showed astrogliosis, perhaps reflecting the relative absence of CD107b in murine brain. CD107b knockout mice showed vacuolar cardioskeletal myopathy and vacuolation of pancreatic, liver, and endothelial cells as well as leukocytes. In humans, CD107b deficiency causes a similar syndrome and is known as Danon disease.

Ligands

The carbohydrates borne by CD107a and b are bound by lectins such as the selectins (CD62 L, E, and P) and galectins.

Expression

CD107a and b are abundant and ubiquitous lysosomal membrane glycoproteins, expressed by metabolically active cells. Approximately 1–2% of total CD107 is expressed at the cell surface and released into the blood.

Applications

Increased expression on tumors may be associated with metastasis.

Soluble forms of LAMP-1 and LAMP-2 are found in circulation. Potential markers for screening for lysosomal storage diseases in neonates, with CD107 levels elevated in the plasma from 72% of neonatal patients.

Gene Name	Entrez Gene#
LAMP1	3916
LAMP2	3920

Selected Monoclonal Antibodies

CD107a: ED11 (Fukuda; La Jolla); H4A3 (August; New York).

CD107b: CD3 (Fukuda; La Jolla); H4B4 (August; New York).

CD108

Other Names

GPI-gp80, John Milton Hagen (JMH) human blood group antigen, Sema L, Sema K1.

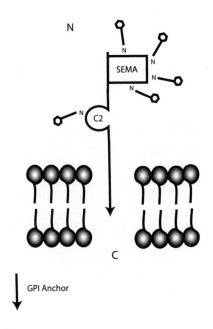

GPI Anchor

Molecular Structure

CD108 is a 602 amino acid glycosylphosphatidylinositol (GPI)—anchored cell membrane glycoprotein and a member of the semaphorin family within the Ig superfamily.

The extracellular domain contains one semaphorin domain and one Ig C2 domain, an RGD (Arg-Gly-Asp) cell attachment sequence, and five potential N-linked glycosylation sites.

Proteolytic release of CD108 from the cell surface is possible; however, soluble CD108 is not normally present in plasma.

Mol Wt: Reduced, 80kDa; unreduced, 76kDa.

Function

The function of CD108 has not been clearly demonstrated, but it is thought to play a role in inflammation.

Recombinant soluble CD108 was found to induce production of inflammatory cytokines such as TNFα, IL-6, and IL-8 and to be chemotactic for monocytes.

Ligands

CD108 binds CD232 (plexin-C1).

Expression

Expressed by erythrocytes, at low levels on circulating lymphocytes and at moderately high levels on lymphoblasts and lymphoblastic cell lines.

Gene Name	Entrez Gene#
SEMA7A	8482

Selected Monoclonal Antibodies

MEM-121 (Horejsi; Praha); MEM-150 (Horejsi; Praha).

CD109

Other Names

Platelet activation factor; 8A3, E123.

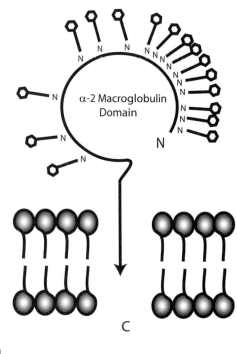

C

GPI Anchor

Molecular Structure

A 170-kDa GPI-linked glycoprotein containing 17 N-linked carbohydrate moieties. Additional Mol Wt forms are seen, which appear to derive from the 170-kDa molecules by partial proteolysis or by having shorter carbohydrate side-chains.

Member of the $\alpha(2)$ macroglobulin/C3, C4, C5 family of thioester-containing proteins.

CD109 carries the Gov a/b platelet alloantigens and possibly the ABH blood group antigen.

Function

Not known. Carries the Gov a/b alloantigens on platelets.

Expression

Expressed on a subset of CD34-positive progenitors, megakaryoblasts, and some myeloid cell lines (megakaryoblastic cell lines and KG1A, HEL), as well as chronic myeloid leukemia in megakaryoblastic crisis. Absent from unstimulated blood leukocytes but expressed on activated platelets and activated T cells. Expressed on vascular endothelium and some epithelial tumors.

Applications

Research reagent for study of progenitor cell subsets.

Gene Name	Entrez Gene#
CD109	135228

Selected Monoclonal Antibodies

7D1 (Sutherland; Toronto); 8A3 (Sutherland; Toronto).

CD110

Other Names

Thrombopoietin receptor (TPO-R), myeloproliferative leukemia virus onco-gene (c-mpl).

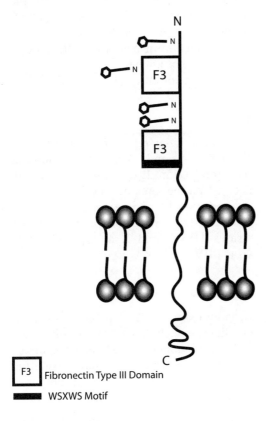

| F3 | Fibronectin Type III Domain |

▬▬ WSXWS Motif

Molecular Structure

CD110 is a 635 amino acid transmembrane protein and a member of the hematopoi-etin receptor family within the cytokine receptor superfamily and therefore the Ig superfamily.

The extracellular domain consists of 466 amino acids and contains 2 fibronectin type III-like (cytokine receptor) domains and has 4 potential N-linked glycosylation sites.

The protein has a 22 amino acid trans-membrane domain and 122 amino acid cytoplasmic domain with 2 cytokine recep-tor box motifs.

CD110 dimerizes upon binding of thrombopoietin (TPO) enabling the intra-cellular binding of JAK2 to the box 1 motif, which results in tyrosine phosphorylation of CD110.

Mol Wt: 85–92 kDa.

Function

Receptor for thrombopoietin (TPO), the main regulator of megakaryocyte and platelet formation.

The binding of TPO to CD110 results in proliferation and differentiation and the prevention of apoptosis.

Knockout mice have severely decreased numbers of megakaryocytes and platelets as well as diminished counts of all other hematopoietic progenitors but normal hemoglobin and leukocyte counts.

Mutations in CD110 are found in some patients with congenital amegakaryocytic thrombocytopenia.

Ligands

CD110 binds thrombopoietin (TPO).

Expression

Expressed by platelets, hematopoietic stem and progenitor cells, megakaryocyte prog-enitors, and megakaryocytes.

Applications

Oncogene V-mpl (murine myelo-proliferative leukemia virus) can immor-talize BM hematopoietic cells; mpl mutations are associated with congenital thrombocytopenia.

Gene Name	Entrez Gene#
MPL	4352

Selected Monoclonal Antibodies

BAH-1 (Avraham; Boston); SW-1 (Ballmaier; Hanover); 5C6, 3G4, 6E10 (Kerr; Tampa).

CD111

Other Names

Poliovirus receptor related 1 protein (PRR1), Nectin-1, Hve C1.

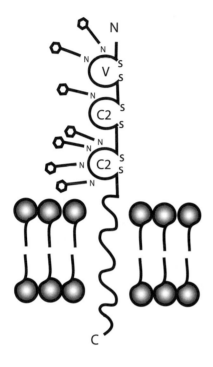

Molecular Structure

A type I transmembrane glycoprotein, member of the Ig gene superfamily. In common with other members of the nectin family, the extracellular region consists of three Ig-like domains (a membrane-distal V-type domain and two C-type domains). Nectin-1 shows approximately 30% homology with Nectins-2 and -3. The predominant isoform is 518 amino acids long, and a shorter isoform (459 amino acids) is also observed.

Nectin-1 has eight potential N-glycosylation sites and an observed Mol Wt of 75 kDa.

Function

Nectin-1, like the other nectins, is an adhesion molecule involved in the formation of adherens junctions between epithelial cells. The intracellular portion of nectins binds to the actin cytoskeleton through afadin. The extracellular portion interacts with the other nectin family members, CD155, Nectin-2, Nectin-3, and Nectin-4.

The function of Nectin-1 on hematopoietic cells is not known.

Receptor for entry of HSV-1, HSV-2.

Ligands

The extracellular region binds the related Nectins-2, -3, and -4 and the poliovirus receptor CD155. It can also interact with nectin-1 on the same or on other cells (i.e., cis- and trans-homo-interaction).

Nectin-1 is a receptor for the α herpes viruses HSV-1 and 2 and pseudorabies virus PRV.

Expression

Broadly expressed within the hematopoietic lineage, including CD34-positive stem cells, myelomonocytic cells, and precursors of red cells and platelets, and outside the hematopoietic lineage in endothelial, epithelial, and neuronal cells.

Applications

A CD111 Fc fusion protein and antibody against CD111 both block viral entry in vitro.

Gene Name	Entrez Gene#
PVRL1	5818

Selected Monoclonal Antibodies

R1.302 (Lopez, Marseille).

CD112

Other Names

Poliovirus receptor related 2 protein (PRR2), Nectin-2, Hve B.

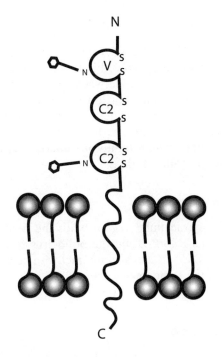

Molecular Structure

A type I transmembrane glycoprotein, member of the Ig gene superfamily. In common with other members of the nectin family, the extracellular region consists of three Ig-like domains (an N-terminal V-type domain followed by two C-type domains). Nectin-2 shows approximately 30% homology with nectins-1 and -3.

Two splice variants have been identified, nectin-2 α and δ, with the latter having a shorter cytoplasmic region. Nectin-2α is 539 amino acids long, and the δ isoform is 479 amino acids long.

The extracellular domains carry two sites for potential N glycosylation.

The observed Mol Wts are 72 and 64 kDa, respectively.

Function

Nectin 2, like the other nectins, is an adhesion molecule involved in the formation of adherens junctions between cells. The intracellular portion of nectins binds to the actin cytoskeleton through afadin. The extracellular portion interacts with the other nectin family members, CD155, nectins-1, -3, and -4.

Nectin-2 is expressed on hematopoietic cells, but its function in hematopiesis is not known.

Nectin-2 functions as a receptor for some Herpes Viruses.

Ligands

The extracellular region binds the related nectins-1 and -3 and the poliovirus receptor CD155. It can also interact with nectin-2 on the same or on other cells (i.e., cis- and trans-homo-interaction).

Nectin-2 is a receptor for the α herpes viruses HSV-1 and pseudorabies virus (PRV).

Expression

Myelomonocytic cells and megakaryocytes, CD34-positive stem cells, as well as endothelial, epithelial, and neuronal cells.

Applications

CD112-Fc fusion has been shown to block infection by HSV in vitro.

Gene Name	Entrez Gene#
PVRL2	5819

Selected Monoclonal Antibodies

R2.525 (Lopez, Marseille); 5-193 (Majdic, Vienna); B-C12 (Ciement, Besencon).

CD113

Other Names

Nectin-3, PVRL3 (poliovirus receptor-like 3).

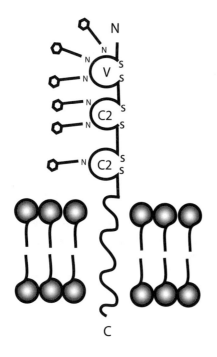

Molecular Structure

A type I transmembrane glycoprotein, member of the Ig gene superfamily. In common with other members of the nectin family, the extracellular region consists of three Ig-like domains (an N-terminal V-type domain followed by two C-type domains). Nectin-3 shows approximately 30% homology with nectins-1 and -2.

Nectin-3 is 549 amino acids long with a predicted Mol Wt of 61 kDa. Two splice variants have been identified, with shorter cytoplasmic regions. The extracellular domains carry six sites for potential N glycosylation. The apparent Mol Wt is 100 kDa, and two bands are seen, possibly reflecting differences in glycosylation.

Function

Nectin-3, like the other nectins, is an adhesion molecule involved in the formation of adherens junctions between epithelial cells. The intracellular portion of nectins binds to the actin cytoskeleton through afadin. The extracellular portion interacts with the other nectin family members, CD155, nectin-1, and nectin-2.

Ligands

The extracellular region binds the related nectins-1 and -2 and the poliovirus receptor CD155. It can also interact with nectin-3 on the same or on other cells (ie cis- and trans-homo-interaction).

Expression

Epithelial cells, in gut, kidney, liver, brain and testis. The different members of the nectin family show different tissue distributions.

Gene Name	Entrez Gene#
PVRL3	25945

Selected Monoclonal Antibodies

N3.12.4, N3.82.5, and N3.81.6, all from del Vecchio (Naples).

CD114

Other Names

Granulocyte colony stimulating factor receptor (G-CSFR), HG-CSFR, CSF3R.

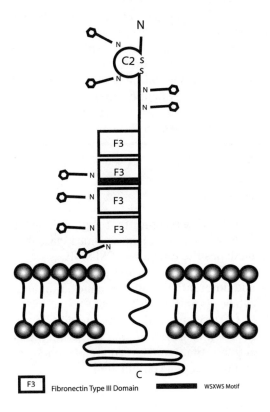

| F3 | Fibronectin Type III Domain | ▬▬ WSXWS Motif |

Molecular Structure

A type I transmembrane glycoprotein of the class 1 cytokine receptor gene family. The protein is 812 residues in size, with a 603 amino acids extracellular domain consisting of an Ig-like domain, 4 fibronectin type III repeats (the second containing a WSXWS motif) and 9 potential N-linked glycosylation sites.

The protein has a 26 amino acid transmembrane region and a 183 amino acid intracellular region with no intrinsic kinase activity.

Alternative splicing yields six splice variants, one of which is a secreted soluble form.

Mol Wt: 130–150 kDa.

Function

CD114 is the cytokine receptor for granulocyte colony stimulating factor (G-CSF) and is a regulator of myeloid differentiation and proliferation. The receptor forms a homodimer when it binds ligand. After dimerization, signal transduction involves the JAK-STAT pathway.

Ligands

Binds the cytokine granulocyte colony stimulating factor (G-CSF).

Expression

Expressed by granulocytes at all stages during differentiation, as well as monocytes, dendritic cells, and mature platelets.

It is also expressed by many non-hematopoietic cells, including endothelial cells, placenta, trophoblasts, and many tumor cell lines.

Applications

Target for stem cell mobilization for blood stem cell transplantation, for enhancing recovery of myelopoiesis following chemotherapy and in the treatment of patients with severe chronic neutropenia.

Gene Name	Entrez Gene#
CSF3R	1441

Selected Monoclonal Antibodies

129 (Kasper; Hannover); LMM741 (Nicholson: Melbourne).

CD115

Other Names

Macrophage colony stimulating factor receptor (M-CSFR), CSF-1R, C-fms.

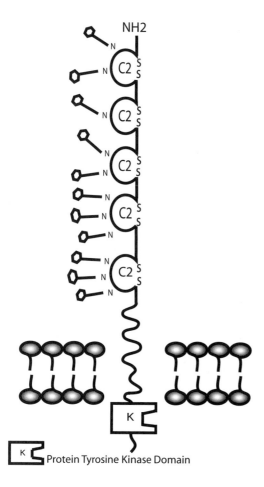

K ⊂ Protein Tyrosine Kinase Domain

Molecular Structure

A type I integral membrane protein, belonging to the Ig domain containing receptor tyrosine kinase (Ig-RTK) family (see CD117, CD135, CD140a, and CD140b).

The extracellular region consists of 492 amino acids, is variably glycosylated, and contains 5 IgC-like domains. The N-terminal 3 Ig-domains are required for high affinity binding of the ligand M-CSF.

The 434 amino acid cytoplasmic region contains a protein tyrosine kinase domain interrupted by a kinase insert domain.

The CD115 molecule is encoded by the c-fms proto-oncogene.

Ligand binding induces and stabilizes dimerization of CD115 and activates the receptor through autophosphorylation in trans.

Phosphorylation of CD115 at several sites generates binding sites for other signaling molecules. Phosphorylation of tyrosine 809 is essential for activity.

Mol Wt: 150 kDa.

Function

CD115 is the receptor for the growth factor M-CSF and is a protein tyrosine kinase that mediates the functions of M-CSF.

It plays a role in the growth, survival, and differentiation of mononuclear phagocytic cells and dendritic cells.

CD115 and CSF-1 are thought to be involved in autocrine and paracrine interactions that may regulate trophoblast and/or decidual cell function.

Ligands

Macrophage-colony stimulating factor (M-CSF, CSF-1).

Expression

Primarily expressed on cells of mononuclear phagocytic lineage. It is also expressed by dendritic cells, osteoclasts, extravillous trophoblastic cells, placenta and decidua, normal and lactating breast tissue, microglia, neurons, and astrocytes.

Myeloid leukemic blasts, vascular smooth muscle in atheroma, and some breast and ovarian cancers express CD115.

Applications

The ligand CSF-1 is used to promote the recovery of myeloid cells following chemotherapy and has been used in the treatment of aplastic anaemia.

Selected Monoclonal Antibodies

3-4A4-E4 (Ashmun; Memphis); 7-7A3-14 (Ashmun; Memphis).

Gene Name	Entrez Gene#
CSF1R	1436

CD116

Other Names

GM-CSF receptor α-subunit.

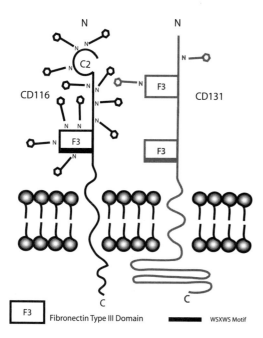

| F3 | Fibronectin Type III Domain | ▬▬▬ WSXWS Motif |

Molecular Structure

CD116 is a 378-residue, type I integral membrane protein belonging to the hematopoietin receptor superfamily within the Ig gene superfamily.

The extracellular region is glycosylated (11 potential N-glycosylation sites) and consists of 298 amino acids containing an N-terminal domain similar to that found in the α chain of CD123 and CD125, followed by a WSXWS motif-containing fibronectin type III domain.

The transmembrane domain consists of 26 amino acids, and the intracellular region of 54 residues has no intrinsic enzymatic activity.

Alternative splicing generates several soluble isoforms, all of which are minor species and have not as yet been found to have any physiological function.

Mol Wt: 80 kDa.

Function

Functions as the primary binding subunit of the granulocyte macrophage colony stimulating factor (GM-CSF) receptor. The functional receptor requires CD116 to be associated with CD131, a β-subunit that also forms part of the IL-3 and IL-5 receptors and is referred to as the common β-subunit.

CD116 has no intrinsic kinase activity, and signal transduction occurs via the JAK-STAT pathway.

Ligands

Binds GM-CSF with low affinity and with high affinity when associated with the common β-subunit CD131.

Expression

Primarily expressed by myeloid cells including macrophages, neutrophils, eosinophils, dendritic cells, and their precursors. Also expressed by endothelial cells.

Expression of CD116 is increased in acute myeloid leukemias (AMLs) and can be very high in some AMLs.

Applications

CD116 is a specific marker of myeloid leukemias.

Gene Name	Entrez Gene#
CSF2RA	1438

Selected Monoclonal Antibodies

hGMCSFR-M1 (Armitage; Seattle).

CD117

Other Names

Stem cell factor receptor (SCFR), c-kit.

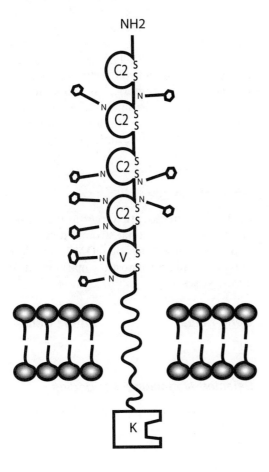

Molecular Structure

A type I integral membrane protein, belonging to subclass III of the receptor tyrosine kinase (RTK) family (see CD115, CD135, CD140a, and CD140b).

The extracellular region consists of 497 amino acids and contains 4 IgC-like and 1 IgV-like domain with 9 potential N-glycosylation sites.

The first three N-terminal Ig-like domains are involved in ligand binding.

Ligand binding leads to dimerization and stabilization of the dimeric complex as well as increasing the local concentration of kinase domains, which assists autophosphorylation and activation of the intrinsic kinase activity of CD117.

The transmembrane domain consists of 23 amino acids. The cytoplasmic region contains a consensus ATP binding site and protein tyrosine kinase domain split by a kinase insert.

Alternative splicing of CD117 results in isoforms with or without four extracellular membrane proximal amino acids (GNNK). The shorter variant has been shown to bind and activate Src family kinases (SFKs) more efficiently.

Other splice variants are characterized by the presence or absence of a serine residue in the kinase insert.

Mol Wt: 145 kDa.

Function

Receptor for the growth factor stem cell factor (SCF) and is required for normal hematopoiesis, pigmentation, gut function, and reproduction.

Ligand binding results in autophosphorylation of intracellular tyrosine residues that in turn become binding sites for signal transduction molecules.

In vitro CD117 can activate several signaling pathways, including the phosphoinositide 3′-kinase (PI3K) pathway, which is involved in adhesion, anti-apoptotic signaling, and proliferation. Loss of the PI3K binding site results in defective gametogenesis.

SCF binding activates the Janus kinase-signal transducers and activators of transcription (JAK-STAT) pathway. In some studies, this was found to be a requirement for maximal SCF-induced proliferation of progenitor cells but not for mast cell proliferation.

CD117 mediated activation of the Ras-Erk pathway is important for hemopoietic differentiation.

Activation of CD117 leads to a rapid increase in Src family kinase (SFK) activity. SFKs are necessary for CD117 internalization after ligand binding and survival and migration of hemopoietic precursors. Mice bearing mutated CD117 SFK binding sites show defective lymphopoeisis, mast cell development and pigmentation, as well as splenomegaly.

Activation of the phospholipase Cγ pathway protects CD117-expressing cells from apoptosis induced by irradiation or the cytotoxin daunorubicin.

CD117 can interact with some cytokine receptors such as the IL-7 receptor and the Epo receptor, which in the presence of SCF results in synergistic signaling.

Negative regulation of CD117 signaling is potentially mediated by serine and threonine kinases belonging to the PKC family, the tyrosine phosphatase SHP-1, and the ubiquitin ligase Cbl.

Ligands

The ligand for CD117 is stem cell factor (SCF).

Expression

Expressed by the earliest hemopoietic stem cells through to committed progenitors of myeloid, erythroid, megakaryocytic, natural killer, and dendritic progenitor cells as well as pro-B and -T cells and tissue mast cells. Expression is weakest in the earliest hemopoietic stem cells and is strongest in the more mature progenitor cells. It is also expressed by cutaneous and choroidal melanocytes.

Expression of CD117 is found in small cell lung, breast and colorectal carcinomas, gynecological tumors, neuroblastoma, gastrointestinal stromal tumor, seminoma germ cell tumors, choroidal melanomas, and acute myeloid leukemias and mastocytosis.

Applications

CD117 is a therapeutic target in the treatment of gastrointestinal stromal tumors.

Somatic mutations of CD117 are phenotypic and prognostic markers for mastocytosis.

Gene Name	Entrez Gene#
KIT	3815

Selected Monoclonal Antibodies

YB5.B8 (Ashman; Adelaide); 95C3 (Bühring; Tübingen).

CD118

Other Names

Leukemia inhibitory factor receptor (LIFR).

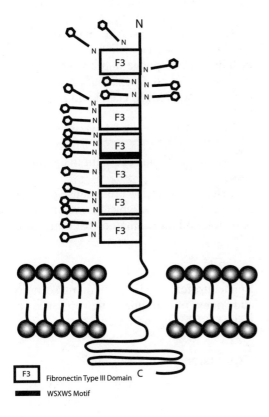

F3 | Fibronectin Type III Domain

■■ WSXWS Motif

Molecular Structure

A type 1 membrane glycoprotein member of the type 1 cytokine receptor family.

Associates noncovalently with CD130 to form the functional LIF receptor.

CD118 is 1097 residues long (including a 44-aa signal sequence), with 6 fibronectin type III domains and 19 potential N-glycosylation in the extracellular region.

A WSXWS motif in the extracellular region is essential for proper folding and expression of the receptor.

Residues 835–857 constitute the membrane-spanning region.

The intracellular region contains a box 1 motif essential for signaling through the JAK system.

A secreted form results from alternative splicing.

Mol Wt: (membrane form) 190 kDa.

Function

LIF and Oncostatin M, which both act through the CD118/CD130 heterodimer, are multifunction cytokines that influence growth and differentiation of a variety of cell types, both in the embryo and in mature individuals.

Ligands

CD118 alone binds LIF with low affinity, but the CD118/CD130 heterodimer binds LIF with high affinity and is the functional receptor. Soluble CD118 binds LIF with low affinity and may have inhibitory effects.

The CD118/CD130 heterodimer also binds oncostatin M.

Expression

Expressed very widely outside the immune system, but not expressed by resting or activated lymphocytes.

Soluble CD118 is found in serum and rises during pregnancy, in parallel with a drop in circulating LIF levels.

Applications

LIF is widely used for the culture of embryonic stem (ES) cells.

Null mutations in LIFR are associated with Stuve–Wiedemann syndrome and Schwartz-Jampel type 2 syndrome.

Gene Name	Entrez Gene#
LIFR	3977

Selected Monoclonal Antibodies

12D3, 7G7 (BD Biosciences; San Jose).

CD119

Other Names

IFN γ receptor α-chain, IFNγR, IFNγRα.

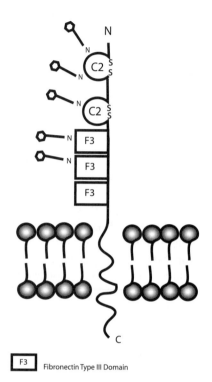

F3   Fibronectin Type III Domain

Molecular Structure

A type I transmembrane glycoprotein and a member of the class II cytokine receptor family within the Ig gene superfamily.

IFNγAF-1 associates with the extracellular region of CD119 to form the functional IFNγ receptor.

The 227 amino acid extracellular domain consists of 2 Ig-like C2 domains, 2 fibronectin type III domains, and 5 potential N-linked glycosylation sites.

The 22 amino acid transmembrane domain is followed by an intracellular domain of 222 amino acids.

Mol Wt: 90–100 kDa.

Function

Forms part of the receptor for IFNγ. Despite being able to bind IFNγ on its own, CD119 must form a complex with IFNγAF-1 for signal transduction to occur.

The receptor plays a role in the initiation and effector phases of immune responses, including macrophage and NK cell activation, B- and T-cell differentiation, as well as upregulation of MHC class I and II in many cell types.

CD119-deficient mice have greater susceptibility to *Listeria monocytogenes* and vaccinia virus but are resistant to endotoxic shock.

Defects in IFNγR1 are a cause of familial disseminated atypical mycobacterial infection and disseminated BCG infection.

Ligands

Binds interferon γ (IFNγ) with high affinity and does not require the presence of IFNγAF-1 for ligand binding.

Expression

Expressed on monocytes, macrophages, T and B cells, NK cells, neutrophils, fibroblasts, epithelial cells, endothelium, and by many tumors.

Gene Name   Entrez Gene#

IFNGR1   3459

Selected Monoclonal Antibodies

GIR-208 (Schreiber; St. Louis).

CD120a

Other Names

TNFRI, TNFRp55, TNFRSF1A.

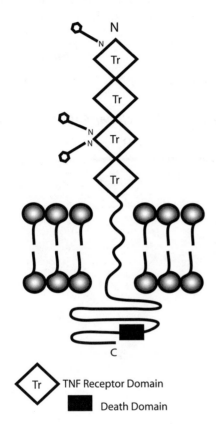

◇ Tr — TNF Receptor Domain

■ — Death Domain

Molecular Structure

CD120a is a type I integral membrane protein and a member of the tumor necrosis factor (TNF)/nerve growth factor (NGF) receptor family (see CD27, CD30, CD40, CD95, CD120b, CD134, and CD137).

The 190 amino acid extracellular region consists of four tandemly repeated cysteine rich motifs and has a pre-ligand-binding assembly domain (PLAD) that promotes the formation of receptor complexes and trimerization of CD120a molecules particularly after activation by ligand binding.

CD120a has three potential N-linked glycosylation sites.

The 221 amino acid intracellular region contains a death domain (DD) motif of approximately 86 amino acids that is crucial for cell death signaling as well as an 11 amino acid neutral sphingomyelinase activation domain (NSD) also known to be involved in apoptotic signaling.

Phosphorylation of CD120 occurs at a consensus mitogen activated protein kinase (MAPK) site within the cytoplasmic domain or at tyrosine residues.

Mol Wt: 50–60 kDa.

Function

CD120a is a receptor for tumor necrosis factor (TNF), binding both membrane-bound and soluble forms of TNFα and TNFβ with high affinity.

Intracellular adaptor proteins known to associate with CD120a are TRADD, RAIDD, RIP, FAN, BRE, SODD, Grb2, MADD, PIP5K, and p60TRAK. Signal transduction via these molecules mediates proinflammatory cellular responses, apoptosis, and anti-viral activity.

CD120a association with TRADD and RAIDD can initiate caspase-dependent cell death. However, CD120a can also mediate anti-apoptotic signaling when TRADD interacts with TNF-associating factor (TRAF) 2, which ultimately leads to NF–kB activation.

Binding of FAN to the NSD motif of CD120a upregulates ceramide production by activating neutral sphingomyelinase ultimately leading to cell death.

CD120a plays a major role in early graft versus host disease and in TNF-mediated insulin resistance seen in type II diabetes mellitus.

Defects in CD120a are a cause of autosomal dominant familial Hibernian fever (FHF) also known as TNF-receptor-associated periodic syndrome (TRAPS).

CD120a knockout mice are more susceptible to infection with *Listeria monocytogenes* but are resistant to TNF- or IL-1-mediated in vivo lethality and are also resistant to LPS- or D-galactosamine induced endotoxic shock.

Ligands

CD120a binds tumor necrosis factor (TNF) α and β with high affinity.

Expression

CD120a is constitutively expressed at a low level by hemopoietic and nonhemopoietic cells. The highest level of expression is found on epithelial cells.

Applications

CD120a is a potential therapeutic target in the treatment of type II diabetes mellitus.

Gene Name	Entrez Gene#
TNFRSF1A	7132

Selected Monoclonal Antibodies

htr-9 (Lesslauer; Basel); MR1-2 (Buurman; Maastricht).

CD120b

Other Names

TNFRII, TNFRp75, TNFRSF1B.

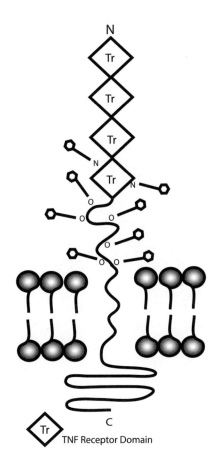

Tr — TNF Receptor Domain

Molecular Structure

CD120b is a type I integral membrane protein and a member of the tumor necrosis factor (TNF)/nerve growth factor (NGF) receptor family (see CD27, CD30, CD40, CD95, CD120a, CD134, and CD137).

The extracellular region consists of 235 amino acid with three potential N-linked glycosylation sites and four tandemly repeated cysteine-rich motifs. The region also has a pre-ligand-binding assembly domain (PLAD) that promotes the formation of receptor complexes and trimerization of CD120b molecules particularly after activation by ligand binding.

The transmembrane region is approximately 30 amino acids in length, and the intracellular region consists of 174 amino acids.

Unlike CD120a, CD120b does not have a death domain.

CD120b is readily cleaved by the metalloprotease TACE into a soluble form that retains the ability to bind TNF.

Mol Wt: 75–85 kDa.

Function

CD120b is a high affinity receptor for TNFα and TNFβ. It is more efficiently activated by membrane-bound rather than soluble TNF.

Unlike CD120a, whose expression is largely unmodulated, the number of CD120b molecules on the cell surface will be determined by the level of expression induced and shedding of the receptor as a result of proteolytic cleavage. This has led to the proposal that a cell's response to TNF is determined by the ratio of CD120a to CD120b.

A common polymorphic variant substituting Met for Arg at position 196 is associated with hyperandrogenism, polycystic ovary syndrome, and systemic lupus erythematosus.

CD120b-deficient mice have shown that the receptor is important in low dose TNF-induced lethality, thymocyte proliferation, and depressed Langerhans cell migration. It also appears to play an important role in models of malaria and microvascular endothelial cell damage and multi-organ inflammation.

Ligands

CD120b binds tumor necrosis factor (TNF) α and β with high affinity.

Expression

CD120b expression is inducible in hemopoietic and nonhemopoietic cells and is highest on myeloid cells.

Gene Name   Entrez Gene#

TNFRSF1B   7133

Selected Monoclonal Antibodies

utr-1 (Lesslauer; Basel); MR2-1 (Buurman; Maastricht).

CD121a

Other Names

Type I IL-1 receptor.

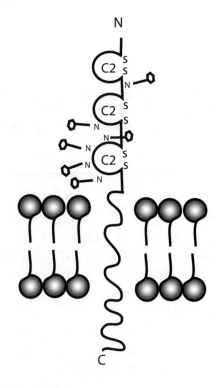

Molecular Structure

CD121a is a type I integral membrane protein member of the Ig gene superfamily.

The 317 amino acid extracellular region consists of three IgC-like domains with six potential N-linked glycosylation sites.

The transmembrane region consists of 19 amino acids, and the cytoplasmic region has 213 amino acids.

Mol Wt: 80 kDa.

Function

CD121a is the IL-1 receptor and mediates all biological effects of IL-1α and IL-1β. It functions in association with the IL-1 receptor accessory protein (AcP), which enhances the affinity for IL-1 and initiates signaling.

CD121a-mediated signaling results in the activation of the transcription factors, including NF-κB, AP-1, and C/EBPb leading to expression of inflammatory proteins such as prostaglandins and inflammatory cytokines.

Binding of the IL-1 receptor antagonist to CD121a prevents IL-1α and IL-1β from binding but does not induce any biological response of its own.

Knockout mice are normal other than they lack IL-1 responsiveness and are deficient in delayed hypersensitivity and contact sensitivity.

Ligands

CD121a binds the three forms of IL-1 [IL-1α, IL-1β, and IL-1ra (IL-1 receptor antagonist)]. Binding to IL-1ra is practically irreversible.

Expression

CD121a is very widely expressed at low levels (50–1000 molecules per cell) in hematopoietic and other tissues.

Applications

Soluble CD121a is a potential anti-inflammatory agent.

Gene Name	*Entrez Gene#*
IL1RI	3554

Selected Monoclonal Antibodies

hIL-1R1-M1 (Armitage; Seattle).

CD121b

Other Names

Type II IL-1 receptor.

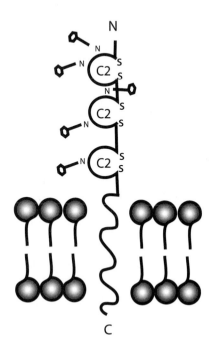

Molecular Structure

CD121b is a type I transmembrane glycoprotein and a member of the Ig gene superfamily.

The extracellular domain consists of 336 residues and contains 3 C2-like Ig domains and 5 sites for N-glycosylation.

The transmembrane domain consists of 20 amino acids, and the cytoplasmic region consists of 29 amino acids.

A soluble form is produced by proteolysis particularly after cell stimulation.

Alternative splicing gives rise to a soluble form.

Soluble CD121b is present at very low concentration, and no biological function has been attributed to it.

Mol Wt: 60–68 kDa.

Function

Unlike CD121a, CD121b does not mediate IL-1 function but acts as a "decoy" receptor reducing the effective concentration of IL-1β.

CD121b may play a role in preventing toxicity in the presence of excessive systemic IL-1β and protect IL-1β producing cells from excessive autocrine stimulation.

Ligands

CD121b binds IL-1β with high affinity and has low affinity for IL-1α and IL-1ra (IL-1 receptor antagonist).

Expression

B cells, monocytes, neutrophils, and basal cells in the epithelium of the skin, female reproductive tract, and ureter.

Applications

CD121b has the potential to be used as an anti-inflammatory agent and may be more effective than soluble CD121a as it has low affinity for the IL-1 receptor antagonist IL-1ra.

Gene Name	Entrez Gene#
IL1R2	7850

Selected Monoclonal Antibodies

hIL-1R2-M2 (Armitage; Seattle).

CD122

Other Names

IL-2 receptor β chain, IL-2/15Rb, p75.

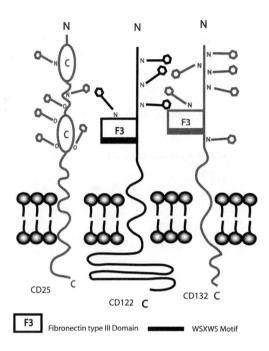

F3 | Fibronectin type III Domain ▬▬▬ WSXWS Motif

CD25   CD122 C   CD132 C

Molecular Structure

A type I transmembrane glycoprotein and a cytokine receptor belonging to the hemopoietin receptor superfamily and the Ig gene superfamily (see also CD123, CD124, CD125, and CD126).

The extracellular domain is characterized by four conserved cysteines and a membrane proximal fibronectin type III domain containing a WSXWS (trp-ser-X-trp-ser) motif.

It is one of three subunits, which in various combinations give rise to receptors capable of binding IL-2 and/or IL-15 with varying affinity.

IL-2 and IL-15 receptors are heterotrimeric or heterodimeric complexes of CD25 (IL-2a subunit), CD122, and CD132 (the common γ chain).

CD122 has a 214 amino acid extracellular region, 25 amino acid transmembrane domain, and 286 amino acid cytoplasmic region.

The cytoplasmic domain contains at least three unique regions, the serine-rich (S), acidic (A), and proline-rich (H) regions. Of the six cytoplasmic tyrosine residues present in the acidic and proline-rich regions, the presence of at least one of three tyrosines, Tyr338, Tyr392 and Tyr510 is sufficient for IL-2-mediated proliferation.

The S region contains box 1 and box 2 motifs that are the binding sites for the Janus kinases Jak1, Jak3 and Syk.

The A region contains binding sites for Src family tyrosine such as Lyn.

Mol Wt: 70–75 kDa.

Function

The biological effect of CD122 ligation will depend on whether IL-2 or IL-15 is bound.

Oligomerization of the receptor subunits activates several tyrosine kinases. The serine-rich region of CD122 has binding sites for Janus-family kinases that induce mitogenic and survival signals.

The acidic-region of the cytoplasmic tail has binding sites required for induction of NK cell cytotoxicity and downregulation of T-cell proliferation.

The proline-rich region is involved in the activation Stat3 and Stat5. When phosphorylated, these factors dimerize and localize to the nucleus and induce the transcription of genes involved in NK-cell and intraepithelial lymphocyte development as well as upregulation of IL-2 expression.

CD122-deficient mice display a dramatic reduction in NK and intraepithelial lymphocytes cells due to impaired differentiation.

These mice develop severe autoimmune disorders and infiltrative granulocytopoiesis.

Ligands

IL-2/IL-15Rβ/γ receptors bind IL-2 and IL-15 with intermediate affinity, whereas IL2/IL-15Rα/β/γ complexes bind both interleukins with high affinity.

Expression

CD122 is constitutively expressed at low levels on lymphocytes and NK cells, and expression is up regulated by activation.

Applications

Combined anti-CD122 and anti-CD25 therapy has been used in the treatment of autoimmune disorders and allograft rejection.

Anti-CD122 monoclonal antibody has been used in clinical trials as a treatment for large granular lymphocytic leukemia.

Gene Name	Entrez Gene#
IL2RB	3560

Selected Monoclonal Antibodies

MiK-β1 (Miyasaka; Tokyo); TU27 (Sugamura; Sendai); CF1 (van Agthoven; Marseille).

CD123

Other Names

Interleukin-3 receptor α-chain (IL-3Rα).

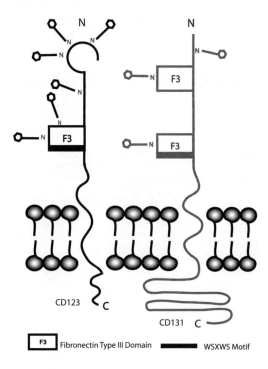

F3 | Fibronectin Type III Domain   ■ WSXWS Motif

Molecular Structure

A type I integral membrane glycoprotein and a cytokine receptor belonging to the hemopoietin receptor superfamily and the Ig gene superfamily (see also CD122, CD124, CD125, and CD126).

It is the α subunit of the human interleukin-3 receptor (IL-3R).

The extracellular region consists of 288 amino acids and contains an N-terminal domain (similar to that found in CD116 and CD125), followed by a 200 amino acid cytokine receptor domain (fibronectin type III domain) containing a WSXWS motif Both of these domains are required for IL-3 binding.

There are nine potential N-glycosylation sites.

The single transmembrane domain consists of 20 amino acids.

The intracellular region consists of 52 residues and is essential for signal propagation.

Mol Wt: 70 kDa.

Function

Associates with CD131 (common to IL-5 and GM-CSF receptors) to form the functional interleukin-3 receptor (IL-3R). The ligation of IL-3R by IL-3 promotes differentiation and proliferation of multipotential stem/progenitor cells as well as monocyte, neutrophil, basophil, and eosinophil bone marrow precursors. IL-3 binding to IL-3R stimulates the proliferation of erythroid and megakaryocyte committed precursors and induces activation of neutrophils and monocytes.

The membrane proximal cytoplasmic region of CD123 is involved in the activation of STAT5 and proliferation, whereas the distal region is linked to cell survival.

Several strains of naturally CD123-deficient mice exist that are hyporesponsive to IL-3 but do not show any overt abnormality in hematopoiesis even when challenged with parasites or bacterial pathogens.

Similarly CD123 knockout mice have no gross abnormalities, which suggests that there is functional redundancy of cytokines, allowing the maintenance of hematopoiesis.

Ligands

Binds IL-3 with low affinity and forms a high affinity IL-3 receptor in association with CD131.

Expression

Constitutively expressed by committed hemopoietic stem/progenitor cells.

It is also expressed by monocyte, granulocyte, megakaryocyte, and erythroid precursors, mast cells, macrophages, and a subpopulation of CD5+ B cells.

Some endothelial cells, Leydig cells of the testis, placenta, and brain express CD123.

Applications

CD123 is a useful phenotypic marker particularly for stem cell populations and assists in the diagnosis of acute myeloid leukemias and B lymphoproliferative disorders.

It is a therapeutic target in the treatment of various tumors, using IL-3R antagonists, anti-CD123 mAb conjugated to cytotoxic agents, or by stimulating leukemic cells into the cell cycle, thereby making them the more susceptible to cytotoxic agents.

CD123 is the target of IL-3 therapy aimed at improving multilineage hematopoietic recovery in myelosuppression or after myeloablative chemotherapy.

Gene Name	Entrez Gene#
IL3RA	3563

Selected Monoclonal Antibodies

9F5 (Lopez; Adelaide).

CD124

Other Names

IL-4 R α-chain, IL-4Rα.

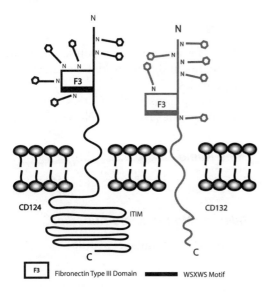

F3 — Fibronectin Type III Domain   ▬ WSXWS Motif

Molecular Structure

A type I integral membrane glycoprotein and a member of the hemopoietin receptor superfamily and the Ig gene superfamily (see also CD122, CD123, CD125, and CD126).

The 207 amino acid extracellular region consists of a cytokine receptor domain with four conserved cysteines and a WSXWS (trp-ser-X-trp-ser) containing fibronectin type III domain.

There are six potential N-glycoslyation sites in the extracellular domain.

CD124 has a single transmembrane domain of 24 amino acids.

The cytoplasmic tail consists of 569 amino acids rich in serines and has a proline-rich box region required for the constitutive association of Janus tyrosine kinases (JAK) that recruit downstream signaling molecules, and five conserved tyrosines.

Tyr497 is a critical component of a motif that recruits insulin receptor substrates 1 and 2 (IRS1/IRS2) to the cytoplasmic domain.

Tyr575, Tyr603, and Tyr631 are STAT 6 docking sites, and providing at least one of these tyrosines is present, IL-4 dependent gene induction can occur.

Tyr713 is part of an immunotyrosine-based inhibitory motif (ITIM) important in the negative regulation of IL-4 and IL-13 responses.

Mol Wt: 140 kDa.

Function

CD124 associates with CD132 (the common γ chain) to form the type I IL-4 receptor. The association of CD124 with IL-13 receptor α1 chain (IL-13Rα1) forms the type II IL-4 receptor and the functional IL-13 receptor. Although CD124 is part of the IL-13 receptor, IL-13 binds IL-13Ra1 not CD124.

IL-4 and IL-13 signaling is mediated via CD124, resulting in the activation of the JAK/STAT and insulin receptor substrate 1 and 2 (IRS-1/IRS-2) pathways.

IL-4 and IL-13 have similar effects on B cells, including proliferation, IgE and IgG4 class switching, in combination with CD40/CD40 ligand costimulation, and induce expression of surface antigens, including CD23 (low affinity IgE receptor) and MHC class II.

IL-4 is important in inducing Th2 cells and contributes to allergic bronchial inflammation.

IL-13 promotes inflammation in allergic disorders.

In monocytes and macrophages, IL-13 enhances the expression of MHC class II, CD23, and integrins involved in adhesion, including CD11b and c, CD18, and CD29.

IL-13 inhibits the production of several pro-inflammatory mediators, including prostaglandins, reactive oxygen, nitrogen intermediates, IL-1, IL-6, IL-8, TNF-α, and IL-12 by monocytes and macrophages.

IL-13 is a potent inducer of VCAM-1 expression by endothelial cells, induces proliferation and cholinergic contraction of smooth muscle cells in vitro, and promotes type 1 collagen synthesis in human dermal fibroblasts.

IL-13-mediated stimulation of respiratory epithelial cells results in chemokine expression, altered mucociliary differentiation, decreased ciliary beat frequency of ciliated epithelium, and goblet cell metaplasia, demonstrating IL-13 to be an important effector molecule in asthma and obstructive pulmonary diseases.

Apart from its role in asthma, IL-13 contributes to the control of helminth infections and suppresses inflammation associated with bacterial and viral infection.

Ligands

CD124 binds IL-4 with high affinity.

Expression

CD124 is constitutively and ubiquitously expressed at very low levels in humans. Expression is upregulated in activated T and B lymphocytes.

Applications

CD124 is a potential therapeutic target in the treatment of bronchial asthma and malignancies.

Polymorphisms in the CD124 gene are associated with severity of allergic disease.

Gene Name	Entrez Gene#
IL4R	3566

Selected Monoclonal Antibodies

hIL-4R-M57 (Armitage; Seattle).

CD125

Other Names

Interleukin-5 receptor α-chain, IL-5Rα.

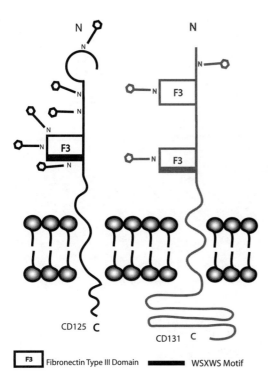

F3　Fibronectin Type III Domain　▬▬ WSXWS Motif

Molecular Structure

A type I integral membrane glycoprotein and a member of the hemopoietin receptor superfamily and the Ig gene superfamily (see CD122, CD123, CD124, and CD126).

The 322 amino acid extracellular region consists of an N-terminal domain (similar to that found in CD116 and CD123), followed by a cytokine receptor domain (fibronectin type III domain) containing four conserved cysteines and a WSXWS motif.

CD125 has six potential N-linked glycosylation sites.

The transmembrane domain consists of 20 amino acids. The 58 amino acid cytoplasmic domain contains a membrane—proximal box 1 motif and the DC3 subregion, both of which are critical for signal transduction.

Alternative mRNA splicing gives rise to a membrane bound form and two soluble forms.

Mol Wt: 60 kDa.

Function

Associates with CD131 β chain common to GM-CSF and IL-3 receptors to form the functional interleukin-5 receptor.

The box 1 motif of CD125 mediates activation of Bruton agammaglobulinaemia tyrosine kinase (Btk) and the JAK2/STAT5 pathway and has been shown in vivo to be essential for IL-5-induced proliferation and differentiation of B-1 and CD125[+] B-2 cells.

The DC3 subregion is important for both IL-5-induced IgM production and the IgM to IgG1 switch recombination in B cells.

IL-5-mediated activation of CD125 plays a central role in eosinophil and basophil differentiation, functional activation, and survival.

Ligands

CD125 binds IL-5 with low affinity and when associated with CD131 binds IL-5 with high affinity.

Expression

CD125 is constitutively expressed on all B1 cells and by 2–4% of resting B-2 cells in the spleen. It is also expressed by eosinophils, basophils, and mast cells.

Applications

CD125 is a potential therapeutic target in the treatment of allergic inflammatory conditions.

Selected Monoclonal Antibodies

KM1257 (Takatsu; Tokyo); KM1266 (Takatsu; Tokyo).

Gene Name	Entrez Gene#
IL5RA	3568

CD126

Other Names

IL-6 receptor α-chain, IL-6Rα.

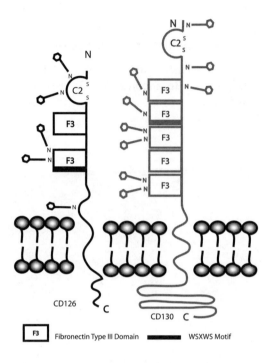

F3 : Fibronectin Type III Domain   ▬▬▬ : WSXWS Motif

Molecular Structure

A type I integral membrane glycoprotein and a member of the hematopoietin receptor superfamily and the Ig gene superfamily (see CD122, CD123, CD124, and CD125).

The 339 amino acid extracellular region consists of an N-terminal IgC-like domain followed by two fibronectin type III (FNIII) modules, which form the cytokine binding domain (CBD). The CBD has conserved cysteines in the N-terminal FNIII domain and a WSXWS motif located within the membrane proximal FNIII domain.

There are four potential N-linked glycosylation sites.

The 82 amino acid cytoplasmic domain is nonessential for receptor complex formation and signal transduction but does contain a tyrosine-based and dileucine-type motif required for direct sorting of CD126 to the basolateral membrane of polarized cells.

Alternative RNA splicing and proteolytic cleavage generates soluble forms of CD126 that retain the capacity to bind IL-6 and associate with CD130.

Mol Wt: 80 kDa.

Function

Binds the cytokine IL-6 and then associates with CD130 homodimers to form the functional IL-6 receptor (IL-6R), which mediates the biological activities of IL-6.

The ability of soluble CD126 to bind IL-6 and associate with membrane-bound CD130 to form a functional receptor is a rare example of a soluble receptor–cytokine complex capable of acting as an agonist rather than antagonistically. However, this complex can act antagonistically when it binds soluble CD130.

IL-6 is essential for differentiation of normal B cells into plasma cells and is an essential survival factor for circulating plasma cell precursors.

IL-6 is a growth factor for myelomas (including hybridomas) and a stimulus for the acute-phase response in the liver.

Ligands

CD126 alone binds IL-6 with low affinity. The CD126/CD130 complex binds IL-6 with high affinity.

Expression

Expressed by normal B cells, T lymphocytes monocytes, and hepatocytes.

Neoplastic plasma cells but not normal plasma cells express CD126.

Applications

CD126 is an endothelial marker used to separate circulating endothelial cells (CECs) from blood, a subset of which are endothelial progenitors that are involved in angiogenesis and are a promising tool in the diagnosis, prognosis, and therapy of vascular disorders.

Humanized anti-IL-6R antibody is a therapeutic agent for chronic inflammatory conditions, including Crohn's disease, rheumatoid arthritis, Castleman's disease, and juvenile idiopathic arthritis.

Gene Name	Entrez Gene#
ILR6	3570

Selected Monoclonal Antibodies

MT-18 (Kishimoto; Osaka); B-C22 (Wijdenes; Besancon); M113 (Brochier; Suzhou).

CD127

Other Names

IL-7 receptor α-chain, IL-7Rα, p90.

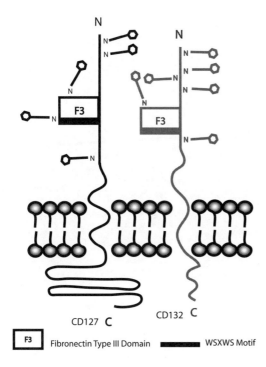

| F3 | Fibronectin Type III Domain | ▬▬▬ WSXWS Motif |

Molecular Structure

A type I integral membrane protein and a member of the hematopoietin receptor superfamily and the Ig gene superfamily (see also CD122, CD123, CD124, CD125, and CD126).

The 220 amino acid extracellular region consists of an N-terminal fibronectin type III (FNIII) domain containing four conserved cysteines and a WSXWS motif.

The 195 amino acid intracellular domain is essential for signal transduction and has structural and functional motifs that

recruit signal-transducing molecules. These include a membrane proximal acidic (A) region followed by a serine-containing (S) domain with a box 1 motif and a tyrosine-containing (T) domain.

Alternative RNA splicing gives rise to a soluble form of CD127.

Mol Wt: 80 kDa.

Function

Associates with CD132 (common γ chain) to form the high affinity IL-7 receptor and mediates all biological effects of IL-7.

The intracellular A region associates with the Src family tyrosine kinases p56lck and p59fyn.

The intracellular S domain is thought to bind Janus tyrosine kinase 1 (JAK1), which promotes cell survival.

When phosphorylated the tyrosine-containing (T) domain is a binding site for the signal transducer and activator of transcription 5 (STAT5), which plays a role in thymocyte differentiation.

Phosphorylation of Tyr449 in the T domain is required for IL-7-dependent activation of phosphatidylinositol 3-kinase (PI3K), which is essential for the survival and proliferation of thymocytes.

CD127 can complex with thymic stromal lymphopoietin receptor subunit (TSLPR) to form the receptor for TSLP. Ligand binding results in phosphorylation of STAT5 but not proliferation.

CD127 knockout mice have severe defects in B- and T-cell development.

Ligands

CD127 binds IL-7 with high affinity when associated with CD132.

Thymic stromal lymphopoietin (TSLP) is an IL-7 homologue and binds to CD127 complexed with a TSLP specific subunit (TSLPR).

Expression

B-cell precursors and the majority of T cells express CD127. The activation of T cells leads to the downregulation of CD127 expression. It is also expressed by foetal liver and bone marrow common lymphoid progenitors.

Gene Name	Entrez Gene#
IL7R	3575

Selected Monoclonal Antibodies

hIL-7R-M20 (Armitage; Seattle).

CD128

Other Names

CD128A: IL-8 receptor α, CXCR1. Reassigned CD181.

CD128B: IL8 receptor β, CXCR2. Reassigned CD182.

Gene Name	Entrez Gene#
IL8RA	3577
IL8RB	3579

CD129

Other Names

IL-9 receptor α-chain, IL-9Rα.

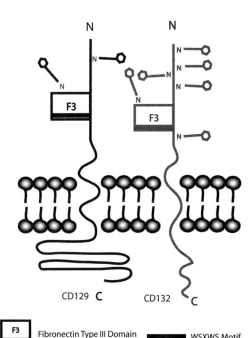

F3 — Fibronectin Type III Domain ▬▬▬ WSXWS Motif

Molecular Structure

A type I transmembrane glycoprotein and a member of the type 1 cytokine receptor (hemopoietin) superfamily.

The protein consists of 521 amino acids and has an N-terminal cytokine receptor domain containing a WSXWS motif (also referred to as a fibronectin type III domain), a single transmembrane domain, and a long cytoplasmic tail.

The cytoplasmic domain lacks tyrosine kinase activity but has a membrane proximal, proline-rich box1 motif required for constitutive association with Janus kinase JAK1.

Tyrosine 407 within a STAT-3 consensus sequence is required for STAT-1, -3, and -5 activation.

CD129 forms heterodimers with the common γ chain (CD132), which is shared by the receptors for IL-2, IL-4, IL-7, IL-15, and IL-21.

Mol Wt: 64 kDa.

Function

Associates with CD132 (common γ chain) to form the functional receptor for IL-9, a growth factor for erythroid and myeloid progenitor cells.

IL-9 binding to CD129/CD132 complex results in phosphorylation of JAK1 bound to CD129 and JAK-3 bound to CD132 and activation of the STAT, IRS-PI3 Kinase, and MAP kinase pathways.

CD129 signaling is important for intrathymic T-cell development and promotes proliferation of Th clones.

IL-9R signaling may play a role in tumorigenesis.

Ligands

CD129, in conjunction with the common γ chain CD132, binds IL-9.

Expression

Expressed by T cells, B cells, mast cells, eosinophils, hematopoietic progenitors, macrophages, epithelial cells, and neurons.

Gene Name	Entrez Gene#
IL9R	3581

Selected Monoclonal Antibodies

Reserved—no antibodies submitted.

CD130

Other Names

gp130.

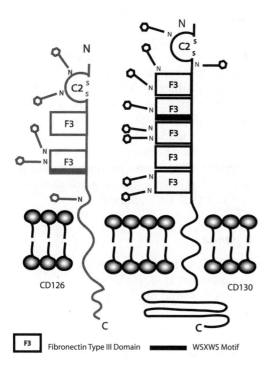

F3 Fibronectin Type III Domain ▬▬ WSXWS Motif

Molecular Structure

A type I integral membrane glycoprotein. Member of the cytokine receptor (hematopoietin) superfamily. The extracellular region consists of an IgC-like domain, followed by five fibronectin type III domains, the second of which contains the WSXWS motif. The molecule is 896 residues long, comprising a 597aa extracellular region, a 22aa membrane-spanning sequence, and a 227aa intracellular domain.

A splice variant lacking the transmembrane sequence is found in serum.

Mol Wt: 130–140 kDa (reduced and unreduced).

Function

Common and signaling chain for IL-6, oncostatin M, LIF, IL-11, ciliary neurotrophic factor, and cardiotrophin-1 receptors.

Knockout mice die as embryos.

The soluble splice variant can act as a competitive inhibitor, by binding with the cytokine-specific receptor chain complexed with the cytokine.

Ligands

CD130 provides the signaling chain for several two-chain cytokine receptors (see Function). Of the ligands that use CD130, only oncostatin M binds CD130 directly.

Expression

Broadly expressed on leukocytes and other tissues.

Applications

Multiple myeloma appears to involve CD130 and autocrine stimulation by IL-6 and oncostatin M.

Gene Name   Entrez Gene#

IL6ST   3572

Selected Monoclonal Antibodies

AM64 (Kishimoto; Osaka).

CD131

Other Names

Common β-chain.

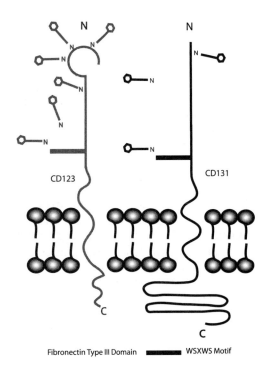

Fibronectin Type III Domain ▬▬▬ WSXWS Motif

CD123

CD131

Molecular Structure

A type I transmembrane glycoprotein member of the cytokine receptor super-family with 897 amino acids, including the signal sequence, two cytokine receptor domains (members of the fibronectin type III domain family), and a long cytoplasmic sequence with proline-rich and serine-rich regions.

Mol Wt: Unreduced, 120–140 kDa.

Function

A key signal transducing molecule of the IL-3, GM-CSF, and IL-5 receptors. It is termed the common β chain, because it associates either with the CD116, CD123, or CD125 molecule to form the appropriate functional receptor. See the individual entries for biological functions.

On binding of cytokine to the two-chain receptor, CD131 is tyrosine-phosphorylated and initiates a signaling cascade based on the JAK/STAT pathway.

Ligands

CD131 is a component of the two-chain receptors for IL-3, IL-5, and GM-CSF, but it does not bind any of these cytokines by itself.

Expression

Myeloid cells, pre-B cells, stem cells, and more differentiated progenitors.

Gene Name	Entrez Gene#
CSF2RB	1439

Selected Monoclonal Antibodies

3D7 (Lopez Adelaide).

CD132

Other Names

Common γ-chain; IL-2R γ-chain.

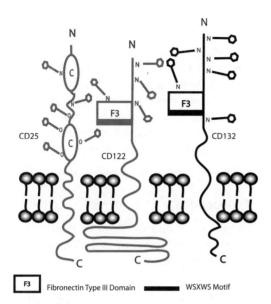

F3 Fibronectin Type III Domain ▬▬▬ WSXWS Motif

Molecular Structure

A type I transmembrane glycoprotein member of the cytokine receptor superfamily comprising 369 residues, including the 22aa signal sequence. The extracellular region consists of one fibronectin type III domain with the WSXWS motif. The 86aa cytoplasmic tail has four tyrosines and an SH2 homology region.

Mol Wt: Unreduced, 64–70 kDa.

Function

Essential component of several cytokine receptors: IL-2, 4, 7, 9, and 15. Mutation causes X-linked severe combined immunodeficiency disease. Knockout mice show a similar broad-ranging immune deficiency, involving T-, B-, and NK-cell lineages. Mutations in any of the individual cytokines or specific receptor chains are associated with mild symptoms, suggesting redundancy in function, but the CD132 chain is critical to the development of the immune system.

Ligand binding induces tyrosine phosphorylation and initiates signaling through a JAK/STAT pathway.

Ligands

Forms part of the three-chain functional receptor for IL-2, IL-4, IL-7, IL-9, and IL-15, with low-to-negative binding affinity on its own.

Expression

Broadly expressed on leukocytes, including T, B, and NK cells, monocytes, and granulocytes.

Mutation in CD132 results in X-linked severe combined immune deficiency (XSCID), and the gene is consequently a target for gene therapy.

Gene Name	Entrez Gene#
IL2RG	3561

Selected Monoclonal Antibodies

TUGh (Sugamura; Sendai); 3BU (Ritz; Boston); 3G11 (Ritz; Boston).

CD133

Other Names

AC133, PROML1.

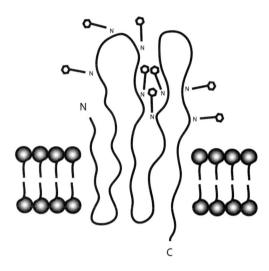

C

Molecular Structure

A 5-transmembrane glycoprotein with the N-terminus outside the cell, two short intracellular sequences interspersed with two long extracellular loops, and the C terminus inside the cell. CD133 and the similar mouse molecule prominin established a new family, referred to as the prominin family.

The extracellular sequences contain eight potential N-glycosylation sites.

Mol Wt: 120 kDa reduced or unreduced.

Function

No known function. A naturally occurring mutation is associated with degenerative disease in the retina of affected patients.

Expression

Expression pattern in progenitor cells is similar to CD34, i.e., hematopoietic stem cells in bone marrow, cord blood, and "mobilized" blood cells. Epithelial cells and endothelial precursor cells express CD133, but not mature endothelial cells. Also found on neural stem cells and in retinoblastoma.

Applications

Identification and isolation of hematopoietic stem cells, including isolation for stem cell transplantation.

Gene Name	Entrez Gene#
PROM1	8842

Selected Monoclonal Antibodies

AC133 and AC141 (Buck; Sunnyvale); W6B3C1 and 293C3 (Bühring; Tübingen).

CD134

Other Names

OX 40, CD252.

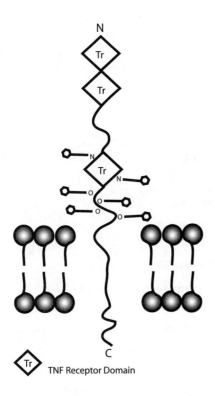

TNF Receptor Domain

Molecular Structure

A type I integral membrane glycoprotein. Member of the TNF/NGF receptor family (see CD27, CD30, CD40, CD95, CD120a, CD120b, and CD137). The extracellular region contains three cysteine-rich repeats.

277 residues long, with calculated Mol Wt 29341 Da. Two sites for N-glycosylation; measured Mol Wt of the glycoprotein is 48 kDa.

Function

Costimulatory molecule of T cells, binding to OX 40 ligand on antigen-presenting cells, including B cells. Ligation of the receptor is inhibitory for apoptosis, and the receptor also appears to be involved in B-cell responses to T-dependent antigens.

Interacts with the adaptor proteins TRAF2, TRAF3, and TRAF5, leading to activation of NF-κB.

Ligands

TNFSF4, also known as Ox 40 ligand or gp 34.

Expression

Activated T cells, fibroblasts, and hematopoietic precursors.

Applications

Upregulated at sites of inflammation in multiple sclerosis and in psoriatic lesions.

Gene Name

Gene Name	Entrez Gene#
TNFRSF4	7293

Selected Monoclonal Antibodies

BER-ACT35 (Stein; Berlin); L106 (Warner; San Jose).

CD135

Other Names

FLT3, STK-1, flk-2.

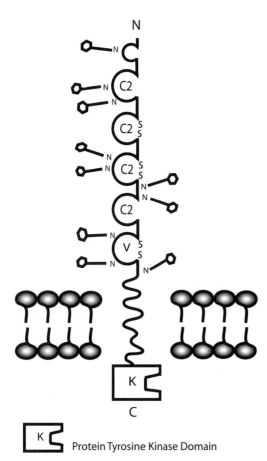

K ⊏ Protein Tyrosine Kinase Domain

Molecular Structure

A type I integral membrane protein, belonging to the Ig and receptor tyrosine kinase family (see CD115, CD117, CD140a, and CD140b). The 541-aa extracellular region consists of five Ig-like domains.

A 21-aa transmembrane domain is followed by a 431-aa cytoplasmic region, with a hydrophilic kinase insertion dividing the intracellular catalytic region in two domains.

Function

Receptor for FLT3 ligand, important in hematopoiesis and differentiation.

Ligands

FLT3 ligand.

Expression

Hematopoietic progenitor cells.

Gene Name	Entrez Gene#
FLT3	2322

Selected Monoclonal Antibodies

4G8 (Bühring; Tübingen); BV10 (Bühring; Tübingen); SF1.340 (Rosnet; Marseille).

CD136

Other Names

Macrophage stimulating protein receptor, MSP-R, RON.

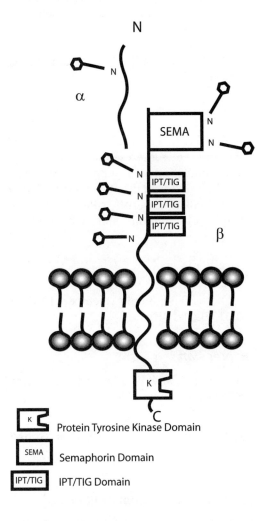

Protein Tyrosine Kinase Domain
Semaphorin Domain
IPT/TIG Domain

Molecular Structure

A 185-kDa protein kinase (35-kDa α chain, 150-kDa β chain) disulphide-linked heterodimer.

The α and β chains are cleaved from a single gene product.

The α chain is extracellular, whereas the β chain spans the membrane. Member of the hepatocyte growth factor receptor subgroup of the receptor tyrosine kinase family.

Has 3 IPT/TIG domains that have immunoglobulin like folds.

Function

Receptor for macrophage stimulating protein (MSP). Ligation-induced receptor dimerization induces cell migration and proliferation.

Tyrosine protein kinase; transmits apoptosis as well as growth signals.

Involved in the regulation of production of blood cells, and in the development of epithelial tissue.

CD136 null mice fail to survive the peri-implantation period. CD136$^{+/-}$ mice are highly susceptible to endotoxic shock.

Ligands

Macrophage stimulating protein (MSP).

Expression

Monocytes, granulocytes, resident macrophages, and epithelial cells.

Gene Name	Entrez Gene#
MST1R	4486

Selected Monoclonal Antibodies

ID1 (van Agthoven; Marseille); ID2 (van Agthoven; Marseille).

CD137

Other Names

4-1BB, Induced by lymphocyte activation (ILA), TNFRSF9.

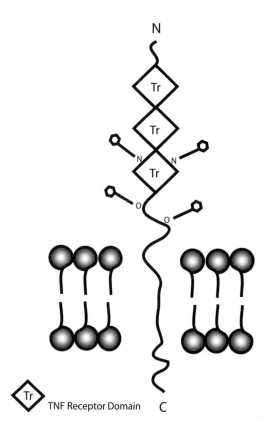

TNF Receptor Domain

Molecular Structure

A type I integral membrane protein that forms disulfide-linked homodimers. Member of the TNF/NGF receptor family (see CD27, CD30, CD40, CD95, CD120a, CD120b, and CD134). The extracellular region is 186 aa long and contains three cysteine-rich repeats and two potential N-glycosylation sites. The 22 aa membrane-spanning sequence is followed by a 47 aa cytoplasmic domain.

Differential splicing leads to the release of a 16-kDa soluble form from activated T cells.

Mol Wt: Reduced, 39 kDa; unreduced, 83 kDa.

Function

T-cell CD137 interacts with the CD137 ligand on antigen-presenting cells, leading to costimulation and apoptosis. Similarly, B-cell CD137 ligand interacts with CD137 on follicular dendritic cells, leading to B-cell proliferation and increased Ig synthesis.

Ligands

Ligand is TNF family member TNFSF9 (CD137L, 4-1BBL).

Expression

Activated T and B cells and monocytes, follicular dendritic cells.

Gene Name	Entrez Gene#
TNFRSF9	3604

Selected Monoclonal Antibodies

4B4 (Kwon; Indianapolis); CAT 13.4G9 (Hadam; Hannover).

CD138

Other Names

Syndecan-1, B-B4.

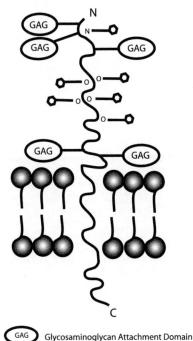

GAG Glycosaminoglycan Attachment Domain

Molecular Structure

A type I integral transmembrane glyco-protein, with a 65–70-kDa protein core and extensive glycosylation.

The core protein is composed of 251 residues for the extracellular region (including signal peptide), 34aa for the membrane-spanning region, and 25aa for the intracellular domain.

The extracellular domain contains two serine clusters, the proximal cluster bearing chondroitin sulfate while the distal cluster bears heparan sulfate.

The membrane-spanning and cytoplas-mic domains of syndecans 1–4 are highly conserved.

The cytoplasmic domain interacts with cytoskeletal components.

The extracellular region contains five potential glycosaminoglycan attachment sites and a protease cleavage site at its C-terminus.

Mol Wt: Varies widely depending on gly-cosylation, and a broad smear is seen ranging from 100 kDa to over 200 kDa.

Function

Involved in the control of cell shape in mature and developing epithelia. It is also involved in adhesion, with the ligand depending on the cell bearing the molecule.

Extracellular heparan sulfate binds growth factors and extracellular matrix constituents, including the basic fibroblast growth factor, collagens, thrombospondin, and fibronectin. CD138 thus is thought to have roles in growth factor action, extra-cellular matrix adhesion, and cytoskeletal organization that controls cell morphology.

Ligands

The CD138-bound heparan sulphate binds growth factors and extracellular matrix constituents, including basic fibroblast growth factor, collagens, thrombospondin, and fibronectin.

Expression

CD138 is expressed by epithelial cells and B-lineage cells; In the B lineage, bone marrow B-cell precursors express CD138, which is lost prior to maturation and release of B lymphocytes into the circula-tion. CD138 is expressed again on plasma cells, including the malignant plasma cells of multiple myeloma, and on some lymphomas.

CD138 is expressed on endothelial cells and on keratinocytes during wound healing and on malignant keratinocytes; it is also expressed on endothelia during embryogenesis.

Applications

Used as marker of plasma cells and for Reed–Sternberg cells.

Potentially useful as a therapeutic agent for destruction of multiple myeloma cells.

Selected Monoclonal Antibodies

MI15 (Brochier; Montpellier); B-B2 (Vermot-Desroches; Lyon); B-B4 (Vermot-Desroches; Lyon).

Gene Name	Entrez Gene#
SDC1	6382

CD139

Molecular Structure

CD139 has not been cloned, and little information is available.

Antibodies precipitate bands of Mol Wt: 209 and 238 kDa.

Expression

CD139 is expressed by B lymphocytes, monocytes, granulocytes, follicular dendritic cells, and weakly on erythrocytes. Also stains renal glomeruli strongly and blood vessel muscle.

Applications

CD139$^+$ CLL may have an improved outcome.

Gene Name   Entrez Gene#

CD139   23448

Selected Monoclonal Antibodies

CAT14.4G9 (Hadam; Hannover); BU30 (Hardie; Birmingham).

CD140a

Other Names

Platelet-derived growth factor (PDGF) receptor.

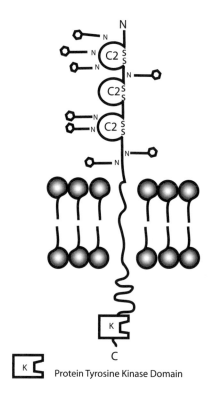

Protein Tyrosine Kinase Domain

Molecular Structure

CD140a is a type I integral membrane protein belonging to the Ig-domain containing receptor tyrosine kinase (Ig-RTK) family (see CD115, CD117, CD135, and CD140b).

The extracellular domain consists of 501 amino acids and contains 3 Ig-like C2-type domains and 8 potential N-linked glycosylation sites.

The protein has a single transmembrane region of 25 amino acids.

The cytoplasmic domain consists of 540 amino acids and contains the tyrosine kinase domain split in two by an insert domain, a membrane-proximal serine-rich region, and two ATP-binding sites and is autophosphorylated at tyrosine 849.

PDGF binding induces either homodimerization or heterodimerization with the CD140b, activation, and autophosphorylation.

Mol Wt: 180 kDa (dimer).

Function

CD140a is a receptor for platelet-derived growth factor (PDGF).

Activation and autophosphorylation of CD140a leads to the recruitment of SH-2 domain containing signal transduction proteins and activation of signaling enzymes, including Src, PI3K, and phospholipase Cγ (PLCγ) resulting in a complex series of signaling events that have not been fully characterized.

The major biochemical difference between CD140a and CD140b is the preferential binding of RasGAP to CD140b but not to CD140a and Crk association with CD140a but not CD140b. Both RasGAP and Crk have negatively regulatory effects.

The predominant role of CD140a is to promote the proliferation of precursor populations of various cell types, including lung alveolar smooth muscle cells, oligodendrocytes, intestinal villae, and dermal papillae.

Deletion of CD140a results in embryonic lethality.

Ligands

CD140a binds platelet-derived growth factor (PDGF)-AA, PDGF-AB, PDGF-BB, and PDGF-CC. Heterodimeric CD140a/CD140b complexes can bind PDGF-AB, PDGF-BB, and PDGF-CC.

Expression

CD140a is expressed by erythroid and myeloid precursors in bone marrow, monocytes, megakaryocytes, fibroblasts, endothelial cells, osteoblasts, and glial cells.

Applications

CD140a is a promising therapeutic target in the treatment of several tumors, particularly those tumors where autocrine PDGFR stimulation is important. Several PDGFR antagonists are currently being investigated.

Gene Name	Entrez Gene#
PDGFRA	5156

Selected Monoclonal Antibodies

6A1 (Bühring; Tübingen); α-R1 (LaRochelle; Bethesda).

CD140b

Other Names

Platelet-derived growth factor (PDGF) receptor.

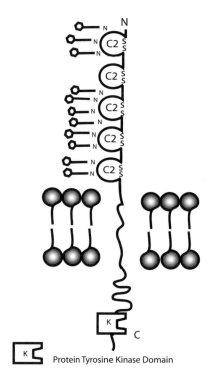

Protein Tyrosine Kinase Domain

Molecular Structure

CD140b is a type I integral membrane protein belonging to the Ig domain-containing receptor tyrosine kinase (Ig-RTK) family (see CD115, CD117, CD135, and CD140a).

The 499 amino acid extracellular region consists of 5 Ig-like C2-type domains and has 11 potential N-linked glycosylation sites.

The single transmembrane domain consists of 25 amino acids.

The intracellular portion comprises 550 amino acids and contains a tyrosine kinase domain split in two by an insert domain and two ATP-binding sites and is autophosphorylated at Tyr751 and Tyr857.

PDGF binding induces either homodimerization or heterdimerization with the CD140a molecule.

Mol Wt: 180 kDa (dimer).

Function

CD140b is a receptor for the platelet-derived growth factor (PDGF).

The major biochemical difference between CD140a and CD140b is the preferential binding of RasGAP to CD140b but not to CD140a and Crk association with CD140a but not CD140b.

CD140b-mediated PI3K signaling is essential for cell migration and chemotaxis.

CD140b knockout mice have defective smooth muscle cell production with the most affected cell types being vascular smooth muscle and pericytes.

The vascular endothelium of the brain, heart, kidney, skin, and eye rely on CD140b signal transduction, and it is probably involved in proliferation of these vascular endothelia.

CD140b plays an important role in wound healing as it mediates chemotaxis/motility of fibroblasts.

The E5 protein of bovine papilloma virus binds the transmembrane domain of CD140b and induces dimerization and activation of the receptor.

Ligands

CD140b binds platelet derived-growth factors (PDGF)-BB and PDGF-DD. Heterodimeric CD140a/CD140b complexes can bind PDGF-AB, PDGF-BB, and PDGF-CC.

Expression

CD140b is expressed by focal endothelial cells and stromal cell lines.

Applications

CD140b is a promising therapeutic target in the treatment of several tumors, particularly those tumors where autocrine PDGFR stimulation is important. Several PDGFR antagonists are currently being investigated.

Gene Name   **Entrez Gene#**

PDGFRB   5159

Selected Monoclonal Antibodies

28D4 (Bühring; Tübingen); PR2712 (Hart; Seattle).

CD141

Other Names

Thrombomodulin (TM), fetomodulin.

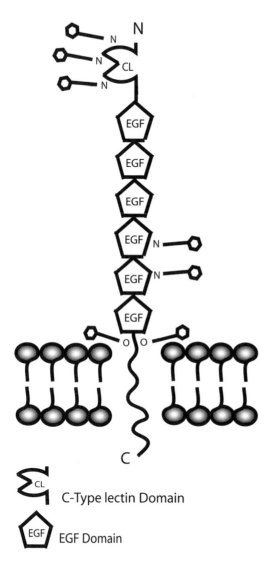

CL C-Type lectin Domain

EGF EGF Domain

Molecular Structure

A type 1 transmembrane glycoprotein, 575 residues long.

The extracellular domain contains an N-terminal C-type lectin domain followed by six EGF-like repeats. The membrane-prox-imal region contains potential O-glycosyla-tion sites and a glycosaminoglycan attach-ment site.

The short cytoplasmic region carries potential phosphorylation sites.

Mol Wt: Reduced, 75 kDa; (unreduced, 105 kDa).

Function

CD141 binds thrombin at the fifth and sixth EGF-like domains, inhibiting its fibri-nolytic activity. CD141 with bound throm-bin then binds protein C at the third and fourth EGF-like domain, and the thrombin then activates Protein C.

Knockout mice die in utero, indicating a vital role in embryogenesis.

Ligands

Thrombin, protein C.

Expression

Endothelium of blood vessels and lym-phatics, smooth muscle cells, epidermal squamous epithelium, mesothelial cells, and syncytiotrophoblasts. Myeloid cells and platelets.

Applications

Plasma CD141 is increased in diabetes mel-litus, SLE, and disseminated intravascular coagulation. Mutations in CD141 may be associated with an increased risk of throm-bosis. Plasma CD141 may be a useful marker of endothelial damage.

Gene Name	Entrez Gene#
THBD	7056

Selected Monoclonal Antibodies

DAKO M0617; 1A4 (Bird; Box Hill); TMmAb20 (Ishi; Kanagawa); KA-4 (Aoki; Saitama); DY12 (Boumsell; Paris); DY35 (Bensussan; Paris).

CD142

Other Names

Tissue factor, thromboplastin, coagulation factor III.

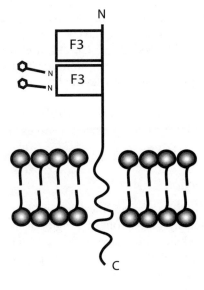

F3   Fibronectin Type III Domain

Molecular Structure

A type I transmembrane protein and a member of the class II cytokine receptor family.

It is related to the IFN-α receptor.

CD142 consists of a 219 amino acid extracellular region comprising two fibronectin type III (FNIII) domains, a 23 amino acid transmembrane region, and a 21 amino acid cytoplasmic domain.

The two FNIII domains are the binding site for Factors VII and VIIa.

The interaction of Factor VIIa with CD142 ensures the active site of Factor VIIa is in the correct conformation for optimal catalytic activity.

Mol Wt: 45–47 kDa.

Function

CD142 is the high affinity receptor for coagulation Factor VII, which when bound to CD142 is converted to Factor VIIa by a variety of serine proteases.

CD142 is the essential cofactor for the serine protease Factor VIIa.

The CD142/Factor VIIa complex initiates the extrinsic coagulation cascade.

CD142 gene knockout in mice is lethal and is associated with severe bleeding and defective development of the cardiovascular system.

Inappropriate expression of CD142 may play a role in tumor biology promoting metastasis and angiogenesis.

Ligands

CD142 can bind blood coagulation Factor VII and Factor VIIa.

Factor Xa/TFPI binds to and inhibits the activity of the CD142/Factor VIIa complex.

Expression

Expressed at high levels in epidermal keratinocytes, various epithelia, adventitial cells of blood vessels, astrocytes, myocardium, Schwann cells of peripheral nerves, and stromal cells of organs such as the liver, pancreas, spleen, and thyroid.

CD142 expression can be induced in monocytes and endothelial cells by inflammatory mediators.

Applications

CD142 is a potential therapeutic target in the treatment and prevention of thrombosis.

Gene Name	Entrez Gene#
F3	2152

Selected Monoclonal Antibodies

MTFH-1 (Morrissey; Oklahoma); TF9-5B7 (Morrissey; Oklahoma); TF9-10H10 (Morrissey; Oklahoma).

CD143

Other Names

Angiotensin-converting enzyme (ACE), peptidyl dipeptidase A.

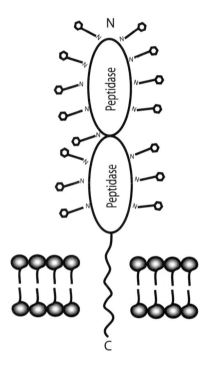

Molecular Structure

A type I transmembrane protein and a zinc metallopeptidase, which occurs in two forms.

The two forms are encoded by a single gene but are transcribed from different promoters.

The somatic form (1306 residues) has highly homologous internal N-terminal and C-terminal domains each with a catalytic site.

Despite their homology, the two domains of somatic CD143 have different conformations and differ immunologically and in their substrate specificity and affinity for various inhibitors.

Somatic CD143 has 15 potential N-linked glycosylation sites.

The germinal (testicular) form (732 amino acids) has a single catalytic site that corresponds to the C-terminal catalytic site of the somatic form.

Germinal CD143 has seven potential N-linked glycosylation sites and has a Serine/Threonine-rich region in the N terminus, which is O-glycosylated.

Soluble forms of CD143 are detectable in plasma, urine, amniotic and cerebrospinal fluids, and seminal plasma.

Mol Wt: Somatic CD143: 170 kDa; germinal CD143: 90 kDa.

Function

CD143 is a zinc metallopeptidase that primarily metabolizes angiotensin and bradykinin but also cleaves C-terminal dipeptides from various oligopeptides as well as various oligopeptides from substance P and LH-RH.

CD143 is important for the efficient binding of spermatozoa to an egg and subsequent penetration.

The fertility of homozygous male mice mutants with disrupted CD143 gene was greatly reduced, whereas all homozygous female mutants were fertile.

Expression

The somatic form of CD143 is expressed by endothelia, brush border epithelium of proximal renal tubules, the brush borders of small intestinal enterocytes, the microvilli of ductuli efferentia of epididymis, neuronal cells, fibroblasts, activated macrophages, Kupfer cells, $CD2^+$ T cells, and immature chondrocytes.

The germinal form of CD143 is expressed exclusively by differentiating germinal cells.

Applications

CD143 activity and concentration are useful prognostic indicators of cardiovascular complications.

Gene Name

ACE

Entrez Gene#

1636

Selected Monoclonal Antibodies

9B9 (Danilov; Chicago); 3A5 (Danilov; Chicago); anti-ACE 3.1.1 (Auerbach; Madison).

CD144

Other Names

VE-cadherin, cadherin-5.

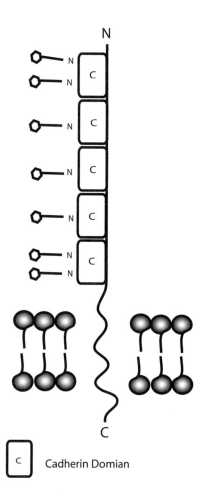

C   Cadherin Domian

Molecular Structure

A type I transmembrane protein and a member of the type II cadherin subfamily within the cadherin superfamily.

The extracellular region consists of 593 amino acids arranged as five cadherin homologue repeats that form a rigid rod-like structure stabilized by the binding of Ca2+ ions between the repeats.

In vitro studies suggest CD144 homotypic binding in cis and trans contribute to cell–cell adhesion.

There are seven potential N-linked glycosylation sites.

The cytoplasmic domain consists of 164 amino acids, and at the distal end has a catenin-binding domain.

Mol Wt: Reduced, 130 kDa; unreduced, 135 kDa.

Function

CD144 is a Ca^{++}-dependent homophilic cell adhesion molecule found in adherens junctions and controls cell-to-cell adhesion and migration of vascular endothelial cells as well as the permeability of microvascular endothelium.

CD144 plays a role in the contact inhibition of endothelial cell growth.

The functions of CD144 are modulated by various catenins, which are critical to its interaction with the cell cytoskeleton and its own intracellular trafficking.

β-catenin and γ-catenin (plakoglobin) associate directly with the catenin binding domain of the CD144 cytoplasmic tail and via α-catenin link the cadherin to the actin cytoskeleton. Plakoglobin can bind desmoplakin, which in turn mediates associates with the vimentin/intermediate filament cytoskeleton.

p120-catenin associates with the juxtamembrane region of the CD144 cytoplasmic domain and plays a regulatory role in cadherin trafficking.

Another catenin, p0071 (plakophilin-4), binds the same region of CD144 as p120-catenin and can bind desmoplakin and ultimately link CD144 to the intermediate filament cytoskeleton.

Ligands

Displays homotypic binding only.

Expression

Expressed by endothelial cells only.

Applications

CD144 expression is reduced in human angiosarcomas.

Gene Name

CDH5

Entrez Gene#

1003

Selected Monoclonal Antibodies

BV9 (Dejana; Milan); BV6 (Dejana; Milan); TEA 1/31 (van Agthoven; Marseille).

CDw145

Molecular Structure

Not characterized or cloned.
Mol Wt: 25 kDa, 90 kDa, 100 kDa.

Expression

CDw145 is expressed by endothelial cells in many tissues, including kidney, lung, spleen, liver, and HUVEC.

Gene Name

none assigned

Entrez Gene#

none assigned

Selected Monoclonal Antibodies

7E9 (Paulie; Stockholm); P7A5 (Paulie; Stockholm).

CD146

Other Names

Muc 18, MCAM, Mel-CAM, s-endo.

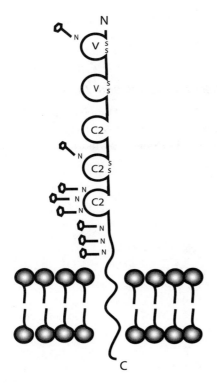

Molecular Structure

A type I transmembrane glycoprotein and a member of the Ig gene superfamily.

The extracellular region consists of two V-type and three C2-type Ig-like domains and is heavily glycosylated.

The carbohydrate moieties present on CD146 are cell-type-specific.

The cytoplasmic tail consists of 63 amino acids and has potential recognition sites for protein kinases.

CD146 forms dimers.

Mol Wt: Reduced, 130 kDa; unreduced, 118 kDa.

Function

Potential adhesion molecule as it is localized at the cell–cell junction.

It is possibly involved in neural crest formation during embryonic development.

CD146 may be involved in tumorigenesis and metastasis of melanoma and prostate cancer through interaction with vascular endothelium.

Cross-linking of CD146 with anti-CD146 antibody results in the phosphorylation of several intracellular proteins. Activated CD146 complexes with Src family kinase p59fyn, which in turn phosphorylates p125FAK. Phosphorylated p125FAK associates with the cytoskeletal protein paxillin, and this complex is thought to promote focal adhesion assembly.

Ligands

Evidence suggests CD146 mediates heterotypic binding to an as yet unknown ligand.

Expression

Expressed by endothelial cells, smooth muscle, melanoma cells, Schwann cells, ganglion cells, myofibroblasts and bone marrow fibroblasts, cerebellar cortex, external root sheath of hair follicles, mammary ductal and lobular epithelium myoepithelium, subcapsular epithelium of thymus, follicular dendritic reticulum cells, and extravillous trophoblast.

CD146 is variably expressed in parathyroid glands and basal cells of bronchial epithelium.

CD146 has been detected on a subpopulation of activated T cells from delayed-type hypersensitivity lesions of the skin and in sinovial fluid of rheumatoid arthritis patients.

Almost all melanomas, angiosarcomas, Kaposi's sarcomas, leiomyosarcomas, placental trophoblastic tumors and chorio-carcinomas, and prostate carcinomas express CD146. Focal and variable CD146 expression is detectable in some squamous cell and small cell lung carcinomas, some breast carcinomas, mucoepidermoid carcinomas of the salivary gland, and between 15% and 43% of leukemias.

Applications

CD146 is a diagnostic and prognostic marker of endothelial cell activation and injury related to coronary artery disease, chronic renal failure, and peritoneally dialysed patients.

It is an endothelial progenitor cell and circulating endothelial cell marker.

CD146 is a prognostic marker of metastatic potential of prostate cancer and melanoma.

Gene Name	Entrez Gene#
MCAM	4162

Selected Monoclonal Antibodies

F4-35H7 (Dignat-George/Sampol; Marseille); 541/10B2 (Knapp; Vienna); TEA 1/34 (Sanchez; Madrid).

CD147

Other Names

Basigin, M6, extracellular metalloproteinase inducer (EMMPRIN).

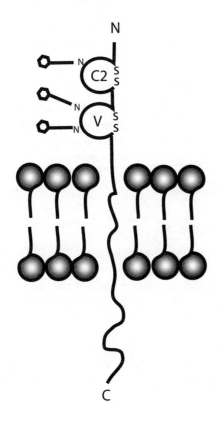

Molecular Structure

A type I integral transmembrane glycoprotein with an extracellular portion containing two Ig superfamily domains (one V and one C2 domain).

Heavily N-glycosylated, with an apparent Mol Wt of 54 kDa reducing to 28 kDa after treatment with Endoglycosidase F. CD147 bears the high frequency blood group antigen Oka.

Highly conserved 21-residue membrane-spanning sequence, containing a glutamic acid residue and a leucine zipper motif, suggesting it is involved in protein–protein interactions.

Function

Knockout mice are infertile and suggest a variety of additional functions, showing differences in memory and learning, odor perception, and immunological function (increased MLR response).

In vitro studies suggest CD147 is involved in adhesion, because CD147 antibodies inhibit homotypic aggregation and CD147 is coimmunoprecipitated with integrins. Soluble CD147 protein stimulates collagen production, suggesting a regulatory activity on metalloproteinases.

Ligands

Adhesion and coimmunoprecipitation suggest CD147 binds to integrins.

Expression

Expressed widely within and outside the hematopoietic system. Expressed strongly on cancer cells in small cell lung cancer and hepatocellular carcinoma. Widely expressed on leukocytes, endothelium, platelets, and red blood cells. Expressed strongly on thymocytes and activated peripheral T cells and less strongly on resting peripheral T cells.

Applications

Potential application in pathology (differentially expressed by granulocytes from patients with inflammatory conditions).

Gene Name	Entrez Gene#
BSG	682

Selected Monoclonal Antibodies

AAA6 (Knapp; Vienna); UM-8D6 (Fox; Michigan); HI197 (Shen; Tianjin), HIM6 (BD Biosciences; San Jose).

CD148

Other Names

DEP-1, HPTP-η.

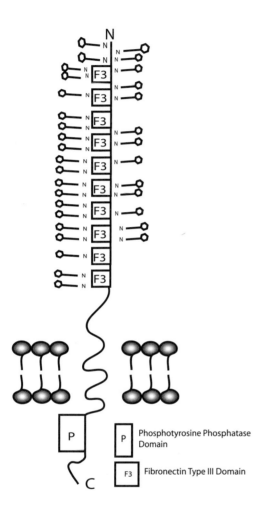

Molecular Structure

A type I transmembrane glycoprotein of apparent Mol Wt 200–250 kDa, with an extracellular portion of 970 aa, a 25 aa transmembrane region, and a 342 aa intra- cytoplasmic tail. The extracellular domain of CD148 has 10 fibronectin III motifs, and the cytoplasmic C-terminal region has a single protein tyrosine phosphatase domain. These features are characteristic of type III receptor tyrosine phosphatases.

The extracellular domain of CD148 contains 34 potential N-linked glycosylation sites as well as O-glycosylation sites.

Function

Tyrosine phosphatase. Role in immune system unclear, but engagement with antibody leads to cytokine secretion.

Natural ligand unknown.

May have a role in arresting cell growth at confluence.

Expression

Among hematopoietic cells, CD148 is expressed strongly on monocytes, granulocytes (especially at sites of inflammation), and dendritic cells. Resting lymphocytes express low levels, but expression is up-regulated after lymphocyte activation and CD45RO-positive express higher levels than naive cells. CD148 is expressed on platelets, nerve cells, Kupffer cells and fibroblasts.

Applications

Research reagent.

Gene Name	Entrez Gene#
5795	PTPRJ

Selected Monoclonal Antibodies

143-41 (Vilella; Barcelona); A3 (Aversa; Vienna).

CDw149

Now CD47R—see CD47.

CD150

Other Names

SLAM, signaling lymphocyte activation molecule, IPO-3.

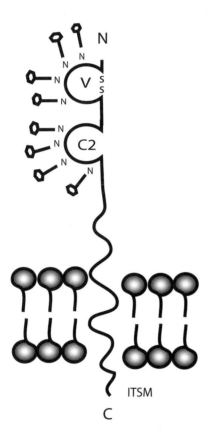

Molecular Structure

A type I integral transmembrane glycoprotein of 335 aa residues. The 209-residue extracellular region consists of one V and one C2 immunoglobulin superfamily domains with 8 potential N-glycosylation sites. Member of the CD2 subfamily.

The intracytoplasmic region consists of 77 residues with several potential sites for tyrosine and serine/threonine phosphorylation. An ITSM (immunoreceptor tyrosine switch motif) is characteristic of this family of proteins and allows interaction with SH2 adaptor proteins.

Three additional isoforms have been described: a variant membrane form with a truncated cytoplasmic domain, a soluble secreted form lacking 30 amino acids encompassing the entire transmembrane domain, and a cytoplasmic form lacking the leader sequence.

Apparent Mol Wt ranges from 70 kDa from T cells to 75–95 kDa for B cells, under reducing conditions. Under nonreducing conditions, apparent Mol Wt is 65–85 kDa. Variation in Mol Wts from different cells attributable to variable N-glycosylation and enzymatic removal of carbohydrate reduces Mol Wt to 40 kDa (reduced).

Function

In vitro studies suggest CD150 may bind homophilically, leading to cellular activation. However, the physiological function is unknown. Ligation of CD150 leads to interferon γ production, and this appears to be physiologically relevant, because several viruses have evolved strategies for modulating CD150-mediated activation.

High-affinity self-ligation considered important in T/B cell stimulation. Consequences of ligation differ in T and B cells.

Receptor for measles virus.

Ligands

Possibly CD150 itself.
 Measles virus.

Expression

Resting CD45RO-positive T cells, a subset of B cells, dendritic cells; upregulated in activated T, B, and dendritic cells. In tissue, thymocytes and endothelial cells are also stained, and germinal center B cells show cytoplasmic staining, whereas follicular mantle B cells show surface staining.

Applications

Research reagent; potential diagnostic applications because CD150 is differentially expressed on monocytes in autoimmune disease.

Gene Name	Entrez Gene#
SLAMF1	6504

Selected Monoclonal Antibodies

IPO3 (Sidorenko; Seattle).

CD151

Other Names

Platelet-endothelial tetra-span antigen, PETA-3, Tspan-24.

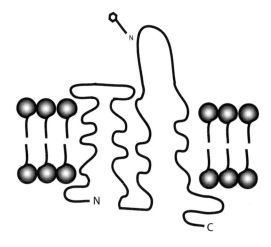

Molecular Structure

Glycoprotein of 253 amino acid residues, member of the transmembrane-4 super-family (TM4SF).

Short cytoplasmic regions at N- (16aa) and C- (5aa) termini.

Two extracellular loops: The first is15aa, and the second is 109aa.

The larger extracellular loop contains a single N-glycosylation site.

Immunoprecipitation shows two bands, with apparent Mol Wt of 28 and 32 kDa, the larger being the glycosylated protein.

Function

CD151 is co-precipitated with β 1 integrins, suggesting involvement in a complex. F(ab')2 fragments of mAb 11B1.G4 cause homotypic adhesion of human ery-throleukemia cell lines HEL and K562 and bring about platelet activation and aggregation.

The in vivo function of CD151 is not known, but it appears to be part of the sig-naling complex of FcγRIIa and to modulate integrin function.

Expression

Endothelium, muscle, epithelial cells, platelets and megakaryocytes, and imma-ture hemopoietic cells. Activated T cells.

Applications

Research reagent. It has been suggested that there are epitope differences between CD151 on malignant and normal cells.

Gene Name	Entrez Gene#
CD151	977

Selected Monoclonal Antibodies

14A2.H and 11B1.G4 (Ashman; Adelaide).

CD152

Other Names

Cytotoxic T lymphocyte antigen, CTLA-4.

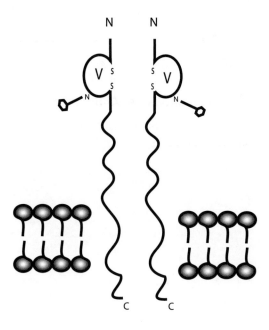

Molecular Structure

A type I integral membrane protein and a member of the Ig gene superfamily.

It is structurally related to the CD28 molecule.

The 124 amino acid extracellular region consists of 1 Ig V-like domain and has 2 potential N-linked glycosylation sites.

The transmembrane region consists of 26 amino acids, and the intracellular region consists of 39 amino acids and contains a phosphatidylinositol 3-kinase (PI3K) binding motif (YVKM) and a tyrosine-containing motif that targets CD152 to Golgi or post-Golgi intracellular membranes.

CD152 is expressed as a homodimer linked by a disulphide bond at Cys120.

Activated T cells produce two transcripts, which have alternative polyadenylation sites.

Restriction fragment length polymorphism (RFLP) is observed with the longer transcript as it contains a repeated -AU-motif and the number of -AU- repeats varies between individuals.

Mol Wt: Reduced, 33 kDa; unreduced, 50 kDa.

Function

CD152 is the inducible receptor for CD80 and CD86, transported from intracellular vesicles to the cell membrane at the immunological synapse after cell activation.

Despite being a homologue of CD28 and binding the same ligands, CD152 antagonizes some functions of CD28 and has an inhibitory effect on T-cell functions.

Unlike CD28, CD152 downregulates IL-2 production and inhibits cell-cycle progression in T cells, thereby depressing T-cell proliferation.

In activated Th2 cells, CD152 mediates anti-apoptotic signaling via PI-3 kinase in a Fas/Fas ligand-dependent manner.

It is postulated that the interaction of CD152+ T cells with CD80 or CD86 on dendritic cells results in the activation of indoleamine 2,3-dioxygenase (IDO), which metabolizes tryptophan. As reduced levels of free tryptophan are associated with decreased T-cell activation, this may represent another mechanism of suppression of T-cell function.

CD152-deficient mice develop a severe lymphoproliferative disorder and die within a few months of birth.

In an experimental model of autoimmune enchephalomyelitis, antibody to CD152 increased the severity of the disease.

CD152 RFLPs appear to be linked to human autoimmune diseases, including type 1 diabetes mellitus, Graves' disease, Hashimoto's thyroiditis, Addison's disease, and multiple sclerosis.

Ligands

CD152 binds CD80 and CD86 with high avidity.

Expression

Expressed on the cell surface by activated T cells only with the exception of regulatory CD4$^+$CD25$^+$ T cells that appear to constitutively express CD152.

The frequency of CD152 expression varies between T-cell subsets; e.g., more Th2 cells express CD152 than Th1.

CD152 expression occurs in some activated B cells.

Applications

Combination therapy of humanized anti-CD152 antibody and vaccination with tumor antigens is being trialed as a potential treatment regime for a variety of tumors.

Gene Name	Entrez Gene#
CTLA4	1493

Selected Monoclonal Antibodies

11D4 (Linsley; Seattle); 10A8 (Linsley; Seattle); 7F8 (Linsley; Seattle).

CD153

Other Names

CD30 Ligand.

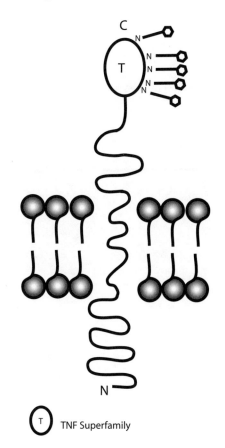

ⓣ TNF Superfamily

Molecular Structure

A type II transmembrane glycoprotein member of the tumour necrosis factor (TNF) superfamily (see also CD70, CD95L, and CD154).

The protein consists of an extracellular domain of 172 amino acids with 5 potential N-linked glycosylation sites and a C terminal region with similarity to TNF, a transmembrane domain of 25 amino acids, and 37 amino acid cytoplasmic domain.

CD153 may form trimers.

Mol Wt: 40 kDa.

Function

Proliferation of peripheral blood T cell is costimulated by CD153, and it enhances antigen-induced proliferation and cytokine production by Th0 and Th2 clones.

CD153 promotes proliferation, cytokine production, and adhesion molecule expression in cell lines derived from Hodgkin's disease and CD30$^+$ T-ALL but has cytostatic and cytotoxic effects on cell lines derived from large-cell anaplastic lymphoma.

CD30 ligation by CD153 induces Fas-independent cell death in T-cell hybridomas.

CD153 signaling via CD30 has been demonstrated to play a role in the negative selection of autoreactive T cells within the thymus.

T cell CD30 ligation of CD153 on IgD$^+$IgM$^+$ B cells specifically inhibits B-cell Ig class switching and plasmacytoid differentiation.

CD153 engagement with CD30 enhances HIV replication in CD4$^+$ T cells from HIV-positive individuals.

CD153 signaling enhances cytokine production by activated neutrophils.

Ligands

CD153 binds CD30 with high affinity.

Expression

CD153 is expressed by activated T cells, activated macrophages, neutrophils, eosinophils, and normal and malignant B cells. CD153 expression is detectable on a proportion of normal bone marrow myeloid precursors, erythroblasts and a subset of megakaryoblasts, and a small subset of lymphoid cells, histiocytes, and granulocytes in reactive lymph nodes and tonsils.

CD153 is widely expressed in hematopoietic malignances. Elevated expression of CD153 by alveolar macrophages is present in sarcoidosis.

Gene Name	Entrez Gene#
TNFSF8	944

Selected Monoclonal Antibodies

M81 anti-CD30L (Armitage; Seattle); M82 anti-CD30L (Armitage; Seattle).

CD154

Other Names

CD40 Ligand; CD40L; gp39; TRAP (TNF-related activation protein)-1; T-BAM.

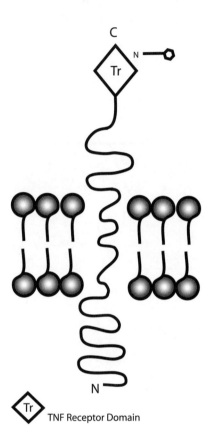

Tr TNF Receptor Domain

Molecular Structure

A type II integral membrane protein belonging to the tumor necrosis factor (TNF) superfamily (see CD70, CD95L, and CD153).

The CD154 is biologically active as a membrane-bound molecule or as soluble multimers (probably homotrimers).

Soluble forms of CD154 are produced as a result of intracellular cleavage by a matrix metalloproteinase in activated cells.

Mol Wt: 33 kDa (membrane form); 18 and 15 kDa (soluble forms).

Function

Ligation of CD154 and CD40 provides a survival signal to CD40$^+$ B cells in germinal centers and is essential for germinal center formation as well as Ig class switching. The CD40/CD154 complex mediates B-cell proliferation in the absence of costimulus as well as IgE production in the presence of IL-4.

Activation of the CD40/CD154 pathway in nonimmune cells leads to the production of pro-inflammatory cytokines, matrix metalloproteases, prostaglandins, and upregulation of adhesion molecules.

The nonfunctional or defective expression of CD154 due to point mutations causes hyper-IgM (HIGM) syndrome.

HIGM patients display elevated circulating levels of IgM and little or no IgG, IgA, and IgE due to the inability of B cells to undergo class switching in response to antigenic challenge. Additionally, these patients display defective T- and B-cell memory responses to recall antigen and are susceptible to opportunistic infections.

CD154-deficient mice display a similar phenotype to HIGM patients but additionally have depressed production of IFNγ and IL-2.

Ligands

CD154 binds CD40.

Expression

Constitutive expression of CD154 occurs on B cells, macrophages, and dendritic cells.

CD154 is transiently expressed by activated CD4$^+$ T cells, variably by CD8$^+$ T cells, mast cells, NK cells, polymorphs, monocytes, and activated platelets.

Applications

Elevated levels of CD154 are found in several autoimmune diseases, including SLE, multiple sclerosis, and inflammatory bowel diseases as well as athersosclerosis.

The potential of CD154 as a therapeutic target in the treatment of these diseases has shown promise in animal models.

Gene Name	Entrez Gene#
TNFSF5	959

Selected Monoclonal Antibodies

5C8 (Lederman; New York); M79, M90, M92 (Armitage; Seattle); HI155 (Shen; Tianjin); TRAP-1 (van Agthoven; Marseille).

CD155

Other Names

Poliovirus receptor (PVR), nectin-like 5.

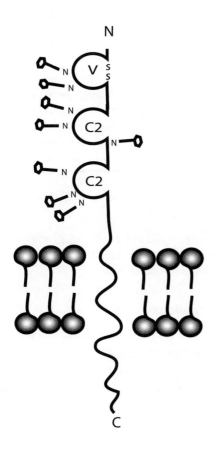

Molecular Structure

A type I transmembrane glycoprotein. Member of the Ig gene superfamily.

The extracellular region consists of three Ig-like domains (an N-terminal V-type domain followed by two C-type domains). This structure is characteristic of the nectin family, and CD155 is designated as a nectin-like molecule.

CD155 is 417 aa long, with a predicted Mol Wt of 45 kDa. There are eight potential N-glycosylation sites.

Function

Adhesion molecule involved in cell–cell and cell–extracellular matrix adhesion. CD155 makes a heterodimer with nectin-3, and the complex binds integrin $\alpha V\beta 3$.

CD155 is thought to regulate CD44 binding to hyaluronan.

CD155 also binds to the matrix protein vitronectin.

Receptor for poliovirus and cytomegalovirus.

Ligands

The complex between PVR and nectin-3 (CD113) binds integrin $\alpha V\beta 3$.

CD155 also appears to bind to vitronectin, CD56 and CD226, to nectin-1 and nectin-2, and to be involved in homotypic adhesion.

Poliovirus and cytomegalovirus bind CD155.

Expression

Endothelial cells, epithelia, central nervous system, and monocytes.

Applications

Research reagent.

Gene Name	Entrez Gene#
PVR	5817

Selected Monoclonal Antibodies

D171 (Freistadt; New Orleans); P44 (Freistadt; New Orleans); PV404-19 (Beckman Coulter/Immunotech, Marseille).

CD156a

Other Names

ADAM 8, MS2.

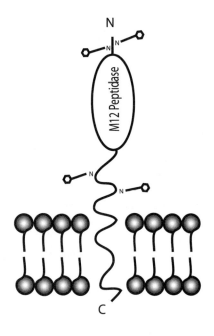

Molecular Structure

A type 1 transmembrane glycoprotein member of the ADAM (a disintegrin and metalloproteinase) family. The protein is 824 residues long, with an extracellular region consisting of disintegrin-, metallo-proteinase-, cysteine-rich-, and EGF domains, and bearing 4 potential N-glyco-sylation sites.

A cytoplasmic region containing a proline-rich Src homology 3 domain follows the membrane-spanning region.

Mol Wt: Predicted, 89 kDa; observed, 69 kDa unreduced.

Function

Probably involved in loosening of cell–cell, cell–matrix contacts, with a possible role in extravasation of leukocytes in inflammation.

A mutant mouse with neurological defects (Wobbler mice) over-expresses CD156a in areas showing neurodegeneration. TNFα induced upregulation of CD156a 15-fold. These findings suggest that ADAM8 may have a role in degenerative disease.

Expression

Monocytes and macrophages, granulocytes; also reported on B-cell lines. Also found in central nervous system.

Applications

Research in inflammation and potentially a target in neurodegenerative disease.

Gene Name	Entrez Gene#
ADAM8	101

Selected Monoclonal Antibodies

2-3-C (Yamamoto; Oita); 1-11-G (Yamamoto; Oita).

CD156b

Other Names

TACE (tumor necrosis factor-α converting enzyme), ADAM 17, snake venom like protease CSVP.

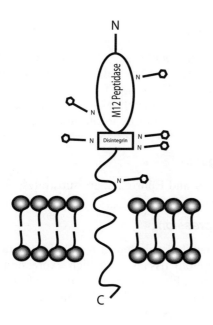

Molecular Structure

A type I transmembrane glycoprotein member of the ADAM (a disintegrin and metalloproteinase) family. The protein is 824 residues long, including a 17-residue signal sequence and a pro-domain (aa18–214) that is cleaved before the molecule becomes catalytically active. The catalytic (zinc-dependent metalloprotease) domain (aa215–473) is followed by a cysteine-rich domain characteristic of disintegrins (aa474–671). There are six potential N-linked glycosylation sites.

A 23-aa membrane-spanning domain is followed by a 129-residue cytoplasmic domain.

Mol Wt: Predicted, 93 kDa; observed, 100 kDa reduced.

Function

A "sheddase" that converts plasma membrane TNFα and TGFα, as well as several other membrane proteins, to soluble forms.

As TNFα is a major mediator of inflammation, and CD156b is essential for its release from cells, CD156b is thought to have a major role in inflammation. Expression by chondrocytes in arthritic joints may release TNF, exacerbating disease.

Deletion of a catalytic domain causes perinatal death.

Ligands

Membrane TNFα and TGFα are substrates.

Expression

Monocytes, macrophages, polymorphonuclear cells, T cells, endothelial cells, and myocytes. Widely expressed in non-lymphoid tissues, including heart, placenta, brain, and muscle. Induced in cartilage in arthritis.

Applications

Possible target for anti-inflammatory and anti-arthritis therapeutics.

Gene Name	*Entrez Gene#*
ADAM17	6868

Selected Monoclonal Antibodies

TACE-M222 (Black; Seattle).

CD156c

Other Names

ADAM 10.

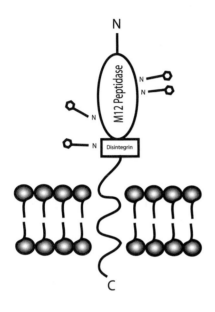

Molecular Structure

A type I transmembrane glycoprotein member of the ADAM (a disintegrin and metalloproteinase) family. The protein is 748 residues long, including a signal sequence and a pro-domain that is cleaved before the molecule becomes catalytically active. The catalytic (zinc-dependent metalloprotease) domain is followed by a cysteine-rich domain characteristic of disintegrins.

There are four potential N-linked glycosylation sites.

A 23-aa membrane-spanning domain is followed by a 129-residue cytoplasmic domain.

Mol Wt: Predicted, 84 kDa; observed, 70 kDa reduced, 65 kDa nonreduced. Precursor is seen at 97 kDa.

Function

An endopeptidase of broad specificity, which releases several membrane proteins, including TNFα and Ephrin A2, as soluble proteins. Although expressed on the cell surface, it is mostly localized in the Golgi.

Ligands

TNFα and Ephrin A2 are substrates.

Expression

Broadly distributed in lymphoid and non-lymphoid tissues, with high expression in thymus, liver, and muscle. It is induced in arthritic tissues and in the inflamed central nervous system.

Applications

ADAM 10 is thought to be involved in myelin degradation in multiple sclerosis, and its upregulation in inflamed CNS and joint tissue makes it a potential therapeutic target.

Gene Name	Entrez Gene#
ADAM10	102

Selected Monoclonal Antibodies

11G2 (Rubinstein E; Paris).

CD157

Other Names

BST-1, BP-3/IF7, Mo5, cADPr hydrolase 2.

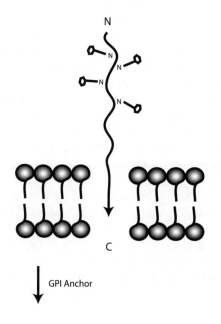

GPI Anchor

Molecular Structure

A GPI-anchored membrane glycoprotein ranging in apparent molecular weight between 42 and 50 kDa due to differential glycosylation in different cells. Removal of N-linked carbohydrate reduces Mol Wt to 31 kDa.

Sequence contains 10 cysteines, which show homology with the structure of CD38.

Function

CD157 is an ectoenzyme, possessing both ADP-ribosyl cyclase and cyclic ADP-ribose hydrolase activities.

CD157 may also function as a signaling molecule, because cross-linking by antibody induces tyrosine phosphorylation of a 130-kDa cytoplasmic protein.

Anti-CD157 mAb IF-7 has synergistic effects on anti-CD3-induced growth of T progenitor cells, and it facilitates the development of α/β T-cell receptor positive cells in fetal thymic organ culture system.

Knockout mice have impaired B-cell function, suggesting CD157 is involved in B-cell development. This is consistent with demonstrated function of bone marrow stromal cell CD157 in supporting pre-B-cell growth.

Ligands

As a bifunctional enzyme, CD157 uses NAD and cyclic ADP-ribose as substrates.

Expression

Expressed on polymorphs and monocytes in blood and on tissue macrophages, follicular dendritic cells, as well as on bone marrow stromal cells and endothelial cells of human umbilical cord veins. Expressed by lymphoid progenitor cells (appears prior to IgH or TCR rearrangement).

Applications

Potential diagnostic value due to elevated CD157 on bone marrow stromal cells and in serum of a subset of rheumatoid arthritis patients with severe disease. Also differentially expressed in the myeloid leukemias.

Gene Name	Entrez Gene#
BST1	683

Selected Monoclonal Antibodies

Mo5 (Todd; Ann Arbor); BEC7 (Hirano; Osaka); RF3 (Kaisho; Osaka); BEC7 (Okuyama; Osaka).

CD158

Other Names

KIR (Killer Inhibitory Receptor) family. Allocated CD 158a, b, c, etc. in centromeric to telomeric sequence, with b1, b2 used for alleles.

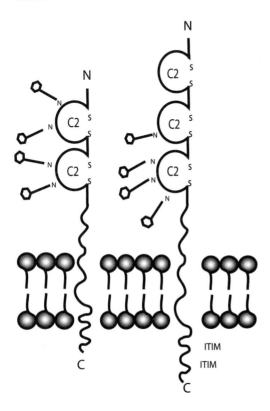

Molecular Structure

CD158 molecules are also known as killer cell immunoglobulin-like receptors (KIRs). The 14 polymorphic genes for these receptors are clustered together on human chromosome 19q13.4.

These molecules have either two (KIR2D, domains D1 and D2) or three (KIR3D, domains D0, D1, and D2) Ig-like domains in their extracellular regions.

CD158 molecules with long cytoplasmic domains have two immunoreceptor tyrosine-based inhibition motifs (ITIMs) and have inhibitory effects, whereas CD158 molecules with a short cytoplasmic region lack ITIMs and have activating functions.

The KIR family can be subdivided into subfamilies based on structure.

KIR2DL subfamily members have two extracellular Ig-like domains and a long cytoplasmic tail of between 76 and 114 amino acids. Its members include CD158a (KIR2DL1), CD158b (KIR2DL2/ KIR2DL3), CD158d (KIR2DL4), and CD158f (KIR2DL5).

KIR2DS subfamily members have two Ig-like domains and a short (39 amino acid) cytoplasmic tail. Its members include CD158h (KIR2DS1), CD158j (KIR2DS2), KIR2DS3, CD158i (KIR2DS4), and CD158g (KIR2DS5).

KIR3DL subfamily members have three Ig-like domains and long cytoplasmic tails of between 84 and 95 amino acids. Members include CD158e 1 and 2 (KIR3DL1) and CD158k (KIR3DL2).

KIR3DS subfamily members have three Ig-like domains and a short cytoplasmic tail of 27 amino acids. Members include KIR3DS1.

Function

The interaction of CD158 molecules on NK cells and some CD8$^+$ T cells with MHC class I molecules on target cells results in either inhibition or activation of cytotoxic function.

NK and T cells may express both inhibitory (ITIM-bearing) and activating (ITAM-coupled) CD158 molecules simultaneously.

Inhibitory CD158 molecules play an important role in self-tolerance by NK cells.

The interaction of inhibitory CD158 on NK and T cells with MHC class I on antigen presenting cells can inhibit cytokine production.

Activating CD158 on T or NK cells can enhance their cytotoxicity toward target cells such as tumor cells and virus-infected cells.

The association of activating CD158 to MHC class I is weak compared with inhibitory CD158, and there is evidence to suggest that activating CD158 may recognize non-MHC class I ligands as well.

Inhibition by ITIM-bearing CD158 over activating CD158 is saturable and proportional to the degree of engagement of both types of receptors.

Ligands

HLA-class 1 allotypes are the ligands for CD158 molecules

Expression

CD158 molecules are expressed by NK cells and a subset of CD8$^+$ T cells. NK cells express between two to six different KIR.

Applications

CD158k is a phenotypic marker of Sezary cells and potential prognostic marker for Sezary syndrome.

CD185k is expressed by the non-MHC restricted cytotoxic T acute lymphoblastic leukemia cell line TALL-104, which is currently being investigated as a potential therapeutic agent in the treatment of various cancers.

Gene Name	Entrez Gene#
KIR3DL1	3811
KIR2DS4	3809
KIR3DL2	3812

Selected Monoclonal Antibodies

CD158e (KIRDL1): Dx9 (Johnson; San Diego); Z27 (van Agthoven; Marseille); AZ158 (Parolini; Brescia).

CD158i (KIR2DS4): PAX180 (Moretta; Genoa); FES 172 (van Agthoven; Marseille).

CD158k (KIR3DL2): AZ158 (Parolini; Brescia); Q66 (van Agthoven; Marseille).

CD159a and c

Other Names

CD159a: NKG 2a, KLRC1 (killer cell lectin-like receptor subfamily C receptor 1).

CD159c: KLRC2, NKG 2C

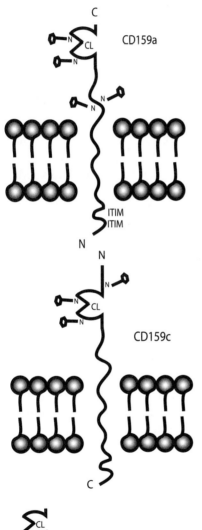

C-Type Lectin Domain

Molecular Structure

Type II transmembrane glycoprotein members of the killer cell lectin-like family, subfamily C. The extracellular regions contain a C-type lectin domain. The cytoplasmic region of CD159a carries two ITIM motifs, but CD159c does not.

The CD159a protein is 233 aa long, whereas CD159 c is 231 aa long.

Both proteins are expressed as disulphide-linked heterodimers with CD94.

The predicted Mol Wt is 26 kDa for both proteins; observed Mol Wts are 43 kDa for CD159a and 36 kDa for CD159c.

Function

CD159a and CD159c, in association with CD94, can bind MHC class I antigen on target cells and inhibit NK cell-mediated cytotoxicity.

CD159c is absent from over 4% of healthy individuals as a result of a homozygous deletion mutant.

Ligands

The complex of CD159a or CD150c with CD94 binds the MHC class I molecule HLA-E.

Expression

NK cells and a few T cells.

Applications

Polymorphism of the CD159a and CD159c coding and noncoding regions have been investigated for association with arthritis, because the gene is in a region associated with rheumatoid disease. Results so far do not show strong associations.

Gene Name	Entrez Gene#
KLRC1	3821
KLRC2	3822

Selected Monoclonal Antibodies

CD159a: Z270 (Moretta; Brescia); p25 (Pende; Italy).

CD159c: R&D Systems 134591 and 134522 (Mortari; St. Paul).

CD160

Other Names

BY55, NK1, NK28.

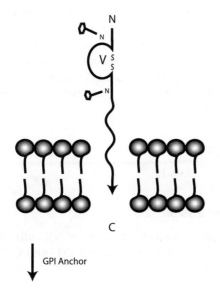

GPI Anchor

Molecular Structure

CD160 is a glycosylphosphatidylinositol (GPI)-anchored glycoprotein and a member of the Ig superfamily.

It is expressed on the cell surface as a disulfide linked multimer.

The 181 amino acid molecule contains 1 Ig-like V domain, has 6 cysteines in the mature polypeptide, and 2 N-linked glycosylation sites.

The Ig-like domain is weakly homologous to CD158d.

Mol Wt: Reduced, 27 kDa; unreduced, 80 kDa.

Function

Cross-linking CD160 with mAb or MHC class I provides a costimulatory signal to CD3-activated CD8$^+$ T lymphocytes, enhancing their proliferation.

After its engagement of an HLA-C molecule on a target cell, CD160 triggers cell cytotoxicity and the release of IFN-γ, TNF-α, and IL-6 by NK cells.

Cell-surface expression of CD160 is downregulated by cytokine-induced NK-cell activation.

The expression of CD160 is altered in patients with paroxysmal nocturnal hemaglobinuria.

Ligands

CD160 displays broad specificity binding to classical and nonclassical MHC class 1 molecules.

Expression

CD160 is expressed by CD56^{dim} CD16$^+$ NK cells, γ/δ T cells, and α/β CD8$^+$ T cells as well as intestinal intraepithelial lymphocytes.

Gene Name	Entrez Gene#
CD160	11126

Selected Monoclonal Antibodies

BY55 (Boumsell; Paris); PAX 71 (Moretta; Genova).

CD161

Other Names

NKR-P1A, killer cell lectin-like receptor subfamily B, member 1.

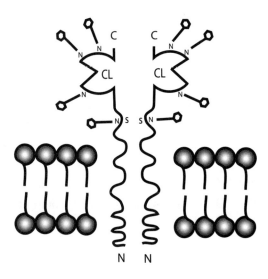

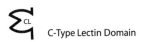

C-Type Lectin Domain

Molecular Structure

A type II transmembrane glycoprotein of 40–44 kDa and 217 amino acid residues. The extracellular domain contains a single C-type lectin domain, and CD161 dimerizes through a disulphide bond. The extracellular domain contains N-linked carbohydrate, and deglycosylation with N-glycosidase F reduces the Mol Wt to 26 kDa.

Member of the Ca^{++}-dependent (C-type) lectin superfamily (see CD23, CD69, CD72, and CD94).

Function

Although a single human NKRP-1 gene has been identified, the mouse has three separate genes, which encode for stimulatory and inhibitory products.

The function of the human protein is not clear. Monoclonal antibodies against CD161 have been reported to either augment or inhibit NK cell-mediated cytotoxicity against certain Fc-receptor bearing targets and induce immature thymocyte proliferation.

Ligands

MHC class I.

Expression

Expressed on the majority of NK cells and 25% of T cells, including CD4- and CD8-positive T cells.

Applications

Research reagent for studies of NK cell function.

Gene Name / Entrez Gene#

Gene Name	Entrez Gene#
KLRB1	3820
NKR-P1A	

Selected Monoclonal Antibodies

191B8 (Poggi; Genova); HP-3G10 (Lopez-Botet; Madrid); DX12 (Lanier; Palo Alto).

CD162, CD162R

Other Names

P selectin glycoprotein ligand 1, PSGL-1. CD162R is also known as PEN5.

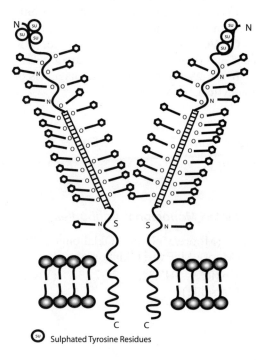

su Sulphated Tyrosine Residues

Molecular Structure

CD162 is a type I transmembrane glycoprotein with mucin-like character and is expressed on the cell surface as a disulfide-linked homodimer.

Electron microscopy studies reveal CD162 molecules to be extended rod-like structures.

The extracellular region consists of 303 amino acids containing 16 repeats of a 10 amino acid sequence, 3 potential N-linked glycosylation sites, as well as complex sialylated and fucosylated O-linked oligosaccharides, some of which appear to contain poly-N-acetyllactosamine.

Most cell lines have CD162 molecules with 15 repeats, whereas CD162 present in most leukocytes have 16 repeats.

In addition to the other post-translational modifications, the sulfation of three tyrosines in the N-terminal region is critical for recognition and binding to CD62P and CD62E.

The transmembrane region consists of 25 amino acids, and the intracellular region contains 69 amino acids.

The interaction of the cytoplasmic domain with the leukocyte cortical cytoskeleton is an essential requirement for leukocyte rolling on CD62P.

Mol Wt: Reduced, 120 kDa; unreduced, 250 kDa and 160 kDa (neutrophils).

CD162R carries the PEN5 epitope, which is a post-translational modification of CD162.

The addition of this sulfated lactosamine epitope creates a unique binding site for L-selectin, independent of tyrosine sulfation.

Mol Wt: Reduced, 110–140 kDa, unreduced, 220–240 kDa.

Function

The calcium-dependent, high affinity interactions of CD162 with selectins mediate adhesion and promote the tethering and rolling of leukocytes on endothelial cells, activated platelets, and other leukocytes at sites of inflammation.

Cross-linking of CD162 with certain mAb has been shown to induce caspase-independent death of activated T cells but not resting T cells and did not interfere with binding to P-selectin. Use of these antibodies in murine models of GVHD and type 1 diabetes mellitus ameliorated the diseases.

CD162 knockout mice have impaired rolling and migration of leukocytes.

CD162R acts as a trafficking and homing receptor for NK cells as it promotes NK-cell tethering and rolling on inflamed endothelium as well as leukocyte–leukocyte interaction at sites of inflammation.

CD162R expression by oligodendrocyte precursor cells (OPCs) is probably involved in the migration of this transient and highly mobile cell population during fetal brain development.

Ligands

Depending on its post-translational modifications, CD162 can bind the selectins CD62P, CD62E, and CD62L.

CD162R binds CD62L.

Expression

CD162 is expressed by most peripheral blood T cells, monocytes, granulocytes, some B cells, and some CD34$^+$ bone marrow cells.

CD162R is expressed by CD56^{dim} CD16$^+$ NK cells, oligodendrocyte precursor cells, a subset of oligodendrogliomas, and all pilocytic astrocytomas.

Applications

CD162 may be a useful marker for differentiating myeloblasts from monoblasts in immunophenotyping of AML subsets.

CD162 is currently being investigated as a potential therapeutic target in the treatment of autoimmune disease and in chronic T-cell-mediated diseases.

CD162R is a specific marker for NK cells and oligodendrocyte precursor cells.

It is a useful marker in the diagnosis of pilocytic astrocytomas.

Gene Name	Entrez Gene#
SELPLG	6404

Selected Monoclonal Antibodies

PL1 (Moore/McEver; Oklahoma); PL2 (Moore/McEver; Oklahoma).

CD162R: 3H3.32, 2G7.13 (Vivier; Marseille).

CD163

Other Names

GHI/61, D11, RM3/1, M130.

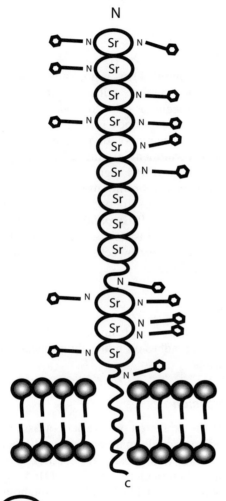

Sr   Scavenger Receptor Cysteine Rich

Molecular Structure

A type 1 integral transmembrane glyco-protein. The extracellular domain consists of 1003 residues forming 12 SRCR (scavenger receptor cysteine-rich) domains of 110 aa each.

A 24aa membrane-spanning sequence is followed by a cytoplasmic sequence that varies through alternative mRNA splicing. The major form has 49aa in the cytoplasmic region, whereas the splice variants have 84- and 89-residue cytoplasmic regions.

CD163 has an apparent Mol Wt of 130 kDa (reduced) and 110kDa (unreduced).

Function

Function unknown, but may have a role in anti-inflammatory response of monocytes.

Expression

Expressed on monocytes and most macrophages and upregulated on monocytes after activation. Dendritic cells and follicular dendritic cells are negative.

Applications

Research reagent.

Gene Name	Entrez Gene#
CD163	9332

Selected Monoclonal Antibodies

GHI/61 (Pulford; Oxford); Ber-Mac3 (Stein; Berlin).

CD164

Other Names

MUC-24, MGC 24, multi-glycosylated core protein 24.

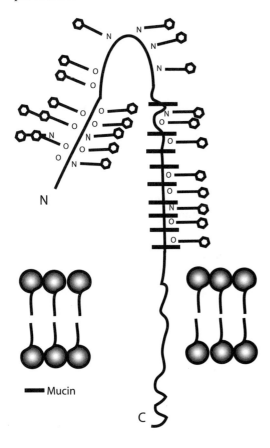

— Mucin

Molecular Structure

A type I integral membrane sialomucin-like glycoprotein (see CD34, CD43, and CD68), which forms disulfide linked homodimers. The dimer has an apparent Mol Wt of 170–180 kDa, reducing to 80–90 kDa for the monomeric chain.

CD164 is a highly glycosylated member of the sialomucin family, with a protein core of 19 kDa and 16 sites for O-glycosylation and 9 sites for N-glycosylation.

Alternative splicing leads to three isoforms. The predominantly expressed isoform consists of 178 residues with two mucin domains separated by a cysteine-rich domain. A soluble isoform lacks the membrane-insertion sequence and is a disulphide-linked homodimer called MGC-24 (Multi-Glycosylated Core protein of 24 kDa).

Function

The function of CD164 is not known, but it appears to mediate adhesion of hemopoietic progenitor cells to bone marrow stromal cells. Antibody ligation of CD164 on primitive hemopoietic progenitor cells reduces recruitment into the cell cycle, suggesting that CD164 signaling suppresses hemopoietic cell proliferation.

CD164 appears to be involved in the adherence of *Plasmodium falciparum* sexual-stage parasites (gametocytes) to human bone marrow cells of stromal and endothelial origin.

Ligands

Physiological ligand unknown. May be used as an adhesion molecule by malarial parasites.

Expression

CD164 is expressed on a variety of tissues, including ectodermal and mesodermal embryonic and post-natal tissues. On human hemopoietic cells, CD164 is expressed by CD34+ cells throughout ontogeny, including CD34+ hemopoietic stem cells in fetal liver, cord blood, and adult bone marrow. CD164 is expressed by committed myeloid and erythroid colony forming cells and their progeny, including monocytes and maturing erythroid precursors. CD164 is expressed by bone marrow stromal and endothelial cells. Mature B cells express CD24, whereas immature B cells and granulocytes are negative and other lymphoid cells weakly positive.

Applications

Highly expressed on T-cell ALL, and may be useful in the analysis of gut tumors.

Selected Monoclonal Antibodies

105A5 (Bühring; Tübingen); 9E10 (Simmons; Adelaide), 103B2 (BD Biosciences; San Jose).

Gene Name

Gene Name	Entrez Gene#
CD164	8763

CD165

Other Names

AD2, gp 37, SN2.

Molecular Structure

Transmembrane protein as yet poorly characterized. Apparent Mol Wt 42kDa (reduced) and 37kDa (nonreduced).

Function

Not known, but in vitro studies suggest a role in adhesion between thymocytes and thymic epithelial cells.

Expression

Highly expressed on platelets, T-ALL cells, and several cell lines; expressed at lower levels on a proportion of circulating T cells and monocytes. Also expressed on thymic epithelium, fibroblasts, epidermal keratinocytes, pancreatic islet cells, and some neurones.

Applications

May be useful as a marker of T-type acute lymphoblastic leukemia, and as a marker for tumor progression.

Gene Name	Entrez Gene#
CD165	23449

Selected Monoclonal Antibodies

AD2 (Patel/Haynes; Durham); SN2 (Seon; Buffalo).

CD166

Other Names

ALCAM, KG-CAM, neurolin (zebra fish), BEN (chicken), DM-GRASP (chicken), activated leukocyte cell adhesion molecule.

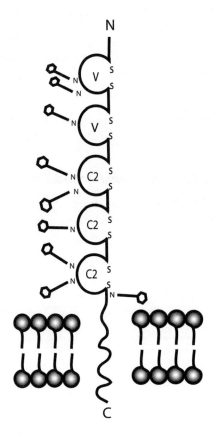

Molecular Structure

A type 1 transmembrane glycoprotein and a member of the Ig gene superfamily and of a subfamily of three glycoproteins (CD146, CD166, and CD239), which share the same extracellular organization of five Ig-like domains (VVC2C2C2).

The mature protein consists of 556 residues, and the extracellular domain consists of 5 Ig-like domains and 9 potential N-linked glycosylation sites, a hydrophobic membrane spanning region of 21 amino acids, and a 32-residue cytoplasmic tail with no known motifs.

The two amino-terminal V-type Ig-like domains are followed by three C2-type Ig-loops.

CD166 is anchored to the actin cytoskeleton via the intracellular domain, but the receptors involved in this interaction are unknown.

The N-terminal Ig domain is the binding site for both homophilic and CD166-CD6 interactions.

Soluble CD166 is produced by proteolytic cleavage of extracellular domains or by alternative splicing.

A recently described soluble isoform produced by alternative splicing has the N-terminal IgV-like domain only and retains the ligand binding capacity of CD166.

Mol Wt: 100–105 kDa.

Function

CD166 is an adhesion molecule whose expression has been found in the development of many organs as well as in hematopoiesis, endothelial and epithelial linings, and the central and peripheral nervous systems.

Murine studies suggest a role for CD166 in hematopoietic cell and endothelial cell differentiation and migration.

Blocking the interaction of CD166$^+$ APCs and CD6$^+$ T cells with soluble monomeric CD166 or CD6 in vitro was found to reduce antigen-specific T-cell proliferation and IL-2 production. This suggests the CD166-CD6 interaction enhances antigen-specific T-cell responses during an immune response.

CD166 is involved in neurite extension by neurons via heterophilic and homophilic interactions.

CD166 knockout mice have motor and retinal ganglion cell axons that fasciculate poorly and are occasionally misdirected and have retinal exvaginated or invaginated regions with photoreceptor ectopias similar to those found in some human retinopathies.

Ligands

CD166 displays homophilic binding and binds CD6.

Expression

Expressed by neurons, activated T cells, activated monocytes, endothelium, epithelium, fibroblasts, and primitive subsets of hematopoietic cells, including pluripotent stem cells, blastocysts, and endometrium.

Stage specific expression of CD166 is observed in a number of tumors, including malignant melanoma, colorectal, prostate, bladder, and breast cancers.

Applications

CD166 is a marker used to select pluripotent stem cells from mesenchymal progenitor populations by flow cytometry.

Expression levels of CD166 are used as a prognostic indicator for melanoma, bladder, prostate, colorectal, and breast cancer. Increased expression generally correlates with more aggressive disease and a poorer prognosis, with the exception of breast cancer, where decreased CD166 expression is indicative of tumor metastasis and poor prognosis.

Gene Name	Entrez Gene#
ALCAM	214

Selected Monoclonal Antibodies

J3-119 (Pesando; Seattle); 3A6 (Patel; Durham).

CD167a, CD167b

Other Names

Discoidin domain receptor (DDR)1 (CD167a).

Discoidin domain receptor (DDR)2 (CD167b).

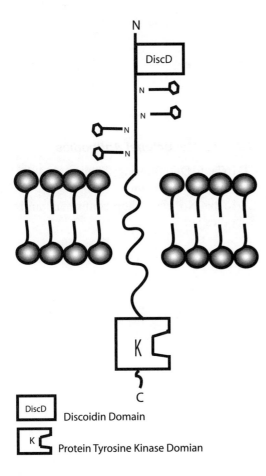

DiscD — Discoidin Domain

K — Protein Tyrosine Kinase Domian

Molecular Structure

CD167a and CD167b are membrane glycoproteins and receptor tyrosine kinases (RTK) belonging to a subfamily of RTKs with a discoidin motif in the extracellular domain.

CD167a and CD167b are both characterized by the 155 amino acid discoidin homology domain (DiscD) followed by a 200 amino acid stalk, a single transmembrane region, and a juxtamembrane region and catalytic tyrosine kinase domain in the intracellular region.

The DiscD domain is sufficient for collagen binding, but the presence of the stalk region enhances this interaction.

Three isoforms of CD167a, DDR1a, DDR1b, and DDR1c are generated by alternative splicing. The longest transcript is DDR1c, and the shortest is DDR1a.

In both CD167a and b, ligand binding is thought to trigger receptor dimerization, which would enable transphosphorylation of tyrosine residues.

Tyrosine 513 has been mapped as a phosphorylation site of DDR1b.

Approximately 10% of CD167a is proteolytically cleaved, resulting in a 52-kDa soluble protein (a-subunit) and a 62-kDa transmembrane protein.

The protease furin may be responsible for shedding of the a-subunit as there is a furin recognition site (amino acids 304–307).

Mol Wt: 125 kDa (CD167a), 130 kDa (CD167b).

Function

CD167a binds and is activated by triple helical collagens and plays a role in cell morphogenesis, differentiation, and collagen synthesis.

Activation of CD167a induces expression of the metalloproteases MMP1 (collagenase 1) and MMP2 (gelatinase 1), which degrade collagen and regulate ECM remodeling.

Overexpression of CD167a in epithelial tumors suggests a role in tumor invasion and metastasis.

CD167a knockout mice are consistently smaller than wild type, and females are frequently infertile as blastocysts are often unable to implant in the endometrium.

Those females that have litters are unable to feed their offspring because their mammary gland epithelium fails to secrete milk.

CD167b is also a tyrosine kinase activated by triple helical fibrillar glycosylated collagen.

When activated, CD167b induces the expression of MMP1 and MMP2.

It is involved in the regulation of cell proliferation and ECM remodeling mediated by metalloproteases MMP1 (collagenase 1) and MMP2 (gelatinase A).

CD167b knockout mice are smaller than wild type and have delayed healing of epidermal wounds.

Ligands

DDR1 binds all types of collagen tested (type I-VI and VIII).

DDR2 binds fibrillar collagens (type I–III and V).

Expression

DDR1 expressed weakly on B cells and immature dendritic cells. It is widely expressed on epithelia, particularly those found in mammary gland, brain, kidney, lung, and colonic mucosa as well as epithelial tumors.

DDR2 is widely expressed but has higher expression in skeletal and heart muscle, kidney, and skin.

Gene Name	Entrez Gene#
DDR1	780
DDR2	4921

Selected Monoclonal Antibodies

CD167a: 51D6 (Bühring; Tübingen); 48B3 (Bühring; Tübingen).

CD167b: No workshop-confirmed antibodies yet.

CD168

Other Names

RHAMM (receptor for hyaluronan involved in migration and motility).

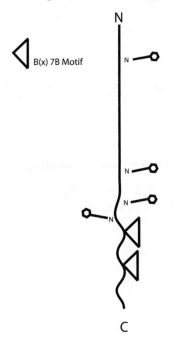

N

B(x) 7B Motif

C

Molecular Structure

CD168 is an acidic coiled coil protein and the original member of the B(X)7B hyaladherin protein family.

It is functionally related to the transforming acidic coiled coil (TACC) proteins, and the CD168 gene is located near other TACC gene loci on human chromosome 5.

Although lacking a signal sequence and a transmembrane domain, CD168 acts as a cell-surface and intracellular hyaluronan binding protein.

The extensive coiled coil structure has a basic amino terminal globular domain and interacts with hyaluronan through carboxy-terminal basic 9-11 amino acid B(x)7B motifs.

Two B(x)7B motifs in the globular domain are binding motifs for interphase and mitotic microtubules.

Three splice variants occur in leukocytes. These are the full-length form of 725 amino acids, a variant lacking exon 4 and another lacking exon 13.

Mol Wt: 80, 84, and 88 kDa.

Function

CD168 is an oncogene with both extracellular and intracellular functions.

It mediates hylauronan-specific motility in a variety of cell types, regulates progression through the G2M of the cell cycle, and is required for both hyaluronan and PDGF-mediated activation of erk kinase.

CD168 plays a role in ras transformation, tumor progression, and metastasis.

It has been shown to interact with the mitotic spindle assembly factors dynein and TPX2. Expression of CD168 and TXP2 is increased during mitosis, and together they maintain spindle integrity after spindle assembly. However, if CD168 is over-expressed, spindle architecture is affected. This finding has lead to the hypothesis that over-expression of CD168 in human tumors affects the centrosomal structure and spindle integrity and potentially modulates apoptotic and cell cycle progression pathways.

Ligands

CD168 binds hyaluronan.

Expression

Expressed at low-to-moderate levels in most CD3$^+$ CD4$^+$/CD8$^+$ thymocytes and some single positive thymocytes.

Resting peripheral blood B cells do not express CD168, whereas 10–30% of peripheral blood T cells are CD168$^+$. Activation leads to transient upregulation of expression in both T cells and B cells.

Most peripheral blood monocytes have a moderate-to-strong expression of CD168.

CD34+CD45lo hematopoietic progenitors have weak surface expression of CD168 but high intracellular levels.

Most hematopoietic cell lines express CD168; however, expression levels vary when the cells are passaged.

CD168 is expressed strongly by B-cell malignancies, acute myeloid leukemias, and breast cancer cells.

Expression of CD168 has also been detected in neuronal cells, fibroblasts, sperm, respiratory epithelium, endothelium, and smooth muscle cells.

Applications

CD168 is a potential therapeutic target in the treatment of acute myeloid leukemias and other CD168-expressing malignancies.

Increased overall CD168 expression and an increase in the ratio of CD168 variant lacking exon 4 to full-length CD168 are indicators of disease progression and a poor prognosis for multiple myeloma patients. Hyper-expression of CD168 correlates with a poor prognosis for colorectal, stomach, and breast cancer patients.

Gene Name	Entrez Gene#
HMMR	3161

Selected Monoclonal Antibodies

3T3.5 (Pilarski; Edmonton); 3T3.9 (Pilarski; Edmonton).

CD169

Other Names

Sialoadhesin (Sn), Siglec-1.

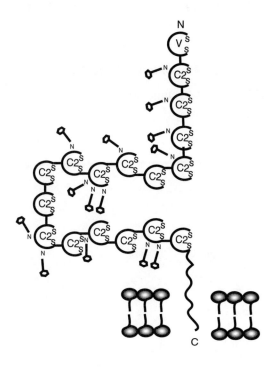

Molecular Structure

A type I transmembrane glycoprotein and the prototypic and largest member of the sialic acid binding Ig-like lectins (Siglec) family (see also CD22 and CD33) within the Ig gene superfamily.

The structure of CD169 is predicted to be an elongated rod-like structure of 40 nm in length.

Its extracellular domain consists of a 1 N-terminal V-set Ig-like domain that mediates binding to sialic acid followed by 16 C2-set Ig-like domains. A conserved Arg residue on the F-strand of the V-set Ig-like domain is essential for sialic acid binding.

The extracellular domain has 14 potential N-linked glycosylation sites, but the predicted and actual molecular weights are similar, which suggests the protein is not heavily glycosylated.

Unlike all other known siglecs, CD169 lacks cytoplasmic immunoreceptor tyrosine-based motifs. Its short cytoplasmic domain has single PTK and CK2 phosphorylation sites.

The CD169 gene is the only known siglec not found on human chromosome 19.

Mol Wt: Reduced, ca. 200 kDa; unreduced, 180 kDa.

Function

CD169 is an adhesion molecule, binding particularly glycolipids and glycoproteins with terminal α-2 sialyl residues.

The extension of CD169 from the macrophage cell surface enables it to interact with sialic acids without interference from sialic acid expressed by the same cell.

High level expression of CD169 by stromal macrophages interacting with developing myeloid cells, particularly erythroid cells in bone marrow, suggests a role in myeloid cell development and erythropoiesis.

Murine studies of allogenic tumor rejection indicate that CD169 may play a role in leukocyte trafficking and in T-cell effector functions.

Expression of CD169 by inflammatory macrophages in rheumatoid arthritis suggests a role in inflammation.

CD169 recognizes sialic acids expressed by some microbial pathogens such as *Neisseria* sp. CD169-deficient macrophages have a reduced capacity to bind *Neisseria*.

Ligands

CD169 preferentially binds α2-3 sialyllactosamines over α2-6-sialyllactosamines and under certain conditions can bind α2-8-linked sialic acids on glycolipids.

There are two known counter-receptors for CD169. The mucin CD227 on breast cancer cells and erythroid cells act as a counter-receptor as does CD43 (leukosialin) on T cells.

Expression

Only expressed by macrophages with a strong expression by perifollicular macrophages in the spleen, sinusoidal and subcapsular macrophages in lymph nodes, stromal macrophages in bone marrow, and inflammatory macrophages associated with rheumatoid arthritis and atherosclerosis. Resident macrophages of liver, gut, and lung display moderate expression of CD169.

Gene Name	Entrez Gene#
SN	6614

Selected Monoclonal Antibodies

7D2 (Croker; Dundee).

CD170

Other Names

Siglec 5 (sialic acid binding Ig-like lectin 5).

Molecular Structure

A type 1 transmembrane protein and a member of the CD33-related subfamily of the sialic acid binding Ig-like lectins (Siglecs) and the Ig gene superfamily (see also CDw327, CDw328, and CDw329).

The extracellular domain consists of an N-terminal V-set Ig-like domain followed by three C2-set Ig-like domains.

The cytoplasmic domain contains two cytoplasmic immunoreceptor tyrosine inhibitory motifs (ITIMs). By comparison with the equivalent motifs of CD33, the membrane proximal ITIM is likely to interact with both SHP-1 and SHP-2 tyrosine phosphatases, whereas the membrane distal ITIM may selectively interact with SHP-1 only.

The protein forms homodimers.

Four isoforms of CD170 have been described having three (hSiglec-5-3L and -3C) or four (hSiglec-5-4L and -4S) extracellular domains linked to either long (hSiglec-5-4L and 3L) or short (hSiglec-5-4S) cytoplasmic tails or occuring as a soluble form (hSiglec-5-3C).

Mol Wt: 140kDa (homodimer).

Function

CD170 acts as an inhibitory receptor able to downregulate cell activation and suppress its own sialic acid binding activity in vitro.

Selective binding of CD170 to sialic acids on *Neisseria meningitidis* has been shown in vitro to enhance bacterial phagocytosis by macrophages implying a role for CD170 in host defences.

Ligands

CD170 binds $\alpha2,3$- and $\alpha2,6$-linked sialic acid with equal avidity and glycophorin A on human erythrocytes.

Expression

Expressed strongly by neutrophils. Macrophages activated during bacterial and viral infections, monocytes, and dendritic cells express CD170.

Aberrant expression of CD170 by CD34[+] progenitor cells is often present in acute myeloid leukemias.

The hSiglec-5-4L isoform has the broadest expression.

Gene Name

Entrez Gene#

SIGLEC5

8778

Selected Monoclonal Antibodies

8H2 (Croker; Dundee); 1A5 (Croker; Dundee).

CD171

Other Names

Neuronal adhesion molecule, LI.

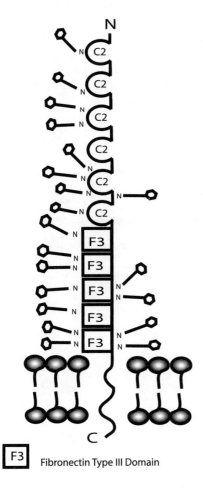

F3   Fibronectin Type III Domain

Molecular Structure

A type I transmembrane glycoprotein and a member of the Ig-gene superfamily.

The extracellular region consists of 6 C2-like Ig domains followed by 5 type III fibronectin domains and has 21 potential N-linked glycosylation sites.

Conserved dibasic sequences in the third fibronectin-like domain are susceptible to serine protease cleavage. The CD171 ectodomain can be shed as a result of post-translational cleavage by disintegrin metalloproteinase (ADAM). Plasmin can also cleave CD170 at the same site.

The cytoplasmic domain consists of either 114 or 110 amino acids and contains 6 potential phosphorylation sites.

Mol Wt: 200–230 kDa depending on the cell type.

Function

CD171 is an adhesion molecule, showing homotypic adhesion and binding laminin, integrins, and proteoglycans containing chondroitin sulphate.

Signaling as a result of CD171 ligation can occur via CD171 or through cis interactions and involves phosphorylation and binding of cytoskeletal ankyrin and can involve pertussis-sensitive g-proteins, protein kinase C, arachidonic acid release, and the influx of intracellular Ca^{++}.

Internalization of CD171 activates the MAP kinase cascade.

CD171 is reported to play a role in haptotactic migration and invasion of tumor cells.

CD171 can function as a T-cell costimulatory molecule in vitro.

It mediates neural cell migration, neurite extension, Schwann cell–axon interaction, synaptogenesis, myelination, and neuronal cell survival and induces long-term potentiation.

Memory consolidation may be linked to changes in neuronal expression and glycosylation of CD171 and CD54.

CD171-deficient mice have dilated brain ventricles, a reduction in the size of the corticospinal tract, and errors in corticospinal axon guidance, abnormal morphogenesis of cortical dendrites, and developmental defects in the hippocampus and corpus callosum as well as defective interaction between axons and Schwann cells.

The neuropathologies seen in CD171-deficient mice are consistent with the human X-linked recessive neurological disorder CRASH syndrome.

Excessive alcohol consumption during pregnancy can disrupt CD171-mediated processes leading to neurodevelopmental disorders in the fetus.

CD171 in cis interactions have been described with CD9, CD24, CD56 and Axonin-1/TAG-1.

Ligands

CD171 binds itself, neurocan, phosphocan, laminin, and the integrins αVβ3 (CD51/CD61), αIIbβ3 (CD41/CD61), α5β1 (CD49e/CD29), and α9β1.

Expression

Strongly expressed by post-mitotic neurons of the CNS and PNS, pre- or non-myelinating Schwann cells of the PNS, and glial cells.

Intermediate to low expression is present on CD4$^+$ T cells, a subet of B cells, monocytes, monocyte-derived and follicular dendritic cells, and renal, urogenital, and intestinal epithelial cells.

Strong to intermediate expression has been found in melanoma and neuroblastoma cell lines; renal, skin, and lung carcinomas, and monocytic leukemias.

Gene Name	Entrez Gene#
L1CAM	3897

Selected Monoclonal Antibodies

5G3 (Montgomery; California).

CD172a

Other Names

SIRPα, SHPS-1, signal regulatory protein α.

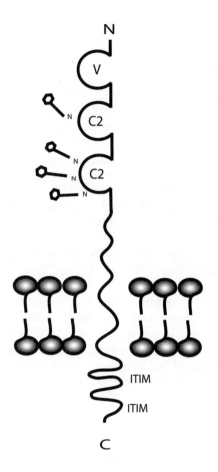

Molecular Structure

CD172a is a transmembrane glycoprotein member of the signal regulatory protein (SIRP) family and a member of the Ig-gene superfamily. The SIRP family can be subdivided into SIRPα and SIRPβ (see CD172b) subfamilies based on the length of their cytoplasmic tails. SIRPα has long cytoplasmic tails of approximately 100 amino acids, whereas SIRPβ members lack an intracellular domain.

The CD172a extracellular domain consists of an amino terminal V-set Ig-like domain followed by two C2-set Ig-like domains and has four N-linked glycosylation sites and several potential O-linked glycosylation sites.

The cytoplasmic domain has two immunoreceptor tyrosine-based inhibitory motifs (ITIMs) and a C-terminal proline-rich region. When these ITIMs are phosphorylated, the protein tyrosine phosphatases SHP-1 and SHP-2 can bind and are activated.

Mol Wt: 85–90 kDa.

Function

CD172a is a signal transduction molecule involved in the negative regulation of several biological processes, including suppression of anchorage-independent cell growth, negative regulation of immune cells, self-recognition of erythrocytes, mediation of macrophage multinucleation, skeletal muscle differentiation, entrainment of circadian clock, neuronal survival, and synaptogenesis.

Ligands

CD172a binds CD47 and the lung surfactant proteins SP-A and SP-D.

Expression

Monocytes, macrophages, hematopoietic precursors, and neuronal tissue express CD172a.

Gene Name   Entrez Gene#

PTPNS1   140885

Selected Monoclonal Antibodies

SE5A4 (Bühring; Tübingen); P3C4 (Bühring; Tübingen).

CD172b

Other Names

SIRPβ1, Signal regulatory protein β1.

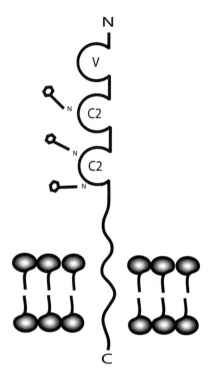

Molecular Structure

CD172b is a transmembrane glycoprotein and a member of the SIRPβ subfamily of the signal regulatory protein family (SIRP) within the Ig gene superfamily (see also CD172a and CD172g).

The extracellular domain of CD172b is 90% identical to CD172a (excluding the signal peptide). It has an amino terminal IgV-like domain followed by two IgC-like domains.

The transmembrane domain has a positively charged lysine residue that is critical to its interaction with DAP-12 (KARAP).

The cytoplasmic portion consists of only a few intracellular residues and is functionally insignificant.

The protein forms disulphide-linked homodimers in the cell membrane.

Mol Wt: 110–120 kDa (homodimer).

Function

CD172b has activating functions in macrophages via constitutive association with DAP-12 (KARAP) homodimers.

Phosphorylation of DAP-12 intracellular immunoreceptor tyrosine-based activating motif (ITAM) enables association with the tyrosine kinase Syk. This complex activates MAPK–MEK pathways and contributes to cellular activation in myeloid cells.

Ligation of CD172b on mouse peritoneal macrophages with mAb-induced phagocytosis.

In a recent study, mAb ligation of CD172b was found to enhance transmigration of polymorphonuclear cells. However, in this study, no association with DAP-12 was found but a smaller protein of 10-kDa coprecipitated with CD172b.

Expression

CD172b is expressed by myeloid cells.

Gene Name	Entrez Gene#
SIRB1	10326

Selected Monoclonal Antibodies

B1D5, B4B6 (Bühring; Tübingen).

CD172g

Other Names

SIRPγ, SIRPβ 2, Signal regulatory protein β 2.

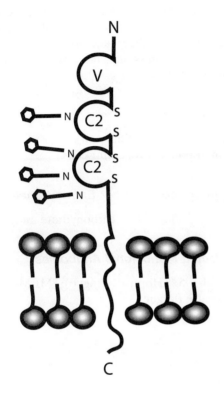

Molecular Structure

CD172g is a transmembrane glycoprotein and a member of the SIRPβ subfamily of signal regulatory proteins (SIRP) within the Ig gene superfamily (see also CD172a and CD172b).

The extracellular region has an N-terminal IgV-like domain followed by two IgC-like domains.

The protein is similar in structure to CD172b in that it has a truncated cytoplas-mic tail with no known motifs, but it lacks the charged lysine residue required for interaction with DAP-12.

Two transcript variants have been described. Variant 1 has three IgC-like domains, whereas variant 2 lacks the two IgC-like domains and does not appear to be expressed on the cell surface.

Mol Wt: ca. 55 kDa.

Function

CD172g may play a role in T-cell–T-cell signaling via CD47 and thus influence T-cell behavior.

Ligation of CD47 by CD172g was shown to induce apoptosis of T-cell lines although not as efficiently as CD172a.

Binding of CD172g was also found to be dependent on the level of CD47 expression on target cells.

Ligands

CD172g binds CD47 but with lower affinity than CD172a.

Expression

CD172g is expressed on the majority of T cells and a proportion of B cells.

Gene Name	Entrez Gene#
SIRPB2	55423

Selected Monoclonal Antibodies

Ox116 (Barclay; Oxford).

CD173

Other Names

Blood Group H2.

$$Gal\,\beta1 \longrightarrow 4Glc\,NAc\,\beta - R$$

Molecular Structure

CD173 is the monofucosylated form of the precursor carbohydrate chain α1-2 Galβ1-4GlcNA expressed on glycosphingolipid or protein and belongs to the A,B,H, Lewis blood group family

CD173 is generated by β-D-galactoside2-L-fucosyl transferase (FUT 1).

Function

Fucose is known to be involved in the adhesion of hematopoietic progenitor cells and bone marrow stromal cells. The expression of CD173 by hematopoietic progenitors suggests a role in the homing process of immature stem cells to the bone marrow.

Expression

CD173 is expressed by CD34$^+$ hematopoietic precursors and CD34$^+$ leukemic cell lines, endothelial cells, basal cells of the bronchial epithelium, and erythocytes.

CD173 expression is increased in a wide variety of carcinomas.

Applications

CD173 is a specific marker of CD34$^+$ hematopoietic progenitor cells.

Gene Name	Entrez Gene#
carbohydrate antigen	

Selected Monoclonal Antibodies

MEM-195 (Horejsi; Prague); MEM-197 (Horejsi; Prague).

CD174

Other Names

Lewis Y blood group, LeY.

$$Fuc\,\alpha1 \longrightarrow 2Gal\,\beta1 \longrightarrow 4\,Glc\,NAc\,\beta1\text{-}R$$
$$3$$
$$\uparrow$$
$$Fuc\,\alpha1$$

Molecular Structure

CD174 is the difucosylated form of the type 2 precursor chain carbohydrate, $\alpha1\text{-}2Gal\beta1\text{-}4GlcNAc$, and is a member of the A,B,H, Lewis blood group family.

It is the product of epistatic interaction of the precursor chains of 1-2 fucosyltransferases encoded by the H gene and the $\alpha1\text{-}3$ fucosyl-transferases encoded by the LeX gene.

CD174 is present either in the plasma membrane linked to glycolipids or to surface receptors such as members of the ErbB family.

Function

CD174 is implicated as a cofactor to pro-coagulant y activity of cancer cells and may play a role in early commitment to apoptosis.

In both in vitro and in vivo studies, soluble CD174 was found to be a potent angiogenic mediator.

The selective increase in CD174 expression by synovial fluid granulocytes from patients with rheumatoid arthritis, spondyloarthritis, and osteoarthritis suggests a role in granulocyte trafficking and inflammatory responses.

Expression

CD174 is expressed by $CD34^+$ hematopoietic progenitor cells and $CD34^+$ leukaemic cell lines.

Overexpression of CD174 occurs in a wide variety of carcinomas, including breast, prostate, pancreas, colon, and non-small cell lung cancers.

LeY is also expressed by *Helicobactor pylori*.

Applications

Anti Lewis Y mAb conjugated with doxorubicin is being trialed for the therapy of epithelial tumors.

CD174 is a specific marker for $CD34^+$ hematopoietic progenitor cells and $CD34^+$ leukemic cell lines.

Gene Name	Entrez Gene#
FUT3	2525

Selected Monoclonal Antibodies

A70-C/C8 (Karsten; Berlin).

CD175, CD175s

Other Names

CD175: Tn Antigen (T-antigen novelle),
CD175s: Sialyl-Tn.

$$GlcNAc\,\alpha1 \longrightarrow Ser/Thr$$

Molecular Structure

CD175 is the monosaccharide GalNAcα1-O-R expressed on glycosphingolipids or O-linked to proteins.

CD175s is the sialylated epitope on O-linked monosaccharide GalNAcα1-O-R, expressed on glycosphingolipid or glycoprotein.

Sialyl-CD175 is synthesized by ST6GalNAc1, which catalyses the transfer of the sialic acid residue in the α2,6 linkage to the CD175 structure. The resulting disaccharide cannot be further elongated.

Function

CD175 is the precursor for ABO antigens and the Thomsen–Friedenreich (TF) antigen (CD176).

It is a tumor-associated carbohydrate antigen (TACA) that arises from aberrant O-linked glycosylation and is not found on differentiated cells.

An exception is the rare Tn syndrome where CD175 is expressed by a proportion of CD34$^+$ hematopoietic stem cells and their progeny due to the absence of UDP-Gal:N-acetylgalactosaminideβ1-3galactosyltransferase activity. Most patients appear healthy but usually have moderate thrombocytopenia and leukopenia and some indicators of hemolytic anemia.

Cytotoxic CD8$^+$ T cells are capable of recognizing CD175 and CD175s in a MHC class 1 restricted manner.

CD175s has been implicated in the induction of metastasis and invasiveness of tumors. It is over-expressed in several carcinomas and is associated with poor prognosis.

Transfection of CD175s-ve breast cancer cell lines with ST6GalNAc1 cDNA results in expression of CD175s and decreased adhesion and increased migration of cells.

Expression

CD175 and CD175s are expressed by breast, ovary, colorectal, gastrointestinal, bladder, larynx, and lung carcinoma cells.

CD175 is also expressed on various T-, B-, and myeloid lineage leukemias and epithelial tumors.

CD175 is expressed by a proportion of CD34$^+$ hematopoietic progenitor cells and in all hematopoietic cells arising from these progenitors in Tn syndrome.

Applications

CD175 is a vaccine candidate in the prevention and treatment of mucin-expressing tumors particularly carcinomas.

CD175-specific mAb have been used for prognostic and therapeutic applications.

CD175s conjugated to keyhole limpet hemocyanin (Theratope) is being trialed as a vaccine for colorectal and non-small cell lung cancer.

A large-scale phase III clinical trial of Theratope in breast cancer patients was completed in 2003, and it is currently being assessed in patients with metastatic breast cancer.

Gene Name   Entrez Gene#

carbohydrate antigen

Selected Monoclonal Antibodies

CD175: HB-Tn-1 (Dako Cytomation; Glostrup).

CD175s: HB-STn1 (Dako Cytomation; Glostrup).

CD176

Other Names

Thomsen–Friedenreich antigen (TF).

$$Gal\,\beta 1 \longrightarrow 3\,Gal\,NAc\,\alpha 1 - R$$

Molecular Structure

CD176 is the carbohydrate Galβ1-3GalNAcα 1-O-R, expressed on glycosphingolipids or glycoproteins.

Function

CD176 is highly immunogenic as evidenced by the presence of anti-CD176 antibody in the serum of carcinoma patients.

CD176 has been implicated in the induction of metastasis and invasiveness of tumors.

Expression

CD176 is broadly expressed by carcinoma cells.

It is also expressed by the syncytium and extravillous trophoblast cells.

Helicobacter pylori express CD176.

Applications

CD176-specific antibodies have been used for prognostic and therapeutic applications.

CD176 is a potentially useful component of a vaccine against prostate cancer.

Gene Name   Entrez Gene#

carbohydrate antigen

Selected Monoclonal Antibodies

A78-G/A7 (Karsten; Berlin).

CD177

Other Names

NB1, HNA-2a, PRV1 (polycythemia vera rubra 1).

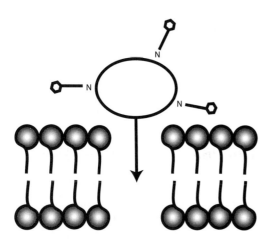

GPI Anchor

Molecular Structure

CD177 encodes the GPI-anchored NB1 glycoprotein also known as HNA-2a. It is a member of the Ly-6 or snake toxin gene superfamily (see also CD87 and CD59).

It is located on secondary granules as well as plasma membranes.

The protein is predicted to have two cysteine-rich regions, 3 N-linked glycosylation sites but no O-linked carbohydrate side chains.

Several single nucleotide polymorphisms that result in amino acid substitutions have been described.

Mol Wt: Reduced, 56–64 kDa; unreduced, 49–55 kDa.

Function

The function of CD177 is not known.

The expression of CD177 is upregulated in response to the chemotactic peptide fMLP.

CD177-negative mothers with CD177-positive neonates can elicit a CD177-specific antibody response that can result in the child experiencing severe neutropenia for several weeks.

Transfusion of blood or blood products containing alloantibodies specific for CD177 can result in severe acute lung injury in the transfusion recipient.

Alloantibodies are sometimes produced in patients receiving CD177-positive granulocyte concentrates and can result in febrile transfusion reactions and reduced survival of the transfused granulocytes.

CD177-positive neutrophils are less adherent to human umbilical vein endothelial cells than CD177-negative neutrophils.

Expression

In healthy individuals, CD177 is expressed by 56–64% of neutrophils as well as neutrophilic metamyelocytes and myelocytes. Expression of CD177 is greater on neutrophils from women than men although CD177 expression decreases in women with age but remains constant in men.

It is overexpressed on neutrophils in patients with polycythemia vera and is transiently increased in patients with severe burns or infections and in healthy subjects given G-CSF.

CD177 expression is reduced on neutrophils of patients with paroxysmal nocturnal hemaglobinuria and chronic myelogenous leukemia.

Gene Name	Entrez Gene#
PRV1	57126

Selected Monoclonal Antibodies

7D8, 1B5 (Clement; Besancon); MEM166 (Horejsi; Prague).

CD178

Other Names

FAS ligand, CD95 ligand.

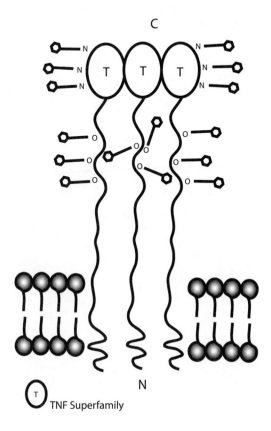

TNF Superfamily

Molecular Structure

A type II (C-terminus extracellular) transmembrane protein member of the TNF family. Expressed in the membrane (and as a soluble cleavage product) as a trimer. The monomeric unit has an apparent Mol Wt of 40 kDa and consists of 281 residues.

The C-terminal domain of FasL (aa103-281) contains the region homologous to TNF and is responsible for the trimeric quaternary organization of TNF ligands. This region is necessary and sufficient for receptor binding. The extracellular region has 3 N-glycosylation sites. The extracellular domain is shed through proteolysis.

The cytoplasmic domain (residues 1–80) is proline-rich and contains a SH3 binding motif.

Function

Induces apoptosis (activation-induced cell death) in cells expressing CD95. Involved in regulation of the immune response as well as many other situations in which Fas-mediated apoptosis is part of homeostasis or pathology. A key mechanism in elimination of virus-infected or transformed cells.

Fas-positive activated T cells can undergo apoptosis as a result of interaction with Fas ligand expressed on other lymphocytes, on other cells (for example, in immune-privileged sites where CD178 expression protects the tissue from T-cell mediated damage), or on the same cell (lymphocyte suicide). CD178 induces activation, not cell death, in Fas-positive dendritic cells.

Knockout mice and humans with CD95L mutation show severe autoimmune disease.

Apart from its activity in killing Fas-bearing cells, engagement of CD178 transmits signals to the cell, inhibiting proliferation or, in some in vitro situations, acting as a costimulator.

The shed soluble domain can induce apoptosis, but it is less active than membrane-bound CD178 and may inhibit cell-mediated apoptosis by competing for FAS sites.

Ligands

FAS (CD95).

Expression

T cells and NK cells, monocytes, neutrophils, and immature dendritic cells. Expressed widely outside the immune system, including sites of "immune privilege," where it provides protection from excessive immune pathology in viral infection. Expressed on some tumors, presumably conferring a degree of protection from immune attack. Induced on many cell types by activation or stress, for example, in the skin by UV radiation.

Applications

Research reagent in studies of apoptosis.

Gene Name	Entrez Gene#
TNFSF6	356

Selected Monoclonal Antibodies

N0K-1 (Shen; Tianjin); Alf-1.2 (Kaplan; Cleveland).

CD179a

Other Names

V pre β, pre lymphocyte gene 1 (VPREB1), immunoglobulin iota chain (IGVPB).

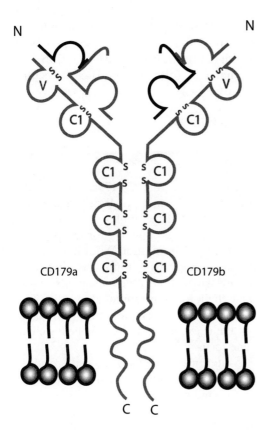

Molecular Structure

CD179a is a member of the Ig gene superfamily.

It has an Ig V-like structure but lacks the last β strand (β7) of a typical V domain.

The mature protein without the leader peptide (19 amino acids) has 126 amino acids.

CD179a associates noncovalently with CD179b to form a surrogate light chain. Within this complex, the incomplete V domain of CD179a appears to be complemented by the extra β7 strand of CD179b carrying a C domain, resulting in the formation of Ig light chain-like structure.

The CD179a/CD179b surrogate light chain is disulphide-linked to membrane bound IgM heavy chain associated with the signal transducing CD79a/CD79b heterodimer to form the pre-B-cell receptor (preBCR).

Mol Wt: 16–18 kDa.

Function

The function of the CD179a/CD179b surrogate light chain in pro-B cells is unclear.

The preBCR complex that contains CD179 mediates signaling for proliferation and differentiation. After limited proliferation, the cells fall into a resting state, during which time rearrangements at the light chain locus are initiated.

The preBCR complex may also signal for allelic exclusion at the IgM heavy chain gene locus.

Expression

CD179a is exclusively expressed in pro-B and early pre-B cells.

Applications

CD179a is a marker of pro-B and early pre-B cells.

Gene Name	Entrez Gene#
VPREB1	7441

Selected Monoclonal Antibodies

VpreB6, VpreB7, VpreB8 (Cooper; Alabama).

CD179b

Other Names

Ig Lambda 5, immunoglobulin omega chain, immunoglobulin lambda-like polypeptide 1.

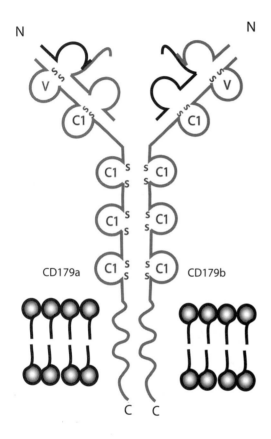

Molecular Structure

CD179b protein is a member of the Ig gene superfamily.

Without the leader peptide (44 aa), the mature protein has 169 aa.

The 50 aa-long N-terminal region shows no sequence homologies to any other proteins.

The 119 aa-long C-terminal region shows homology to the J region (β7-strand of the variable region) and the constant region of the lambda light chain.

In the CD179a/CD179b surrogate light chain, the incomplete V domain of CD179a lacking the last β strand (β7) appears to be complemented by the extra β7 strand of CD179b, resulting in the formation of Ig light chain-like structure.

The CD179a/CD179b surrogate light chain is disulphide-linked to membrane bound IgM heavy chain associated with the signal transducing CD79a/CD79b heterodimer to form the pre-B-cell receptor (preBCR).

Mol Wt: 22 kDa.

Function

The function of the CD179a/CD179b surrogate light chain in pro-B cells is unclear.

The preBCR complex that contains CD179 mediates signaling for the proliferation and differentiation. After limited proliferation, the cells fall into a resting state, during which time rearrangements at the light chain locus are initiated.

The preBCR complex may also signal for allelic exclusion at the IgM heavy chain gene locus.

Mutations in the CD179b gene result in agammaglobulinemia and impaired B-cell development.

CD179b knockout mice have impaired early B-cell development. However, it is not as severe as that seen in humans.

Expression

CD179b is selectively expressed in pro-B and early pre-B cells.

Gene Name	Entrez Gene#
IGLL1	3543

Selected Monoclonal Antibodies

HSL11 (Karasuyama; Tokyo).

CD180

Other Names

RP105, Bgp95, LY64.

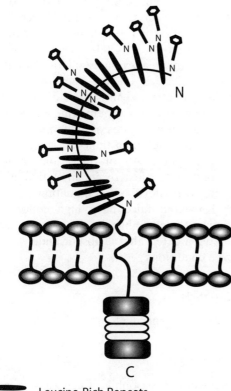

Leucine-Rich Repeats

Toll Interleukin Receptor Domain

Molecular Structure

CD180 is a type I membrane protein that belongs to the Toll-like receptor family.

The extracellular domain contains 17 leucine-rich repeats (LRR) that consist of tandem repeats of a leucine-rich motif (LRM) comprising 24–28 amino acids in which leucines are characteristically positioned.

The cytoplasmic tail is short.

Mol Wt: Reduced, 95–100 kDa; unreduced, 95–100 kDa.

Function

CD180 regulates recognition of LPS and signaling in B cells.

Ligation of CD180 by mAb leads to B-cell activation, upregulation of CD80/CD86, and increase in cell size.

CD180 null mice have an impaired response to LPS-induced proliferation and antibody production.

Expression

CD180 is strongly expressed on mantle zone B cells and marginal zone B cells but very weakly on germinal center B cells.

CD180 expression occurs in peripheral blood monocytes and dendritic cells.

Gene Name	Entrez Gene#
LY64	4064

Selected Monoclonal Antibodies

MHR73 (Kensuke; Miyake).

CD181

Other Names

Formerly assigned CD128A.
CXCR1; IL-8 receptor α.

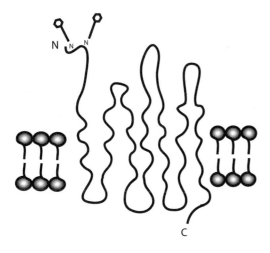

Molecular Structure

Chemokine receptors are G-protein coupled receptors (GPCRs) consisting of an extracellular amino terminal, seven membrane-spanning regions, and a cytoplasmic carboxyl terminal. This structure is shared by several receptor families. The chemokine receptors form a division of the leukocyte chemoattractant subfamily, which is part of the rhodopsin family of GPCRs.

CXCR1 is 350 residues long and has 2 N-glycosylation sites. The two IL-8 receptors CXCR1 and CXCR2 are 77% identical and show most differences in the amino-terminal tail and the second loop, as well as the intracellular C-terminal. The differences in the extracellular region may explain differences in ligand specificity, whereas the intracellular differences suggest there may be differences in signaling mechanisms.

Mice have a single IL-8 receptor, which is most homologous with CXCR2.

Function

CXCR1 is a high affinity receptor for IL-8, and its functions thus reflect the function of this chemotactic pro-inflammatory factor.

Ligation of CXCR1 triggers a signal cascade that leads to upregulation of adhesion molecules on the receptor-bearing cells and directed migration of the cells. The migration, up a chemokine gradient, is generally toward sites of inflammation, the site of production of the chemokine.

The end result of migration of neutrophils into sites of inflammation is to increase the level of inflammation.

Knockout mice have high concentrations of neutrophils in the marrow and blood, a defect that is absent under germ-free conditions.

Ligands

CXCR-1 is specific for IL-8.

Expression

Neutrophils, basophils, T-cell subsets, and at lower levels, monocytes and NK cells. Expressed in myeloid but not lymphocytic leukemias.

Applications

Research reagent in studies of inflammation and with potential as a marker of functional subsets of neutrophils.

Gene Name	Entrez Gene#
IL8RA	3577

Selected Monoclonal Antibodies

MAB330 (R&D Systems; Minneapolis).

CD182

Other Names

Formerly assigned CD128B.
CXCR2; IL8 receptor β;

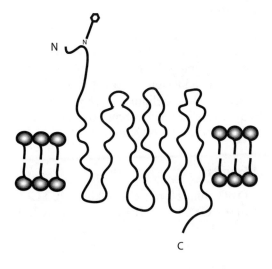

Molecular Structure

Chemokine receptors are G-protein coupled receptors (GPCRs) consisting of an extracellular amino terminal, seven membrane-spanning regions, and a cytoplasmic carboxyl terminal. This structure is shared by several receptor families. The chemokine receptors form a division of the leukocyte chemoattractant subfamily, which is part of the rhodopsin family of GPCRs.

CXRC2 is 355 residues long and has 2 N-glycosylation sites. The two IL-8 receptors CXCR1 and CXCR2 are 77% identical and show most differences in the amino-terminal tail and the second loop, as well as the intracellular C-terminal. The differences in the extracellular region may explain differences in ligand specificity, whereas the intracellular differences suggest there may be differences in signaling mechanisms.

Mice have a single IL-8 receptor, which is most homologous with CXCR2.

Function

CXCR2 is a high affinity receptors for IL-8, and its functions thus reflect the function of this chemotactic pro-inflammatory factor. CXCR2 binds other chemokines in addition to IL-8, so may be expected to have a wider range of functions than CXCR1, which is specific for IL-8.

Ligation of CXCR2 triggers a signal cascade that leads to upregulation of adhesion molecules on the receptor-bearing cells and directed migration of the cells. The migration, up a chemokine gradient, is generally toward sites of inflammation, the site of production of the chemokine.

The end result of migration of neutrophils into sites of inflammation is to increase the level of inflammation.

Knockout mice have high concentrations of neutrophils in the marrow and blood, a defect that is absent under germ-free conditions.

Ligands

CXCR-2 binds, in addition to IL-8, GRO α, β, γ, and NAP-2.

Expression

Neutrophils, basophils, T-cell subsets, and at lower levels, monocytes and NK cells. CXCR2 is also expressed widely outside the hematopoietic system, including the nervous system and various epithelia. Expressed in myeloid but not lymphocytic leukemias.

Applications

Research reagent in studies of inflammation and with potential as a marker of functional subsets of neutrophils.

Gene Name	Entrez Gene#
IL8RB	3579

Selected Monoclonal Antibodies

MAB331 (R&D Systems; Minneapolis).

CD183

Other Names

CXCR3, G protein-coupled receptor 9.

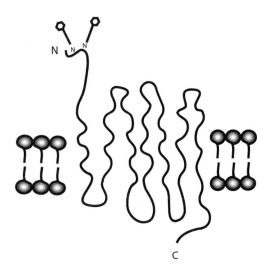

Molecular Structure

Chemokine receptors are G-protein coupled receptors (GPCRs) consisting of an extracellular amino terminal, seven membrane-spanning regions, and a cytoplasmic carboxyl terminal. This structure is shared by several receptor families. The chemokine receptors form a division of the leukocyte chemoattractant subfamily, which is part of the rhodopsin family of GPCRs.

CD183 shares 30% identity with CD181 and CD182 (CXCR1 and 2).

Function

Receptor for chemokines CXCL9, CXCL10, and CXCL11. CD183 mediates CXCL9- and CXCL10-induced integrin-mediated adhesion of effector T cells to vascular endothelium. CD183 may also play a role in augmenting Th1 cell activation and IFN-γ production.

Ligands

CD183 binds the chemokines, CXCL9 (Mig), CXCL10 (IP10), and CXCL11 (I-TAC).

Expression

T cells, activated NK cells, and transformed B cells.

Gene Name	Entrez Gene#
CXCR3	2833

Selected Monoclonal Antibodies

49801 (R&D Systems; Minneapolis).

CD184

Other Names

CXCR4, Fusin.

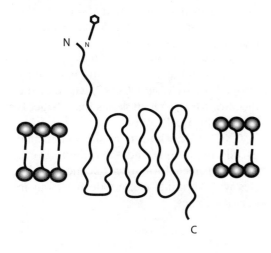

Molecular Structure

Chemokine receptors are G-protein coupled receptors (GPCRs) consisting of an extracellular amino terminal, seven membrane-spanning regions, and a cytoplasmic carboxyl terminal. This structure is shared by several receptor families. The chemokine receptors form a division of the leukocyte chemoattractant subfamily, which is part of the rhodopsin family of GPCRs.

CD184 is found in at least two isoforms; isoform 1 and isoform 2/CXCR4-L0; produced by alternative splicing.

CD184 has two potential N-glycosylation sites.

Function

Receptor for the C-X-C chemokine SDF-1. Tranduces a signal by increasing the intracellular calcium ion level. Involved in hemopoiesis and in cardiac ventricular septum formation.

Plays an essential role in vascularization of the gastrointestinal tract, probably by regulating vascular branching and/or remodeling processes in endothelial cells.

Could be involved in cerebellar development. In the CNS, could mediate hippocampal-neuron survival.

Acts as a primary receptor for some HIV-2 isolates and as a coreceptor with CD4 for HIV-1 X4 viruses.

Ligands

CXCL12 (SDF-1).
CD184 is also a coreceptor for HIV.

Expression

Widely expressed in hematopoietic cells, vascular endothelium, and neural tissue.

Gene Name	Entrez Gene#
CXCR4	7852

Selected Monoclonal Antibodies

B-P27 (Clement; besancon); 12G5 (van Agthoven; Marseille); 44717 (R&D Systems; Minneapolis).

CD185

Other Names

CXCR5 (Chemokine, CXC motif, receptor 5); BLR1 (Burkitt's lymphoma receptor 1).

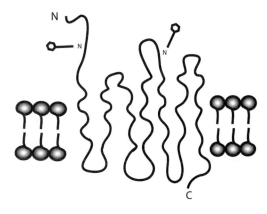

Molecular Structure

Chemokine receptors are G-protein coupled receptors (GPCRs) consisting of an extracellular amino terminal, seven membrane-spanning regions, and a cytoplasmic carboxyl terminal. This structure is shared by several receptor families. The chemokine receptors form a division of the leukocyte chemoattractant subfamily, which is part of the rhodopsin family of GPCRs.

CD185 has two potential N-glycosylation sites.

Two isoforms are seen. One lacks the first 45 aa of the 55-residue first (N-terminal) extracellular region.

Function

Binding of CXCL13 to CD185 induces a chemotactic response.

CD185 is thought to be involved in B-cell migration to and localization of, in particular, B-cell compartments such as the primary or secondary follicles in secondary lymphoid tissues.

The localization of B cells appears to depend on a balance between response by CXCR5 to BCL and CCR7, which is the receptor for two chemokines that attract B cells to the T-cell zones.

CXCR5 Knockout mice show abnormal B-cell migration and disrupted B-cell primary follicle formation. Secondary follicles with germinal centers do form but in abnormal sites.

Ligands

CXCL13 (BLC).

Expression

B cells and monocytes.

Applications

Expression and possible role in Burkitt's lymphoma makes CD185 and its ligand a possible therapeutic target.

Gene Name	Entrez Gene#
BLR1	643

Selected Monoclonal Antibodies

51505 (R&D Systems; Minneapolis).

CD186

Other Names

CXCR6, BONZO, STRL33, TYMSTR.

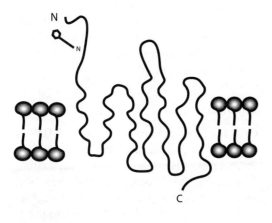

Molecular Structure

Chemokine receptors are G-protein coupled receptors (GPCRs) consisting of an extracellular amino terminal, seven membrane-spanning regions, and a cytoplasmic carboxyl terminal. This structure is shared by several receptor families. The chemokine receptors form a division of the leukocyte chemoattractant subfamily, which is part of the rhodopsin family of GPCRs.

CD186 is a 342-aa long protein and has a single site for N-linked glycosylation, at residue 16 in the 32-residue first (N-terminal) extracellular region.

Mol Wt: 39 kDa (predicted).

Function

CD186 is the cellular receptor for the chemokine CXCL16, and is used as a coreceptor by strains of HIV-1 and HIV-2 and by the monkey virus SIV.

CD186 functions as a G-protein coupled receptor.

Ligands

CXCR6 binds the chemokine CXCL16 (also known as SRPSOX), and is a coreceptor of strains of HIV-1, HIV-2 and the monkey virus SIV.

Expression

Expressed by activated T cells.

Seen in tissue sections, presumably staining activated T cells.

Gene Name	Entrez Gene#
CXCR6	10663

Selected Monoclonal Antibodies

56811 (R&D Systems; Minneapolis).

CD191

Other Names

CCR1 (Chemokine, C-C motif, receptor 1), CC-CKR-1.

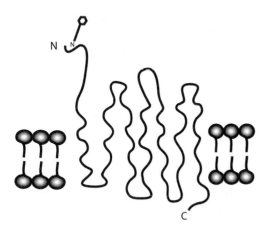

Molecular Structure

Chemokine receptors are G-protein coupled receptors (GPCRs) consisting of an extracellular amino terminal, seven membrane-spanning regions, and a cytoplasmic carboxyl terminal. This structure is shared by several receptor families. The chemokine receptors form a division of the leukocyte chemoattractant subfamily, which is part of the rhodopsin family of GPCRs.

CCR1 is 355 amino acids in length and has a predicted Mol Wt of 41 kDa. The first (N terminal) extracellular sequence bears the single potential N-glycosylation site in the molecule.

Function

Mediates the effects of its several chemokine ligands. Ligand binding causes a calcium flux, but the downstream consequences are not known. Appears to be involved in stem cell proliferation.

A knockout mouse model suggests that CCR1 provides a degree of protection from inflammatory damage and protection from parasitic and viral infection.

Ligands

CCR1 has several ligands: MIP-1α (macrophage inflammatory protein 1α), RANTES (Regulated on Activation, Normal T-cell Expressed and Secreted protein), MCP-3 (monocyte chemoattractant protein 3), and MPIF-1 (myeloid progenitor inhibitory factor 1).

Expression

mRNA expression data show low levels in most tissues, with a high level in caudate nucleus. Antibody-based studies show expression by T lymphocytes, NK cells and monocytes but not B cells and granulocytes. Among T cells memory cells express higher levels of CCR1.

Gene Name	Entrez Gene#
CCR1	1230

Selected Monoclonal Antibodies

53504 (R&D Systems; Minneapolis).

CD192

Other Names

CCR2 (Chemokine, C-C motif, Receptor 2), MCP-1-R (Monocyte chemoattractant protein 1 receptor), CKR2.

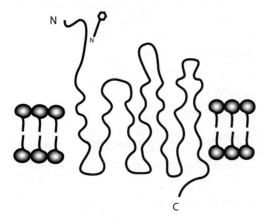

Molecular Structure

Chemokine receptors are G-protein coupled receptors (GPCRs) consisting of an extracellular amino terminal, seven membrane-spanning regions, and a cytoplasmic carboxyl terminal. This structure is shared by several receptor families. The chemokine receptors form a division of the leukocyte chemoattractant subfamily, which is part of the rhodopsin family of GPCRs.

The first (N-terminal) extracellular region is 42 residues long and contains the only potential N-glycosylation site in the molecule.

CCR2 is found in two isoforms differing as a result of alternative splicing at the carboxy terminus.

The best-characterized isoform is 374aa in length and has an apparent Mol Wt of 42 kDa.

Function

Binding of the ligand, MCP-1, mediates Ca flux, leading to chemotactic responses. The ligand attracts monocytes to sites of inflammation and is thought to have a role in localized inflammatory conditions, for example, in involved joints in rheumatoid arthritis.

Apart from the chemotactic effects of the ligand on monocytes, which have been studied extensively, the receptor is expressed by B cells and activated T cells, and may be expected to activate chemotactic responses in these cells.

Ligands

MCP-1 (Monocyte chemoattractant protein 1).

CCR2 is also a co-receptor for HIV.

Expression

Monocytes, activated T cells and B cells.

Applications

Animal models have suggested a major role for CCR2 and its ligand in multiple sclerosis, but human studies have so far not confirmed this.

Coreceptor for HIV, and inhibition of this reaction may have therapeutic potential.

Gene Name	Entrez Gene#
CCR2	1231

Selected Monoclonal Antibodies

48607 (R&D Systems; Minneapolis).

CD193

Other Names

CCR3 (Chemokine, C-C motif, Receptor 3), Eosinophil eotaxin receptor, CKR3.

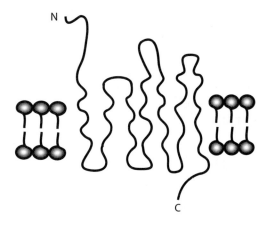

Molecular Structure

Chemokine receptors are G-protein-coupled receptors (GPCRs) consisting of an extracellular amino terminal, seven membrane-spanning regions, and a cytoplasmic carboxyl terminal. This structure is shared by several receptor families. The chemokine receptors form a division of the leukocyte chemoattractant subfamily, which is part of the rhodopsin family of GPCRs.

CD193 is a 355-aa protein of apparent Mol Wt of 41 kDa.

The 34-aa first (N-terminal) extracellular sequence has no N-glycosylation sites, unlike many of the other chemokine receptors.

Function

CCR3 binds eotaxin, and the functions reflect the activities of the ligand. Eotaxin is a chemoattractant for eosinophils and basophils.

The function of the ligand and the cell distribution of CCR3, being expressed on basophils, eosinophils, and the T-cell subset that makes IL-4 and IL-5 (which promote allergic reactions), make it potentially a central agent in allergic reactions. It appears to be involved in accumulation and activation of eosinophils in the airways in allergic lung disease.

Ligands

Eotaxin (CCL11), MCP-4 (macrophage chemoattractant protein 4). Also reported to bind MCP-3 and RANTES.

Also functions as a coreceptor for HIV.

Expression

Eosinophils and basophils, epithelial cells in the airways, and T-cell subset with TH2 pattern of cytokine production.

Applications

Role in allergic responses makes CCR3 and its ligand a potential therapeutic target, and antagonists of the pathway have been synthesized. Useful as a marker for TH2 cells in monitoring immune responses.

Gene Name	Entrez Gene#
CCR3	1232

Selected Monoclonal Antibodies

61828 (R&D Systems; Minneapolis).

CD194

Other Names

CCR4, (Chemokine, C-C motif, Receptor 4). Although CD194 has been reserved for CCR4, no assignment was made at HLDA8 because there were no confirmed antibodies.

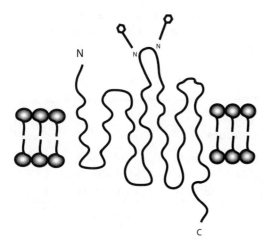

Molecular Structure

Chemokine receptors are G-protein-coupled receptors (GPCRs) consisting of an extracellular amino terminal, seven membrane-spanning regions, and a cytoplasmic carboxyl terminal. This structure is shared by several receptor families. The chemokine receptors form a division of the leukocyte chemoattractant subfamily, which is part of the rhodopsin family of GPCRs.

CCR4 is a 360-aa protein with an apparent Mol Wt of 41.4 kDa.

The 39-residue first (N-terminal) extracellular sequence has no N-glycosylation sites, but two N-glycosylation sites are present in the second extracellular loop, at residues 183 and 194.

Function

CD194 acts as a chemoattractant homing receptor involved in the skin homing of circulating memory lymphocytes and as a coreceptor for some primary HIV-2 isolates.

CD194 may also be involved in the termination of immune reactions because it is expressed on the surface of T regulatory cells.

Ligands

CD194 is a high affinity receptor for C-C type chemokines CCL17 (TARC) and CCL22 (MDC).

Also functions as a coreceptor for HIV.

Expression

CD194 is expressed by all CLA$^+$ T cells regardless of their Th1 or Th2 phenotype, activated Th2 lymphocytes, CD4$^+$ CD25$^+$ regulatory T cells, IL-2 activated NK cells, basophils, and macrophages.

Applications

CD194 blockade has potential as a therapeutic treatment of inflammation.

Gene Name	Entrez Gene#
CCR4	1233

Selected Monoclonal Antibodies

205410 (R&D Systems; Minneapolis); 1G1 (BD Biosciences; San Jose).

CD195

Other Names

CCR5 (Chemokine, C-C motif, Receptor 5), CKR5.

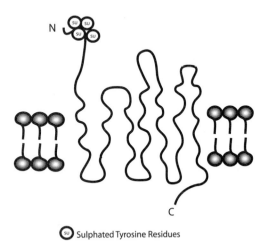

(su) Sulphated Tyrosine Residues

Molecular Structure

Chemokine receptors are G-protein-coupled receptors, (GPCRs) consisting of an extracellular amino terminal, seven membrane-spanning regions, and a cytoplasmic carboxyl terminal. This structure is shared by several receptor families. The chemokine recptors form a division of the leukocyte chemoattractant subfamily, which is part of the rhodopsin family of GPCRs.

CCR5 is a 352-residue glycoprotein with apparent Mol Wt of 37 kDa. It is most closely related to CCR2 (75% identity).

The N-terminal extracellular domain contains 30 residues, whereas the intracellular C-terminus is 50 residues long. The extracellular regions have O-linked carbohydrate and sulphated tyrosine residues.

Function

Chemokine receptors mediate the functions of chemokines, which have several roles as inducers of cell movement and activation. CD195 is involved in regulating both innate and adaptive immune responses. It is also a major coreceptor for HIV, and some individuals with an allele of CD195, which does not bind HIV, are resistant to infection.

Ligation of CD195 induces downstream signaling, including calcium flux and chemotaxis.

Knockout mice are healthy, but they show deficits in handling infections and an increase in delayed hypersensitivity and antibody production, suggesting CCR5 regulates the immune function in a complex way.

Ligands

CD195 binds the chemokines CCL3 (MIP-1α), CCL4 (MIP-1β), and CCL5 (RANTES) with high affinity. It also binds, though with lower affinity, CCL11 (eotaxin), CCL7 (MCP-3), and CCL13 (MCP-4).

Also acts as a coreceptor for HIV.

Expression

Expressed widely on leukocytes, including blood lymphocytes, monocytes, macrophages, and immature dendritic cells. Among T cells, CD195 is expressed preferentially on a subset with the phenotype of activated memory cells with TH1 function.

Applications

There is significant interest in blockade of CCR5 as an approach to HIV treatment.

Gene Name	Entrez Gene#
CXCR5	1234

Selected Monoclonal Antibodies

2D7, 3A9 (San Jose, BD Biosciences).

CD196

Other Names

CCR6 (Chemokine, C-C motif, Receptor 6), CKR6, LARC receptor.

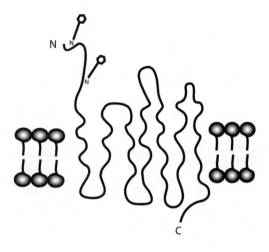

Molecular Structure

Chemokine receptors are G-protein-coupled receptors (GPCRs) consisting of an extracellular amino terminal, seven membrane-spanning regions, and a cytoplasmic carboxyl terminal. This structure is shared by several receptor families. The chemokine receptors form a division of the leukocyte chemoattractant subfamily, which is part of the rhodopsin family of GPCRs.

CCR6 is 374 amino acids long and has a calculated Mol Wt of 42 kDa.

The first (N-terminal) extracellular sequence is 47 amino acids long and bears two potential N-glycosylation sites.

Function

Mediates chemotaxis in response to its ligands, CCL20, and the β defensins.

Involved in maturation of B lineage cells and their antigen-driven differentiation; thought to be involved in dendritic cell maturation and T-cell recruitment in immune and inflammatory processes.

Particularly involved in mucosal immunity.

Interaction with β defensins suggests a role in the immune response to bacterial infection.

Ligands

CCL20, also known as MIP-3α (Macrophage Inflammatory Protein 3 α) and LARC (Liver and Activation-Regulated Chemokine). CCR6 also binds the β defensins, a family of anti-bacterial peptides.

Expression

Memory T cells and immature dendritic cells. B cells, showing selective expression in tissue by marginal zone and follicular mantle B cells.

Expressed selectively by a subset of non-Hodgkin's lymphomas associated with mucosal tissue.

Applications

The selective expression of CCR6 by mucosa-associated non-Hodgkin's lymphoma has a potential diagnostic value, and the interaction between the receptor and its ligand may provide a therapeutic target in these malignancies.

Gene Name	Entrez Gene#
CCR6	1235

Selected Monoclonal Antibodies

53103 (R&D Systems; Minneapolis).

CD197

Other Names

CCR7, Epstein–Barr Induced gene 1 (EBI1), Burkitt's lymphoma receptor 2 (BLR2).

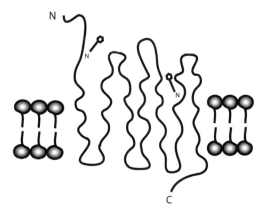

Molecular Structure

Chemokine receptors are G-protein-coupled receptors, (GPCRs) consisting of an extracellular amino terminal, seven membrane-spanning regions, and a cytoplasmic carboxyl terminal. This structure is shared by several receptor families. The chemokine receptors form a division of the leukocyte chemoattractant subfamily, which is part of the rhodopsin family of GPCRs.

CD197 has sites for N-glycosylation in the N-terminal extracellular tail and in the third (N-terminal-distal) extracellular loop. A disulphide bond forms between cysteines in the first (N-terminal proximal) and second extracellular loop.

Function

Chemokine receptors mediate the functions of chemokines, which have several roles as inducers of cell movement and activation. CD197 appears to be essential for correct homing of lymphocytes and dendritic cells.

In addition, CD197-positive T cells activate dendritic cells to produce IL-12.

The T cells of mice lacking CCL21 cannot home to secondary lymphoid tissues. Dendritic cells in these mice also failed to localize in secondary lymphoid tissue.

CD197 knockout mice show similar defects in lymphocytes and DC migration and homing to secondary lymphoid tissue, leading to impaired cell-mediated and antibody responses.

Expression of CD197 identifies a subset of memory T cells, designated central memory T cells, which also express high levels of CD62L. These cells activate dendritic cells and home to secondary lymphoid tissue, but they lack the effector function. This subset is distinguished from CD197$^-$, CD62L^{low} memory T cells, and designated effector memory T cells, which carry out effector functions and migrate into peripheral tissues.

Ligands

CCL19 (ELC) and CCL21 (SLC) are both bound with high affinity.

Expression

Most T cells express CD197, including naive T cells and the CD62L-positive subset of memory T cells. B cells, NK cells, and dendritic cells also express CD197.

Applications

Research reagent, distinguishing central memory from effector memory T cells. Malignant T cells expressing CD197 have a greater tendency to involve secondary lymphoid organs.

Gene Name   Entrez Gene#

CCR7   1236

Selected Monoclonal Antibodies

150503 (R&D Systems; Minneapolis).

CDw198

Other Names

CCR8 (Chemokine, C-C motif, Receptor 8), CKRL1.

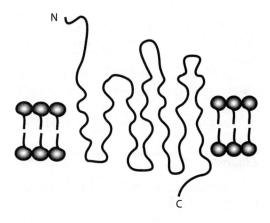

Molecular Structure

Chemokine receptors are G-protein-coupled receptors (GPCRs) consisting of an extracellular amino terminal, seven membrane-spanning regions, and a cytoplasmic carboxyl terminal. This structure is shared by several receptor families. The chemokine receptors form a division of the leukocyte chemoattractant subfamily, which is part of the rhodopsin family of GPCRs.

CCR8 is 355aa in length, with a predicted Mol Wt of 41 kDa.

It has a 35-residue extracellular (N-terminal) sequence and a 51-residue cytoplasmic C terminal sequence. There are no predicted N-glycosylation sites.

Function

Chemokine receptors mediate the functions of chemokines, which have several roles as inducers of cell movement and activation.

CCR8 is the receptor for the chemokine SCYA1/I-309. It is thought to regulate monocyte chemotaxis and thymocyte apoptosis.

It also functions as a coreceptor with CD4 for HIV-1.

Knockout mice showed deficiency in the Th2 arm of the immune system, including deficits in Th2 cytokine (principally IL-4, IL-5, and IL-13) production and reduced eosinophil responses in vitro and in vivo.

Ligands

CCR8 binds the chemokine SCYA1/I-309.

It also functions as a coreceptor with CD4 for HIV-1.

Expression

CCR8 is expressed in the thymus, and by circulating NK cells, monocytes, and monocyte-derived dendritic cells.

CCR8 is also reported to be expressed by IL-10-producing regulatory T cells.

Gene Name	Entrez Gene#
CCR8	1237

Selected Monoclonal Antibodies

191704 (R&D Systems).

CDw199

Other Names

CCR9 (Chemokine, C-C motif, Receptor 9).

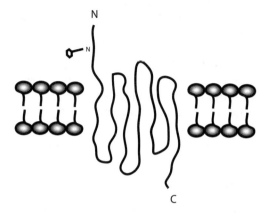

Molecular Structure

Chemokine receptors are G-protein-coupled receptors (GPCRs) consisting of an extracellular amino terminal, seven membrane-spanning regions, and a cytoplasmic carboxyl terminal. This structure is shared by several receptor families. The chemokine receptors form a division of the leukocyte chemoattractant subfamily, which is part of the rhodopsin family of GPCRs.

CCR9 is 369 amino acids long and has a predicted Mol Wt of 42 kDa.

Function

Chemokine receptors mediate the functions of chemokines, which have several roles as inducers of cell movement and activation.

CCR9 is the receptor for the chemokine SCYA25/TECK.

Binding of the ligand leads to an elevation of cytosolic $Ca2^+$ level, which in turn leads to a chemotactic response to the ligand.

CCR9 appears to confer homing properties to the small intestine on memory T cells.

Also functions as a coreceptor for HIV-1.

Ligands

CCR9 binds the chemokine SCYA25 also known as TECK.

Expression

Strong expression in thymus (by cDNA analysis) with weaker expression in bone marrow and spleen.

Expressed on a subset of memory T cells specialized for mucosal homing.

Gene Name	Entrez Gene#
CCR9	10803

Selected Monoclonal Antibodies

112509 (R&D Systems, Minneapolis).

CD200

Other Names

MRC, OX 2.

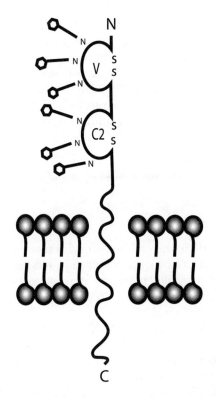

Molecular Structure

CD200 is a type I transmembrane glycoprotein and a member of the Ig superfamily.

The protein has one IgV-like domain followed by an Ig-like C2-set domain in the extracellular region, a single transmembrane domain and a short cytoplasmic domain with no known signaling motifs.

The transmembrane sequence is highly conserved between mouse and human, suggesting a functional role for the membrane-spanning sequence.

The extracellular region contains six potential N-glycosylation sites.

Mol Wt: 33 kDa.

Function

Binding of CD200 to OX2R on cells of macrophage/monocyte lineage results in the recruitment of SH2-containing inositol phosphatase (SHIP) to OX2R and leads to the downregulation of cellular activity.

CD200 knockout mice have a defect in the organization of the mesenteric lymph nodes, increased numbers of macrophages in the spleen, and enhanced endogenous macrophage activation. CD200 null mice display a rapid onset of experimental allergic encephalomyelitis (EAE) and have a greater susceptibility to collagen-induced arthritis and autoimmune diseases compared with wild-type mice.

In a model of nerve damage, microglia from CD200 knockout mice were found to be unusually highly activated.

Several diverse viruses including poxviridae and β- and γ-herpesviridae encode CD200 homologues, some of which have been shown to bind OX2R. This potentially provides these viruses with a means of downregulating myeloid cell activity.

Ligands

CD200 binds OX2R.

Expression

CD200 is expressed on B lymphocytes, thymocytes and T cells, neurons, some dendritic cells, and endothelium.

Gene Name	Entrez Gene#
CD200	4345

Selected Monoclonal Antibodies

MRC OX-104 (Barclay; Oxford).

CD201

Other Names

Endothelial protein C receptor (EPCR).

Molecular Structure

CD201 is a 221 amino acid, type I transmembrane glycoprotein that shares ca. 20% sequence homology with the MHC class 1/CD1 family of molecules.

A characteristic feature for members of the MHC class 1/CD1 family is the presence of a deep hydrophobic groove involved in antigen presentation, formed by two α helices that overlie an eight-stranded β-pleated sheet.

The structure of CD201 resembles that of CD1d but lacks the α3 domain of MHC class 1 molecules and does not associate with β2-microglobulin.

The CD201 groove is occupied by a tightly bound phospholipid whose presence is important for interaction with protein C even though the protein C binding site does not involve the groove and is distal from the cell membrane. It is speculated that the phospholipid is required to maintain the structure of CD201.

A soluble form of CD201 that retains its ligand binding capacity is constitutively shed into plasma. Susceptibility to cleavage is conferred by a genetic polymorphism in exon 4 of the CD201 gene. Thrombin and IL-1 have been shown to induce shedding of CD201 and accumulation of soluble CD201.

Mol Wt: Reduced, 50 kDa.

Function

CD201 is the endothelial cell receptor for protein C, which is involved in the regulation of coagulation and preventing tissue injury during inflammation and Gram-negative sepsis.

The presence of CD201 provides a five-fold enhancement of the thrombin–thrombomodulin mediated activation of protein C on endothelial cell surfaces.

CD201 and PAR1 mediate the anti-inflammatory activities of protein C, including the downregulation of P53 and inhibition of endothelial cell apoptosis.

Furthermore, the CD201-proteinase 3 complex can bind Mac-1 on activated neutrophils and inhibits tight adhesion of neutrophils to endothelium.

Protein C and CD201 inhibit disseminated coagulation and inflammation in Gram-negative sepsis.

Plasma soluble CD201 inhibits protein C activation in vitro, which suggests it may promote thrombosis in vivo.

A large increase in plasma concentration of soluble CD201 occurs during sepsis and Lupus erythematosus. In Lupus erythematosus, vascular dysfunction is associated with increased levels of soluble CD201

CD201 null mice exhibit early embryonic lethality.

Ligands

CD201 binds protein C, proteinase 3, and an unidentified phospholipid.

Expression

CD201 is broadly expressed on endothelium of arteries and capillaries in skin, lung, and heart. Expression of CD201 is much higher on large vessels particularly arteries.

Giant trophoblast cells at the foetomaternal boundary express CD201.

Applications

The presence of autoantibodies to CD201 has been shown to correlate with autoimmune fetal loss.

Patients expressing aberrant CD201 have an increased risk of venous and possibly arterial thrombosis.

Gene Name	Entrez Gene#
PROCR	10544

Selected Monoclonal Antibodies

RCR-42, RCR-252, RCR-49, RCR-121 (Fukudome; Japan).

CD202b

Other Names

TIE2, TEK.

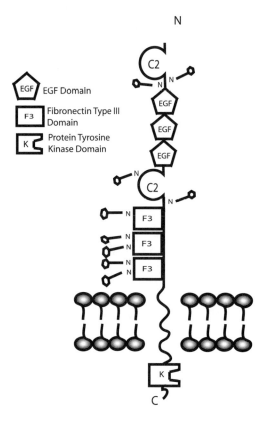

Molecular Structure

CD202b is a type 1 transmembrane protein and member of the receptor tyrosine kinase (RTK) family of proteins.

The extracellular region consists of a C-terminal Ig-like C2-type loop, three EGF-like domains followed by another Ig-like C2-type domain, and three fibronectin type III domains. There are nine potential N-linked glycosylation sites.

A single transmembrane domain of 25aa precedes the intracellular domain, which contains a split tyrosine kinase domain.

Mol Wt: Reduced, 145 kDa.

Function

CD202b is an endothelial-specific membrane receptor tyrosine kinase that plays a crucial role in the secondary stages of blood vessel formation, during which vessels remodel, mature, and form complex hierarchical networks.

Angiopoietin 1 binding to CD202b results in activation and phosphorylation of CD202b and the subsequent activation of the Akt signaling pathway. The Akt pathway is associated with increased survival of endothelial cells under stress conditions.

Angiopoietin 2 (Ang-2) /CD202b signaling appears to be involved in postnatal angiogenesis and vascular and lymphatic remodeling. In some in vitro studies, Ang-2 was found to antagonize the effects of the Ang-1/CD202b interaction.

CD202-deficient mice die during embryogenesis at approximately embryonic day 10.5 because of vascular defects, particularly vascularization and trabeculation of the heart. Aortas of CD200 null mice have fewer endothelial cells and significantly reduced numbers of smooth muscle cells. The smooth muscle cells also fail to properly attach to the blood vessel.

Some familial forms of defective venous formation are associated with point mutations in the tyrosine kinase domain of CD202b resulting in a constitutively active CD202b. These patients typically have large, thin-walled veins with fewer pericytes and smooth muscle cells than the equivalent normal veins.

The interaction of Ang-1 expressing sub-endosteal osteoclasts with CD202b+ hemopoietic stem cells (HSC) has been shown to maintain the HSC in an anti-apoptotic and quiescent state, ensuring their long ability to repopulate the bone marrow.

Ligands

CD202b binds angiopoietins Ang-1, Ang-2, and Ang-4.

Expression

CD202b is expressed by endothelial cells and a subset of CD34$^+$ hematopoietic stem cells.

Applications

CD202b is a useful marker of neo-angiogenesis in tumors and a prognostic indicator of metastasis in breast carcinoma and astrocytomas.

Increased CD202b expression correlates with increased tumor size and stage of differentiation of hepatocarcinomas.

Gene Name	Entrez Gene#
TEK	7010

Selected Monoclonal Antibodies

B-A37, B-D41, B-C38, B-F40, B-H38, B-B48 (Vermot-Desroches, Besancon).

CD203c

Other Names

E-NPP3, PDNP3, PD-1β.

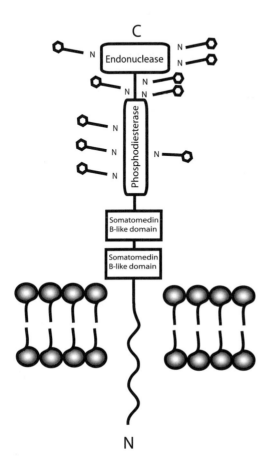

Molecular Structure

CD203c is a type II transmembrane protein and a member of a family of ecto-nucleotide pyrophosphatase/phosphodiesterase (E-NNP) enzymes that catalyze the hydrolysis of oligonucleotides, nucleoside phosphates, and NAD. Other family members include the plasma cell antigen ENPP1 (PC-1) and ENPP2 (autotaxin).

The 833 amino acid extracellular domain contains two membrane proximal cysteine-rich somatomedin B-like domains, an RGD cell adhesion motif, a phosphodiesterase-1 catalytic site, and an EF-hand motif as well as several potential N-linked glycosylation sites.

Mol Wt: Reduced, 130 and 150 kDa; unreduced, 270 kDa.

Function

CD203c is capable of cleaving a variety of phosphodiester and phosphosulfate bonds present in deoxynucleotides, nucleotide sugars, and NAD. Its role may be to clear extracellular nucleotides.

Expression

CD203c is expressed by basophils, mast cells, and CD34+ hematopoietic progenitor cells. CD203c mRNA is detectable in glioma cells, the prostate, and the uterus.

Applications

CD203c is strongly expressed by colon carcinoma cells and is associated with malignant subversion and invasion.

Gene Name	Entrez Gene#
ENPP3	5169

Selected Monoclonal Antibodies

97A6 (Bühring; Tübingen).

CD204

Other Names

MSR, SRA, Macrophage scavenger receptor.

Sr) Scavenger Receptor Cysteine Rich

Molecular Structure

CD204 is a trimeric type II transmembrane protein and a member of the type 1 class A scavenger receptor (SR) family.

The C-terminal extracellular domain consists of 375 amino acids and contains a 102-residue scavenger receptor cysteine-rich domain (SRCR), a collagen-like domain followed by an α-helical coiled coil, and a membrane-proximal spacer. There are 7 potential N-linked glycosylation sites.

The 50-residue cytoplasmic domain is the amino terminal portion of the protein.

Alternative mRNA splicing gives rise to three isoforms.

SR-A1 is the longest and fully functional transcript. SR-AII isoform is shorter than SR-AI, has an alternative 3′ end, and different C terminus but retains the ligand binding capacity.

SR-AIII lacks 65 residues compared with SR-AI and is not exported to the cell surface but remains trapped in the endoplasmic reticulum. When coexpressed with the other CD204 isoforms, it inhibits their function. This suggests a role for SR-AIII in regulating scavenger receptor activity in macrophages.

Mol Wt: 220 kDa (trimer).

Function

CD204 mediates the uptake of a wide variety of negatively charged macromolecules by mononuclear phagocytes and plays a role in both innate and acquired host defences and in the pathology of atherosclerosis and Alzheimer's disease.

CD204 knockout mice are more susceptible to endotoxic shock and infection by some bacterial pathogens such as *Listeria monocytogenes* and do not mount efficient T-cell responses.

Furthermore, CD204-deficient mice are less susceptible to diet-induced atherosclerosis than wild-type mice, suggesting a pro-atherogenic role for CD204.

Ligands

CD204 binds acetylated and oxidized low density lipoproteins, glycated collagen type IV, fibrillar bat-amyloid, advanced glycation end products, chondroitin sulphate, fucoidin, polyinosinic acid, apoptotic cells, myelin, and lipopolysaccharide and lipoteichoic acid.

Expression

CD204 is expressed by mononuclear phagocytes in various tissues, including macrophages, dendritic cells, Kupffer cells, and perivascular macrophages (Mato cells) in human brain. Expression of CD204 by microglia in normal adult human brain is controversial. However, in Alzheimer's disease, CD204 is strongly expressed by microglia associated with amyloid deposits and ischemic lesions.

Applications

Rare germline mutations in MSR1 gene are reported to be associated with an increased risk of prostate cancer.

Gene Name	Entrez Gene#
MSR1	4481

Selected Monoclonal Antibodies

MH1, SRA-C6, SRA-C5 (Takeya; Kumamoto).

CD205

Other Names

DEC-205, lymphocyte antigen 75.

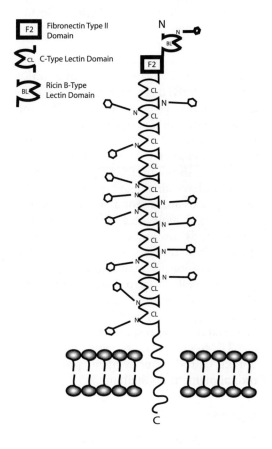

F2 Fibronectin Type II Domain

CL C-Type Lectin Domain

BL Ricin B-Type Lectin Domain

Molecular Structure

CD205 is a type I transmembrane glyco-protein and a C-type lectin receptor.

The 1639-residue extracellular domain contains a ricin B-type lectin domain, an N-proximal fibronectin type II domain followed by 10 C-type lectin domains, and has 14 potential N-linked glycosylation sites.

The protein has a 25 amino acid transmembrane region and 31-residue intracellular domain containing a tyrosine-based motif used to mobilize the clathrin-endocytic pathway.

Mol Wt: 205 kDa.

Function

CD205 is a recycled endocytic receptor that directs bound antigen from the extracellular space to antigen processing machinery for presentation by MHC class I.

Ligands

Binds a variety of antigens, presumably through carbohydrate-binding lectin domains.

Expression

CD205 is expressed by mature dendritic cells, Langerhans cells, thymic epithelium, and at low levels on T and B lymphocytes.

Gene Name	Entrez Gene#
LY75	4065

Selected Monoclonal Antibodies

DEC-205, MMRI-4 (Hart; Brisbane).

CD206

Other Names

Macrophage mannose receptor (MMR).

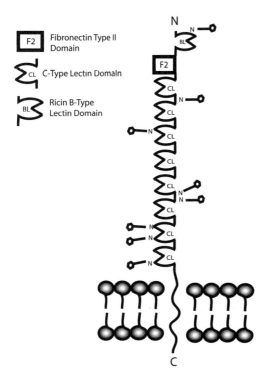

Molecular Structure

CD206 is a type I transmembrane glycoprotein. It is a mannose receptor with C-type lectin activity and belongs to the pattern recognition family of receptors.

The protein consists of an N-terminal, extracellular cysteine-rich domain, ricin B-type lectin domain, followed by a fibronectin type II-like domain and eight C-type lectin carbohydrate recognition domains (CRDs), a single transmembrane domain, and a short cytoplasmic tail.

Secreted forms can occur as a result of proteolytic cleavage.

Mol Wt: Unreduced, 162–175 kDa.

Function

CD206 acts as an antigen receptor that promotes endocytosis and phagocytosis by mononuclear phagocytes. Its function contributes to innate and acquired immunity.

The two distinct extracellular lectin-binding sites have different binding specificities.

The cysteine-rich domain is known to bind sulphated sugars present in anterior pituitary derived glycoprotein hormones and sulphated glycoforms of CD169, and CD45 found in specialized macrophage subpopulations. The second lectin-like activity is mediated by several of its eight CRDs and shows preference for branched sugars with terminal mannose, fucose, or N-acetyl-glucosamine. Binds oligo-mannose-containing molecules and mediates phagocytosis of microorganisms bearing these carbohydrates.

Presentation of mannose-bearing antigens to T cells in vitro is improved in the presence of cultured CD206[hi] dendritic cells. This suggests a role for CD206 in acquired immune responses.

CD206 may also be involved in the uptake of rod outer segment proteins by retinal pigment epithelium.

Ligands

The ligands of CD206 include lysosomal hydrolases, plant glycoprotein, yeast proteins, neoglycoproteins, chitin, bacterial cell wall molecules, viral glycoproteins, glycoforms of sialoadhesin (CD169) and CD45, lutropin, and chondroitin sulphate.

Expression

CD206 is strongly expressed by subsets of mononuclear phagocytes with the exception of circulating monocytes.

It is also expressed by hepatic and lymphatic endothelial cells, immature dendritic cells, retinal pigment epithelium, and mesangial cells.

Expression of CD206 is downregulated in the presence of IFN-γ but increased in the presence of IL-3 and IL-4.

Gene Name	Entrez Gene#
MRC1	4360

Selected Monoclonal Antibodies

3.29B1.10 (van Agthoven; Marseille); 19.2 (Johnson; San Jose); 190.BB3 (Lanzavecchia; Bellinzona); MR15-2 (Rijken; Leiden).

CD207

Other Names

Langerin.

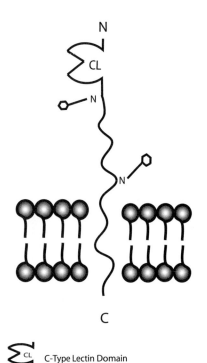

$$\sum_{CL}$$ C-Type Lectin Domain

Molecular Structure

CD207 is a 328-amino acid type II transmembrane and belongs to the C-type lectin family.

The protein has a single extracellular C-type lectin domain featuring an EPN motif with mannose-type specificity and two N-glycosylation sites in the membrane-proximal neck domain.

A proline-rich motif (WPREPPP) in the 43-residue cytoplasmic region is predicted to be a signal transduction site that associates with SH3 domain proteins involved in vesicular trafficking and cytoskeletal movement.

Mol Wt: 40 kDa.

Function

High level expression of CD207 induces membrane superimposition and zippering, which form pentilaminar organelles known as Birbeck granules (BG).

CD207 molecules are an integral part of BG. The mildly acidic content of BG suggests a role in antigen processing and the endocytic pathway.

Ligand binding results in rapid internalization of CD207. However, there is no evidence that CD207 is part of the classic antigen-processing pathway as it does not colocalize with MHC class II molecules.

In vitro studies of Langerhans Cells (LCs) have demonstrated that the mycobacterial antigen lipoarabinomannan is internalized in association with CD207 but is then loaded onto CD1a and presented to T cells.

There is one documented case of a CD207-deficient patient with LC lacking BG. No associated pathology was observed.

Similarly CD207 null mice are phenotypically identical to wild-type mice. LC from CD207$^{-/-}$ mice lack BG but can present antigen to CD4^{+} and CD8^{+} T cells.

Ligands

CD207 binds mannose-bearing glycoproteins and glycolipids found on microbial pathogens, including the gp120 protein of human immunodeficiency virus (HIV).

Expression

CD207 is expressed at high levels in immature LCs and decreases during LC maturation.

Applications

CD207 is a specific marker for Langerhans cells.

Selected Monoclonal Antibodies

DCGM-4 (Saeland; Dardilly).

Gene Name	Entrez Gene#
CD207	50489

CD208

Other Names

DC-LAMP.

Molecular Structure

CD208 is a 416-amino acid type I integral membrane protein and a member of the lysosomal associated membrane protein (LAMP) family.

The 381-residue extracellular region contains two potential disulphide bonds, 7 sites for N-glycosylation, and several O-glycosylation sites, with the potential for extensive O-glycosylation to form a mucin.

The short (10-residue) cytoplasmic sequence has a glycine-tyrosine based lysosome-targeting motif common to all LAMP members.

Mol Wt: 70–79 kDa.

Function

CD208 is transiently expressed by dendritic cells at the limiting membrane of MHC class II-containing intracellular compartments. With further maturation, CD208 becomes concentrated in perinuclear lysosomes.

The intracellular lysosome-targeting motif is recognized by adaptor complexes AP1, AP2, and AP3, which transport CD208 from the trans-Golgi network to the lysosomal membrane.

It is proposed that CD208 plays a role in sorting MHC class II-membrane associated molecules and therefore is important in the processing of exogenous antigen.

Expression

CD208 is expressed by activated dendritic cells and type II pneumocytes. Weak expression is detectable in testis and spleen.

Expression of CD208 is upregulated in carcinomas of oesophagus, colon rectum, ureter, stomach, breast, fallopian tube, thyroid, and parotid tissue but not in corresponding normal tissue from the same patients.

Applications

CD208 is a specific marker for mature dendritic cells.

Gene Name	Entrez Gene#
LAMP3	27074

Selected Monoclonal Antibodies

DC-LAMP (de Saint-Vis; Dardilly).

CD209

Other Names

DC-SIGN.

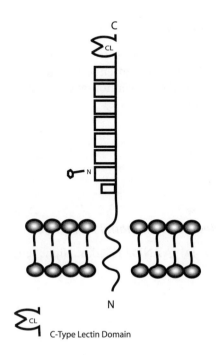

C-Type Lectin Domain

Molecular Structure

CD209 is a 404 amino-acid type II trans-membrane protein and a member of the C-type lectin family.

The extracellular domain consists of 346 amino acids and contains a C-terminal, 126-residue C-type lectin domain followed by 7 complete and 1 incomplete tandem repeats of an 11-residue sequence, which is predicted to mediate the formation of tetramers.

Tetramers of CD209 have been shown to aggregate into well-organized micro-domains on the dendritic cell (DC) surface.

The protein has 6 calcium binding sites, 1 potential N-linked glycosylation site, and 3 disulphide bonds.

The 21-residue transmembrane region is followed by the N-terminal 37 amino acid intracellular region that contains a di-leucine motif essential for internalization as well as a triacidic cluster and tyrosine-based motif, which are potential internalization motifs.

Mol Wt: 44 kDa (monomer).

Function

CD209 binds the mannose-like carbohydrate of ICAM-2 (CD102) and ICAM-3 (CD50).

Ligation of CD209 with CD50 on T cells appears to regulate DC-induced T-cell proliferation.

Interaction with CD102 may enable DC rolling and transendothelial migration from blood to tissues.

The EPN motif in the lectin domain predicts mannose-binding specificity, and it is probable that attachment of a variety of pathogens to immature DC is mediated via CD209 Ca^{2+}-dependent recognition of high mannose N-linked carbohydrates. This interaction leads to endocytosis of pathogens and their subsequent degradation in lysosomal compartments. CD209 is recycled to the cell surface, whereas pathogen-derived antigens are presented to resting T cells via MHC class II proteins to initiate an adaptive immune response.

Entry of pathogens via CD209 has the potential to enable transport of pathogens to other cellular targets as in the case of HIV. Not all endocytosed viral particles are degraded but can be presented to T cells mediating infection in trans.

Other pathogens use engagement of CD209 as a means of suppressing an immune response. Binding of secreted ManLAM from *M. tuberculosis* to CD209 triggers inhibitory signals and suppresses immune activation. Probiotic bacteria such as the *Lactobacillus* species have also been found to induce immune suppression through engagement of CD209.

Ligands

CD209 binds CD50 (ICAM-3) and CD102 (ICAM-2) with high affinity.

It also acts as a receptor for several pathogens, including all four serotypes of Dengue virus, Ebola virus, human cytomegalovirus, Hepatitis C virus E1/E2, gp120 protein of HIV-type1, *Leishmania pifanoi* amastigotes, *Mycobacterium tuberculosis* LPS, Lewis X antigen of *Schistosoma mansoni* and *Lactobacillus* species, *Helicobacter pylori* LPS, and mannose of *Klebsiella pneumoniae* LPS.

Expression

CD209 is expressed by immature dendritic cells (DC) at dermal and mucosal sites and on immature and mature DC in lymphoid tissues as well as a subset of $CD14^+$ DC-like cells found in blood, placental macrophages, and endothelial cells of placental vascular channels.

Applications

As the DC receptor for many pathogens, CD209 warrants attention as a potential target in the prevention and treatment of infection.

Gene Name	Entrez Gene#
CD209	30835

Selected Monoclonal Antibodies

AZN-D1, AZND2 (Figdor; Nijmegen).

CDw210a and b

Other Names

IL-10 receptor, IL-10RA and B, IL-10R1 and 2. CDw210b was also known as CRFB4 before its function was established.

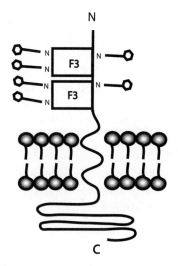

| F3 | Fibronectin Type III Domain |

Molecular Structure

CDw210a is a 578aa type I membrane glycoprotein member of the type II cytokine receptor family, with a calculated Mol Wt of 63 kDa. The extracellular region contains two fibronectin type III domains, and the cytoplasmic tail is 318 residues in length.

CDw210b is a 325aa type I membrane glycoprotein with a calculated Mol Wt of 37 kDa. Like CDw210a, CDw210b is a member of the type II cytokine receptor family with two type III fibronectin domains.

Mol Wt: 90–110 kDa.

Function

CDw210a binds IL-10 and initiates a signaling cascade through the JAK/STAT pathway.

IL-10 is primarily a downregulator of activation, inhibiting, for example, production of interferon γ by T cells, monocytes, and NK cells.

IL-10 also inhibits dendritic cell function, through binding to the IL-10 receptor on dendritic cells. On the other hand, IL-10 can costimulate proliferation of NK cells induced by IL-2.

CDw210b does not bind IL-10 but is essential for signal transduction.

Ligands

CDw210a binds IL-10 with high affinity, and the soluble extracellular portion of CDw210a can bind IL-10. CDw210b does not bind IL-10 directly, but the functional receptor appears to be a tetramer containing two molecules of CDw210a and two of CDw210b.

CDw210b binds IL-22 directly with high affinity, and binding has been reported to IL-26, IL-28A and B, and IL-29.

Expression

T and B cells, NK cells, monocytes, and macrophages.

Applications

Cytomegalovirus (CMV) and Epstein–Barr virus (EBV) make viral IL-10 analogs that bind to the IL-10 receptor.

Gene Name	Entrez Gene#
IL10RA	3587
IL10RB	3588

Selected Monoclonal Antibodies

CDw210a: E10FT (van Agthoven; Marseille); 3FT (Johnson; San Diego).
CDw210b: No antibodies assigned yet.

CD212

Other Names

IL-12 receptor β1-chain.

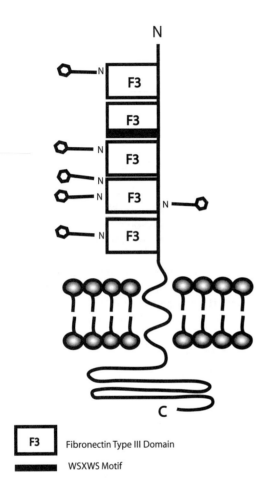

F3 — Fibronectin Type III Domain

▬ — WSXWS Motif

Molecular Structure

Type I transmembrane protein of the cytokine receptor family, with strong homology to CD130.

The extracellular region contains five fibronectin type III-like domains, with the second containing a WSXWS motif required for proper folding and surface expression.

The extracellular region bears six potential N-glycosylation sites.

The 25-residue membrane-spanning sequence is followed by a 92aa cytoplasmic sequence that includes a box-1 motif, essential for activation of the JAK signaling pathway.

Function

CD212 dimerizes with the IL-12 receptor β-2 chain to form the functional IL-12 receptor. IL-12 directs immune responses preferentially toward Th1-type responses.

Defects in CD212 are associated with an inherited susceptibility to mycobacterial disease known as familial disseminated atypical mycobacterial infection.

Ligands

Binds IL-12, but requires dimerization and complexing with the IL-12Rβ2 protein to give high affinity binding.

Expression

Reportedly expressed by Th1 but not by Th2 cells. However, also reported on 72% of blood lymphocytes, indicating the majority of T cells express the receptor.

Also expressed on NK cells and some B-cell lines.

Applications

Identification of Th1 cells. Deficiency in this gene is associated with severe infection by Mycobacteria and other organisms, including some that are weakly pathogenic in normal individuals. On the other hand, CD212 has been reported to be upregulated in the chronic inflammatory disease Crohn's disease.

Gene Name	Entrez Gene#
IL12RB1	3594

Selected Monoclonal Antibodies

IL-12RB.44 (van Agthoven; Marseille); 2.4E6 (Johnson; San Diego).

CD213α1 and 2

Other Names

IL-13 receptor α1- and α2-chains.

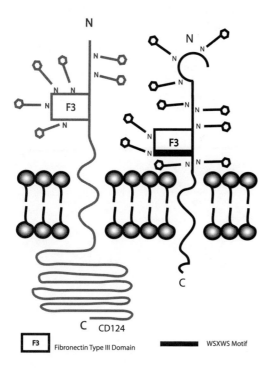

Molecular Structure

Both receptors chains are type I trans-membrane molecules with a membrane proximal fibronectin type III domain. The molecules are classified as members of the hematopoietin family.

Human CD213α1 is 406 residues long, with a 324-residue extracellular domain, a 23aa membrane-spanning sequence, and 50 residues in the cytoplasm. Human CD213α2 is 354aa in length, with 317 residues in the extracellular domain, 20 in the membrane-spanning sequence, and 17 in the intracellular region. The molecules show only 27% homology with each other, whereas homology to the murine equiva-lent chains is much higher (74% and 59% for CD213α1 and 2, respectively).

Function

IL-13 can bind cells through either a com-bination of CD213α1 and CD124 or through CD213α2. In both cases, the common γ chain appears to be necessary for signaling.

IL-13, through its receptors, regulates inflammation and immunity. IL-13 inhibits the production of pro-inflammatory cyto-kines and chemokines from monocytes and macrophages.

IL-13 also upregulates several cell-surface molecules, including MHC class II and CD23, and it can act as a costimulus for B-cell proliferation and Ig synthesis and class switching.

IL-13 is not restricted in function to lym-phocytes and has activities on progenitor cells and endothelial cells. IL-13 can induce airway hyper-responsiveness and may have a role in asthma.

CD213α1 is also a necessary component for IL-4-induced signal transduction in the type II IL-4 receptor system. The cyto-plasmic domain of CD213a1 has been implicated in murine B-cell activation and differentiation.

Ligands

IL-13, a cytokine that has structural and functional similarities with IL-4. CD213α1 binds IL-13 with low affinity, but together with CD124 (IL-4 R α chain) can bind IL-13 with high affinity. CD213α2 binds IL-13 with high affinity.

Expression

CD213α1 is broadly expressed in hema-topoietic tissue, the nervous system, and other tissues.

CD213α2 is expressed by cord blood lymphocytes, a subset of peripheral blood lymphocytes, and immature dendritic cells.

Applications

CD213a1 antibody has potential as a therapeutic target for glioma, whereas soluble CD213α2 can reverse IL-13 airway hyperresponsiveness, suggesting a possible use in asthma.

Gene Name	Entrez Gene#
IL13RA1	3597
IL13RA2	3598

Selected Monoclonal Antibodies

CD213α1: B-K19, B-B30 (Clement; LC).
CD213α2: B-F30, B-P16 (Clement; LC).

CD217

Other Names

IL-17 receptor.

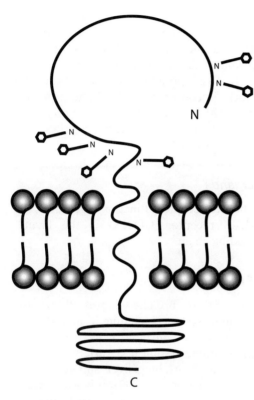

Molecular Structure

Type I transmembrane glycoprotein with no homology with other cytokine receptors. The DNA sequence predicts a 866-residue protein with 293aa in the extracellular domain (including 6 N-glycosylation sites), a 21aa membrane-spanning region, and 525 residues intracellular domain.

Mol Wt: 128–158 kDa.

Function

CD217 binds IL-17 with low affinity, but IL-17 can stimulate cells at low concentrations, suggesting that there is another component to the receptor, which converts the interaction to high affinity.

IL-17 is a pro-inflammatory cytokine, with a variety of effects, including stimulation of IL-6 production.

Ligands

Binds IL-17 with low affinity.

Expression

Broad tissue distribution. Cord blood lymphocytes, peripheral blood lymphocytes, and thymocytes.

Applications

IL-17 is associated with inflammatory disease, including rheumatoid arthritis. Control appears to be at the level of the cytokine rather than at the receptor, because the receptor is expressed widely and equally in health and disease.

Gene Name	Entrez Gene#
IL17R	23765

Selected Monoclonal Antibodies

M204 (Fanslow; Seattle).

CD218a, CD218b

Other Names

CD218a: IL-18 receptor α, IL-1RRP.

CD218b: IL-18 receptor β, IL-18 receptor accessory protein (IL18RAP).

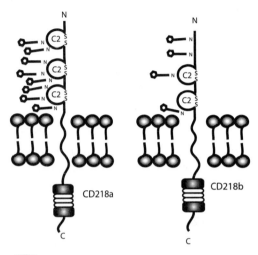

CD218a

CD218b

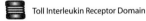
Toll Interleukin Receptor Domain

Molecular Structure

CD218a is a type 1 membrane glycoprotein 523 residues in length. The predicted molecular weight (including the 18aa signal sequence) is 62 kDa.

The extracellular region contains three Ig-C2-type domains and eight potential N-glycosylation sites.

The 21aa membrane-spanning region is followed by a 191aa cytoplasmic sequence, which includes a TIR (Toll/IL-1Receptor like) homologous region. TIR regions are involved in interaction with cellular signaling molecules.

CD218b is a type 1 membrane glycoprotein 580 residues in length. The predicted molecular weight (including the 19aa signal sequence) is 68 kDa.

The extracellular region contains two Ig-C2-type domains and four potential N-glycosylation sites.

The 21aa membrane-spanning region is followed by a 222aa cytoplasmic sequence, which in common with CD218a includes a TIR.

Function

The two receptor chains together bind IL-18 and mediate the activities of IL-18 through the activation of NFκB.

IL-18 is a proinflammatory cytokine that works in concert with IL-12 and promotes both Th1 and Th2 immune responses.

IL-18 induces interferon γ production and activates NK cells.

Ligands

The two receptors function together as the IL-18 receptor. CD218a is the ligand-binding chain.

Expression

CD218a is broadly expressed in the immune system, including T and B cells, NK cells, and myeloid cells, and outside the immune system in a variety of tissues, including heart, lung, liver, and gut.

Information on CD218b is less certain, but it appears to show a more selective distribution, being seen on activated but not on resting helper T cells.

Gene Name	Entrez Gene#
IL18R1	8809
IL18RAP	8807

Selected Monoclonal Antibodies

CD218a: H44 (BD Biosciences; San Jose); B-C41 (Diaclone; Besancon)

CD218b: B-P28, B-K31 (Diaclone; Besancon).

CD220

Other Names

Insulin receptor.

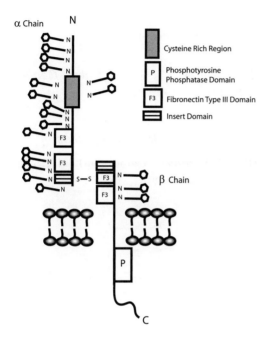

α Chain

Cysteine Rich Region

P Phosphotyrosine Phosphatase Domain

F3 Fibronectin Type III Domain

Insert Domain

β Chain

Molecular Structure

CD220 is a dimeric transmembrane protein and a member of the tyrosine kinase receptor family.

After removal of the signal peptide, the CD220 precursor is post-translationally cleaved into the α and β chains that are then covalently linked.

CD220 is heavily glycosylated and is estimated to contain 58–64kDa of carbohydrate. There are 16 confirmed and 2 potential sites for N-linked glycosylation, 14 on the α chain and 4 on the β chain. O-linked glycosylation has been found on the β chain only.

Ligand binding is mediated by the three fibronectin type III domains (FnIII-1, -2, and -3) present in the C-terminal portion of the CD221 extracellular domain. FnIII-2

has a large insert domain (ID) of between 120–130 residues.

The α chain comprises 731 amino acids, is entirely extracellular, and has two large homologous domains L1 and L2, each comprising 120 residues, separated by a cysteine-rich region containing 25–27 cysteines in three repeating units.

The L1 and L2 domains contain four internal repeats that result in an α-helix/β-strand/turn/β-strand secondary structure.

The FnIII-1 and a portion of FnIII-2 and the ID comprise the C-terminal portion of the α subunit.

The β chain is a transmembrane tyrosine kinase and consists of an extracellular region of 194 residues, which includes a portion of the ID and FnIII-2 domains and the entire FnIII-3 domain, a 26-residue transmembrane region, and a 408-residue C-terminal cytoplasmic region containing a tyrosine kinase domain.

Alternative RNA splicing gives rise to two isoforms: HIR-B or long isoform and HIR-A or short isoform. The longer isoform includes a 122aa sequence at the C terminal of the α chain that is missing in the short isoform.

Mol Wt: Unreduced, 400kDa, 135-kDa α chain and 95-kDa β subunit.

Function

CD220 is the cellular receptor for insulin. Binding of insulin leads to autophosphorylation of the kinase domain and subsequent phosphorylation of insulin receptor substrates and the induction of complex signaling cascades within the cell. It plays a critical role in stimulating glucose uptake.

The insulin/CD220 complex is internalized into endosomes where the acidic environment causes insulin to dissociate and be degraded, thereby preventing insulin-driven re-phosphorylation and enables endosomally associated tyrosine phosphatases to dephosphorylate CD220.

The receiver is then recycled to the cell surface.

Mutation in CD220 leads to insulin-resistant diabetes mellitus, which can vary in severity. Insulin-resistance type A is associated with ancanthosis nigricans, hirsutism, and hyperandrogenism. Rabson–Mendehall syndrome is a severe insulin resistance characterized by severe insulin-resistant diabetes mellitus with pineal hyperplasia and somatic abnormalities. Defects in CD220 are also responsible for the most severe form of insulin-resistance syndrome known as Donohue syndrome or leprechaunsim, which is characterized by interuterine and postnatal growth retardation and death in early infancy. Both Rabson–Mendehall and Donohue syndromes are autosomal recessive inherited disorders.

Ligands

CD220 binds insulin and IGF-2. The short isoform has a higher affinity for insulin than the long isoform.

Expression

CD220 is ubiquitously expressed.

Gene Name	Entrez Gene#
INSR	3643

Selected Monoclonal Antibodies

IR83-7 (Siddle; Cambridge); IR18-44 (Siddle; Cambridge).

CD221

Other Names

IGF I receptor, type I IGF receptor.

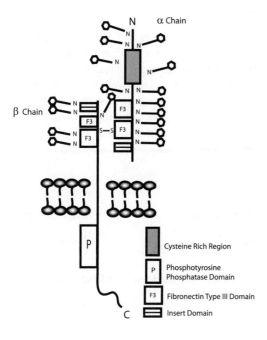

Molecular Structure

CD221 is a heterotetrameric transmembrane tyrosine kinase and thus belongs to the tyrosine kinase receptor family (which includes CD220 and the orphan insulin receptor-related receptor IRR) and is related to the epidermal growth factor receptor (EGFR) family.

CD221 is synthesized as a 180-kDa (1367 amino acids) pre-pro-receptor. After cleavage of the 30 amino acid signal peptide, the polypeptide is further cleaved by furin protease between residues 708 and 711 to produce an α chain (residues 1–707) and a β chain (residues 712–1337).

The α and β chains are disulphide-linked to yield the mature heterotetrameric receptor.

The extracellular portion of CD221 has 16 potential N-linked glycosylation sites, 11 in the α chain and 5 in the β subunit.

Ligand binding is mediated by the three fibronectin type III domains (FnIII-1, -2, and -3) present in the C-terminal portion of the CD221 extracellular domain. FnIII-2 has a large insert domain (ID) of between 120 and 130 residues.

The α chain is entirely extracellular and has two large homologous domains L1 and L2, each comprising 120 residues, separated by a cysteine-rich region containing 25–27 cysteines in three repeating units.

The L1 and L2 domains contain four internal repeats that result in an α-helix/β-strand/turn/β-strand secondary structure.

The FnIII-1 and a portion of FnIII-2 and the ID comprise the C-terminal portion of the α subunit.

The β chain has an extracellular region of 195 residues, which includes a portion of the ID and FnIII-2 domains and the entire FnIII-3 domain.

The β subunit has a single transmembrane sequence (residues 906–929) followed by a 408-residue intracytoplasmic region containing the tyrosine kinase domain between residues 973 and 1229.

The tyrosine kinase domain is flanked by a juxtamembrane region and a C-terminal tail that contains phosphotyrosine binding sites for signaling molecules.

Mol Wt: α subunit 135 kDa; β subunit 90 kDa.

Function

CD221 is the receptor for insulin-like growth factors IGF-I and IGF-II. Activation of CD221 results in the initiation of complex signaling cascades, and the pathways involved remain unclear.

IGF-1 activated CD221 mediates mitogenic signaling and in vitro provides anti-apoptotic signaling in response to a wide range of apoptotic stimuli.

When over-expressed and ligand-activated, CD221 acts as a cellular oncogene and participates in cellular transformation. Over-expression of CD221 and its ligands have been observed in a variety of human tumors.

CD221 knockout mice are born weighing less than half the normal weight and die soon after birth. The development of CD221 null mice is first affected between days 11 and 12.5 of embryogenesis. The growth retardation is characterized by widespread organ hypoplasia as a result of an extended transition through all stages of the cell cycle.

Embryonic fibroblasts derived from CD220 knockout mice cannot be transformed by a variety of viral and cellular oncogenes. Restoration of CD221 expression reverses this effect.

Ligands

CD221 binds IGF-I (insulin-like growth factor 1) with high affinity as well as IGF-II and insulin.

Expression

CD220 is widely expressed among fetal and postnatal tissues and is over-expressed in many tumors.

Applications

The receptor gene is subject to imprinting. Biallelic expression is associated with Beckwith–Wiedemann syndrome.

CD221 expression levels are a prognostic indicator in some tumors, such as breast and gastric cancers, and the receptor is a therapeutic target for the development of anti-tumor agents.

Gene Name	Entrez Gene#
IGF1R	3480

Selected Monoclonal Antibodies

IGFR17-69 (Siddle; Cambridge).

CD222

Other Names

Mannose-6-phosphate receptor, insulin-like growth factor II receptor, IGF2R.

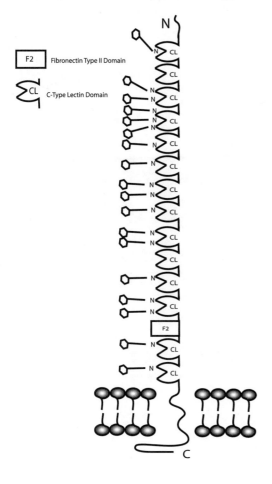

Molecular Structure

CD222 is a type I transmembrane protein and a lectin.

The protein has 15 homologous domains; the thirteenth domain has a 43 amino acid insert that is a fibronectin-like collagen-binding domain.

CD222 has 19 potential N-linked glycosylation sites but not all are used. It is palmitoylated and undergoes cytoplasmic serine phosphorylation.

Cleavage of the extracellular portion gives rise to a soluble form found in human and bovine serum.

The CD222 gene has several microsatellite regions that have a higher frequency of mutation.

A tetranucleotide deletion/insertion polymorphism occurs in the 3′ untranslated region.

In addition to the 250-kDa form of CD222, an incompletely glycosylated form of 230 kDa occurs in monocytes.

Mol Wt: Reduced, 300 kDa; unreduced, 250 kDa.

Function

CD222 binds and internalizes a variety of extracellular ligands and directs them to lysosomes and sorts newly synthesized M6P-containing lysosomal enzymes.

As the receptor for LAP (see Ligands), CD222 plays a role in regulating TGFβ activity.

Latent TGFβ is activated by a complex of CD222, CD87, and plasminogen.

CD222 is used as an anchor by acid lysosomal hydrolases during degradation of pericellular and extracellular proteoglycans.

Activation of CD222 by IGF-II stimulates increased insulin secretion by pancreatic β cells.

Proliferin-induced angiogenesis is mediated by CD222. *Chlamydia pneumoniae* uses CD222 as a receptor and as a means of infecting endothelial cells.

Mutated forms of CD222 are found in many tumor types, leading to the suggestion that CD222 may be a tumor suppressor oncogene.

CD222 null mice exhibit organ and skeletal abnormalities and die at birth.

Ligands

CD222 binds IGF-II, TGFβ latency associated peptide (LAP), leukemia inhibitory factor (LIF), proliferin, prorenin, Herpes simplex virus, retinoic acid, plasminogen, thyroglobulin, and mannose-6-phosphate (M6P)-containing proteins.

Expression

CD222 is expressed ubiquitously. A truncated form is present in human and bovine serum.

Gene Name	Entrez Gene#
IGF2R	3482

Selected Monoclonal Antibodies

MEM-238 (Horejsi; Videnska); MEM-240 (Horejsi; Videnska).

CD223

Other Names

LAG-3 (Lymphocyte activation gene 3).

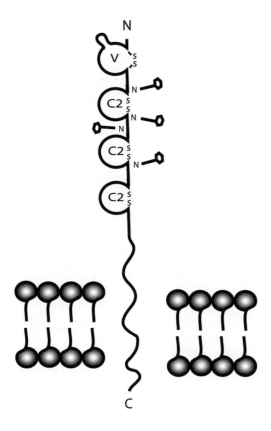

Molecular Structure

CD223 is a type I transmembrane protein that bears homology with CD4 and is a member of the Ig gene superfamily. Comparison of the gene structure and co-localization on the human chromosome indicates CD223 and CD4 are derived from a common ancestor.

To bind ligands, CD223 needs to be dimerized or oligomerized at the cell surface.

The extracellular domain contains an N-terminal V-set Ig-like domain (D1) of approximately 140 amino acids, which includes a 30 amino acid extra-loop and an unusual disulphide linkage followed by 3 C2-set Ig-like domains (D2–D4).

D1 binds the non-polymorphic region of MHC class II molecules and is required for LAG-3 dimerization.

The transmembrane region is followed by a short intracellular region containing a conserved KIEELE motif and a repeated EP motif at the C terminus, which binds LAG-3 associated protein (LAP).

The protein has four N-glycosylation sites.

Three alternatively spliced variants have been described: LAG-3V1 (D1–D2, soluble, 36 kDa); LAG-3V2 (D1–D3, membrane bound, 61 kDa; and LAG-3V3 (D1–D3, soluble, 52 kDa)

Mol Wt: Reduced, 70 kDa; unreduced, 70 kDa.

Function

CD223 binds MHC class II and regulates the homeostatic expansion of T cells in vivo.

It associates with the TCR–CD3 complex and negatively regulates TCR-mediated signal transduction. This function is mediated via the cytoplasmic KIEELE motif.

In contrast to its negative regulatory effects, LAG-3 induced MHC class II signaling in monocytes and dendritic cells leads to activation of the antigen-presenting cell and induction of cytotoxic T cells and CD4 Th1 responses in mice coadministered soluble LAG-3 and antigen.

LAG-3-deficient mice show normal immune responses, but as the mice age, they have increased T-cell numbers compared with wild-type mice.

Ligands

CD223 binds MHC class II molecules with high affinity.

Expression

CD223 is expressed by activated T cells and NK cells. Expression is stronger on CD8$^+$ cells than CD4$^+$ cells.

Gene Name | Entrez Gene#

LAG3   3902

Selected Monoclonal Antibodies

17B4 (Triebel; Villejuif).

CD224

Other Names

γ-glutamyl transferase, GGT, γ-glutamyl transpeptidase.

Molecular Structure

CD224 is a heterodimeric type II transmembrane protein, an ectoenzyme, and a member of the threonine peptidase family.

The enzyme consists of a 380 amino acid heavy chain and a 189 amino acid light chain, which are translated from a single mRNA. The precursor protein is then proteolytically cleaved into the two subunits and assembled into the active enzyme.

The catalytic site for hydrolysis of glutathione comprises residues from both subunits.

There are between five and six potential N-linked glycosylation sites on the heavy chain and two on the light chain. The enzyme also contains hexoses, hexosamines, and sialic acid residues.

Alternative RNA splicing gives rise to three isoforms: GGT1, GGT2, and GGT3. GGT3 is thought to be an inactive form.

Soluble CD224 is detectable in blood and is the result of proteolytic cleavage. The enzyme is also present in lung surfactant, but as this form retains its signal anchor transmembrane region, it is not a product of proteolytic cleavage.

Mol Wt: Reduced, 55–60-kDa heavy subunit, 21–30-kDa light subunit; unreduced, 100 kDa.

Function

CD224 is an integral part of the γ-glutamyl cycle and is essential for maintaining the homeostatic balance of the cellular redox.

It binds the γ-glutamyl portion of GSH, cleaves glutamate from GSH, or transfers the γ-glutamyl residue to another amino acid or dipeptide. The remaining cysteinyl-glycine is further broken down by membrane-associated dipeptidases into individual amino acids, which can be transported into the cell and used for de novo GSH synthesis.

CD224 can convert leukotriene C4 to leukotriene D4 and has been shown to convert the nitric oxide donor, GSNO, to the unstable form s-nitrocysteinyl-glycine, thereby providing nitric oxide to the cell.

CD224 associates with CD37 and CD53 and has been found to noncovalently associate with CD19, CD21, CD81, and CD82 in a B lymphoblastoid cell line.

CD224 knockout mice have elevated levels of glutathione and glutathione conjugates in plasma and urine but decreased levels in tissues. Furthermore, their growth is retarded, they are sexually immature, develop cataracts, and often die between 8 and 12 weeks of age.

The effects of CD224 deficiency can be partially reversed by feeding the mice N-acetyl cysteine.

Autosomal recessive defects in GGT1 are a cause of human glutathionuria.

Expression

CD224 is strongly expressed by renal tubular cells, pancreas, epididymis, seminal vesicles, vascular endothelium, alveolar epithelial type II cells, and nonciliated bronchiolar Clara cells.

Expression of CD224 is found in peripheral blood macrophages and a subset of B cells. Resting CD45RA$^+$ T cells have little or no expression of CD224; however, expression is upregulated upon activation and remains elevated on CD45RO$^+$ T cells.

Very low to no expression is detectable in normal hepatocytes; however, CD224 activity is increased during liver disease.

Applications

CD224 activity is increased in liver disease.

Gene Name	Entrez Gene#
GGT1	2678

Selected Monoclonal Antibodies

158 (Colonna; Basel).

CD225

Other Names

Leu-13, interferon-induced transmembrane protein 1.

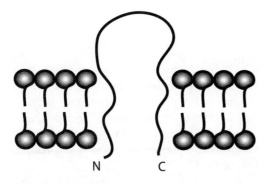

Molecular Structure

CD225 is a transmembrane protein consisting of 125 amino acids and belongs to the interferon-inducible transmembrane protein family.

It coprecipitates with TAPA-1.

The sequence predicts two transmembrane regions, but the structure of the molecule is not well characterized.

Mol Wt: 17 kDa.

Function

CD225 is a component of the CD21/CD19/TAPA-1 complex involved in B-cell activation and control of cell growth.

It noncovalently associates with the tetraspan molecule, CD81, in cells of multiple lineages.

The specific role of CD225 is not clear.

Expression

CD225 is expressed by leukocytes and endothelial cells.

Applications

CD225 is a pan endothelial cell marker.

Gene Name	Entrez Gene#
IFITM1	8519

Selected Monoclonal Antibodies

AntiLeu13 (Evans; Buffalo).

CD226

Other Names

DNAM-1, PTA-1,TLiSA1.

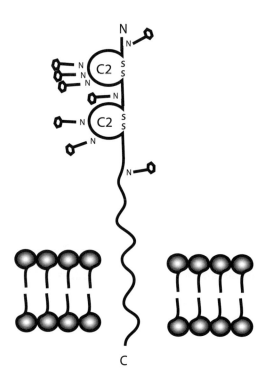

Molecular Structure

CD226 is type I transmembrane glyco-protein and a member of the Ig gene superfamily.

The 232 amino acid extracellular portion contains 2 Ig-like C2-type domains and has 8 potential N-linked and 3 O-linked glycosylation sites.

The 25-residue transmembrane region precedes a 61 amino acid intracellular domain that contains predicted phosphorylation sites for protein kinase C and casein kinase II and Fyn.

Phosphorylation of the cytoplasmic serine 329 residue is required for the interaction of CD226 with CD11a/CD18 (LFA-1).

A 50-kDa soluble form of CD226 is detectable in normal serum and culture supernatant of activated T cells.

Mol Wt: 65 kDa.

Function

CD226 can mediate the attachment of transfected cells to presumed ligand-bearing cells in a process independent of divalent cations but regulated by serine 329 phosphorylation by protein kinase C.

It associates with LFA-1 and actin-binding protein 4.1 G.

Intact antibody and F(ab′)2 fragments of some mAb and polyclonal antibodies to CD226 inhibit the generation of cytotoxic T lymphocytes (CTL) in mixed lymphocyte culture and the restimulation of allergenic cytotoxic T-cell clones.

MAb to CD226 can initiate platelet activation and aggregation in a process dependent on the Fc receptor and protein kinase C activation.

Depending on the experimental conditions, some CD226-specific mAb can trigger NK- or T-cell-mediated cytotoxicity and cytokine production, or they can inhibit the cytolysis of some tumor target cells.

Ligands

CD155 and CD112 are the ligands for CD226.

Expression

Expression of CD226 is induced upon activation on NK cells, platelets, monocytes, and a T-cell subset.

Applications

CD226 expression is increased in patients with some autoimmune diseases and viral infections.

Selected Monoclonal Antibodies

PX11 (Lanier; San Francisco).

Gene Name	Entrez Gene#
CD226	10666

CD227

Other Names

MUC 1, Mucin 1, DF3 antigen, H23 antigen, episialin, peanut reactive urinary mucin (PUM), polymorphic epithelial mucin (PEM), epithelial membrane antigen (EMA).

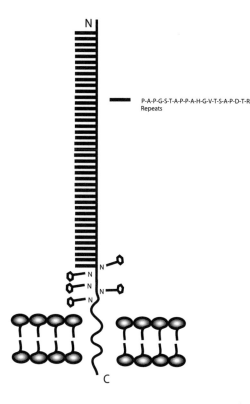

P-A-P-G-S-T-A-P-P-A-H-G-V-T-S-A-P-D-T-R.
Repeats

Molecular Structure

MUC 1 is a large type I transmembrane glycoprotein and belongs to the epithelial mucin family.

The 1255 amino acid protein is cleaved into a C-terminal extracellular peptide and a membrane-bound subunit in the endoplasmic reticulum. The two subunits reassemble to form a heterodimer but can dissociate or be proteolytically cleaved, leading to shedding of the extracellular peptide.

The non-membrane bound subunit has a large tandem repeat domain that is highly polymorphic, varying from 21 to 125 repeats between individuals. Each repeat consists of 20 amino acids rich in serine, threonine, and proline residues and is potentially O-glycosylated at positions 5, 6, 14, 15, and 19. The density of O-glycosylation varies between tissues and with cell differentiation. For example, lactation-associated CD227 is typically 50% glycosylated, but for CD227 produced by various breast carcinomas, the extent of glycosylation is often >90%.

The mucin also has several potential N-linked glycosylation sites.

Although the molecular weight of the core protein ranges from 120 to 225 kDa, the mature glycosylated protein can vary between 250 and 700 kDa.

The mucin is concentrated at the apical surface of epithelial cells and forms a rigid extended structure that protrudes 200–500 nm above the cell surface, exceeding the distance spanned by most cell-surface proteins.

The cytoplasmic portion consists of 72 amino acids and contains 7 tyrosine residues and a potential clathrin-mediated endocytic signal sequence. Several signaling molecules such as β-catenin, Grb/SOS, associate with the cytoplasmic tail.

Alternative RNA splicing gives rise to several isoforms, two of which, isoforms 5 and 9, are secreted.

Isoform 1 and 7 undergo transphosphorylation.

Mol Wt: Reduced, 25 kDa (membrane associated subunit) and 220–700 kDa (variably glycosylated extracellular subunit).

Function

The elongated rigid structure of CD227 extends well beyond other molecules in the glycocalyx and has a protective role by lubricating and hydrating the cell surface, protecting against degradative enzymes and sterically inhibiting microbial access to the cell wall.

CD227 cytoplasmic domain is highly conserved across species and is involved in multiple signal transduction pathways.

Expression of CD227 in epithelial tissues can be highly variable in response to steroid hormones and cytokines.

Very high cell-surface expression can sterically hinder both cell–cell and cell–extracellular matrix interactions and may be a factor that promotes metastasis of tumor cells.

Malignant transformation often leads to CD227 over-expression of altered RNA splice variants with aberrant glycosylation and loss of apical restriction. In some cases, a tumor-specific epitope may arise that may trigger an immune response.

Ligands

CD227 binds CD54, selectins, and CD169.

Expression

CD227 is strongly expressed by epithelia of glands and ducts as well as goblet and columnar cells in epithelial tissues. High level expression occurs in most human adenocarcinomas.

Widely expressed at varying levels among leukocytes and at high levels by many myelomas.

Applications

CD227 is a prognostic marker in adenocarcinoma.

Gene Name	Entrez Gene#
MUC1	4582

Selected Monoclonal Antibodies

BC-3 (Golder; Sydney).

CD228

Other Names

Melanotransferrin, p97.

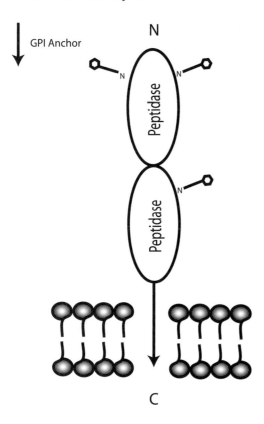

Molecular Structure

CD228 is a GPI-anchored melanoma associated sialoglycoprotein and is a member of the transferrin superfamily.

The gene resides in the same region of human chromosome 3 as members of the transferrin family.

The protein consists of two nonfunctional peptidase S60 domains and has three potential N-linked glycosylation sites.

Alternative RNA splicing gives rise to two transcript variants. Variant 1 is the full-length protein, whereas variant 2 is divergent in the central coding region producing a frameshift that results in a truncated and distinct C-terminus.

Mol Wt: Reduced, 80–90 kDa.

Function

CD228 is presumed to have iron transport function; however, the importance of this function has not been demonstrated. Each subunit binds a single atom of iron with high affinity.

In vitro studies have demonstrated CD228 can interact with pro-UPA and plasminogen and stimulate plasminogen activation.

CD228 influences the migration capacity of endothelial cells and the cell motility and invasiveness of melanoma cells.

Ligands

pro-UPA and plasminogen bind CD228.

Expression

CD228 is strongly expressed in melanomas, stem cells, microglia, intestine, and smooth muscle. It is also found in certain fetal tissues, placenta and umbilical cord, and sweat gland ducts and shows low level expression in leukocytes.

Applications

Expression of CD228 by reactive microglia is increased five- to six-fold in Alzheimer's disease.

Gene Name	Entrez Gene#
MF12	4241

Selected Monoclonal Antibodies

96.5 (Hellstrom; Seattle).

CD229

Other Names

Ly9.

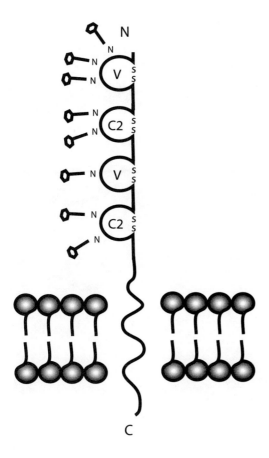

Molecular Structure

CD229 is a type I transmembrane glyco-protein and belongs to the CD150 (SLAM) family (see also CD150, CD84, and CD244) within the Ig gene superfamily.

The 407 amino acid extracellular region contains 2 V-set and 2 C2-set Ig domains arranged (N)-V-C2-V-C2. There are 8 potential N-linked glycosylation sites.

The cytoplasmic region consists of 179 amino acids and contains 16 threonine residues, 17 serine residues, and 8 tyrosines. Two copies of the tyrosine-based motif (TV/IYxxV/I) at Y558 and Y581 are critical for binding of SLAM-associated protein (SAP) in T cells or the EAT-2 protein in B cells.

Y606 is involved in Grb2 association, and Y470 is involved in AP-2 recruitment.

Alternative RNA splicing gives rise to three isoforms.

Mol Wt: 120 kDa.

Function

The function of CD229 is unclear; however, its homophilic binding may contribute to adhesion between T cells and B cells. The protein has been shown to relocate to the contact area between T cells and B cells during antigen-dependent immune synapse formation.

Recent studies have indicated CD229 can negatively regulate TCR signaling.

CD229 is the only member of the CD150 family whose trafficking is regulated by its association with m2, a subunit of the clathrin-associated adaptor complex-2 (AP-2), and its rate of internalization is controlled by Grb2.

MAb-mediated cross-linking of CD229 induces rapid internalization and degradation within lysosomes. This process is further enhanced by coligation of antigen receptors on T and B cells.

Ligands

CD229 participates in homophilic binding.

Expression

CD229 has the most restricted expression of the SLAM receptors and is primarily expressed by T and B cells and thymocytes.

Although CD229 expression is negligible in normal cells of myeloid lineage, a significant number of acute myeloblastic leukemias express CD229.

Gene Name	Entrez Gene#
LY9	4063

Selected Monoclonal Antibodies

Hly9.1.25 (Engel; Barcelona); Hly9.1.84 (Engel; Barcelona).

CD230

Other Names

Prion protein, PrPc, PrPsc (abnormal form).

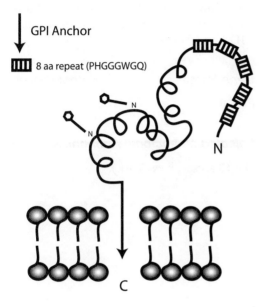

GPI Anchor

8 aa repeat (PHGGGWGQ)

N

N

N

C

Molecular Structure

CD230 is a glycophosphatidylinositol (GPI) anchored sialoglycoprotein.

The mature protein consists of 209 amino acids that in the normal form of the protein (PrPc) are arranged in an α helix with a folded domain between residues 90 and 231 and a flexible, disordered N-terminal region incorporating a series of octapeptide repeat units.

The protein has two N-linked glycosylation sites.

CD230 can be shed from the cell surface by cleavage at the GPI-anchor or is endocytosed and recycled to the cell surface.

Two transmembrane forms have been described that differ in their topology. The C-terminus of CD230 may be directed toward the ER lumen (CtmPrP) or be in the opposite orientation (NtmPrP). The NtmPrP form is not glycosylated, and the GPI-anchor is not added.

PrPc can be endoproteolytically cleaved between residues 110 and 111 giving rise to a peptide known as C1.

Polymorphism is associated with the five tandem repeat sequence, which is unstable, and insertions and deletions within these repeats are associated with prion diseases.

The abnormal and disease-associated isoform, PrPsc, is distinguishable from the normal form by its β-sheet structure, altered glycosylation, relative insolubility, partial resistance to proteinase K digestion, and greater tendency to form aggregates. PrPsc undergoes endoproteolytic cleavage at a different position to PrPc, and a larger peptide (C2) is cleaved.

The generation of unique transmissible spongiform encephalopathies (TSE) strains appears to be related to the available pool of CD230, the strain type of PrPsc, and the infected cell.

Mol Wt: Reduced, 30–40 kDa.

Function

The function of CD230 is unknown, but several studies have implicated CD230 in binding copper, oxidative stress homeostasis, maintenance of circadian rhythms, and cell signal transduction.

Ligation leads to signal transduction through caveolin-1 to the tyrosine kinase Fyn.

The prion protein PrPsc is associated with transmissible spongiform encephalopathies (TSE). Transmission of prions in humans appears to be related to use of infected blood or blood products, cannibalism, or ingestion of prion-infected beef. Prions are delivered to the central nervous system via macrophages, dendritic cells, and T and B cells.

PrPsc aggregates bind cholesterol-rich phospholipid membranes and are cytotoxic. The characteristic neuropathology associated with prion disease includes spongiform degeneration of neurons, severe astrocytic gliosis, and amyloid plaque formation, which is physiologically manifested as progressive dementia and myoclonic seizures and may include insomnia, abnormally high cortical function, and cerebellar and corticospinal disturbances. The disease is fatal within 3–12 months of the onset of symptoms.

CD230 knockout mice remain healthy and have a normal lifespan. Unlike wild-type mice, CD230$^{-/-}$ mice do not become diseased when exposed to prions from any source.

Ligands

CD230 displays homotypic binding.

Expression

CD230 is ubiquitously expressed; however, the abnormal isoform PrPsc is predominantly associated with central nervous system tissue.

Applications

Infective agent in transmissible spongiform encephalopathies, including human Creuzfeldt–Jacob Disease (CJD). Mutations in Prp gene associated with familial CJD-like disorders.

Gene Name	Entrez Gene#
PRNP	5621

Selected Monoclonal Antibodies

3F4 (Kascsac; New York).

CD231

Other Names

TALLA-1, TM4SF2.

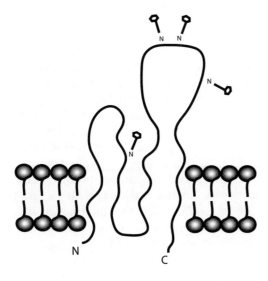

Molecular Structure

CD231 is a glycoprotein belonging to the TM4SF or tetraspanin family (see also CD9, CD37, CD53, CD63, CD81, CD82, and CD151).

The protein consists of 244 amino acids with 4 putative transmembrane domains and 2 extracellular domains.

The 2 extracellular loops are of unequal size. The smaller loop, EC1, consists 16 amino acids and has 1 potential N-glycosylation site.

The second and larger loop, EC2, consists of 101 amino acids and has 4 N-glycosylation sites.

The 2 extracellular loops are divided by an EC1-proximal transmembrane region of 19 amino acids followed by 11 intracellular residues and an EC2-proximal transmembrane region of 26 amino acids.

The N-terminal cytoplasmic tail comprises 16 amino acids and is separated from EC1 by a transmembrane domain of 24 residues.

The C-terminal intracellular domain consists of 15 amino acids and contains a tyrosine-based internalization motif (YxxF) common to all tetraspanins. A 21 amino acid transmembrane region separates the C-terminal cytoplasmic tail from EC2.

Mol Wt: Reduced, 32–45 kDa; unreduced, 150 kDa.

Expression

CD231 is expressed in neuronal tissue and strongly expressed in neuroblastoma and T-type acute lymphoblastic leukemia.

Applications

CD231 mutations are involved in X-linked mental retardation in which TM4SF2 is inactivated by a translocation or point mutations.

CD231 is a specific marker, and CD231 antibody is a potential therapeutic agent in the treatment of T-cell acute lymphoblastic leukemia.

Gene Name	Entrez Gene#
TM4SF2	7102

Selected Monoclonal Antibodies

SN1 (Seon; New York); AZM30.3 (Azorsa; Bethesda).

CD232

Other Names

VESPR, Plexin C1.

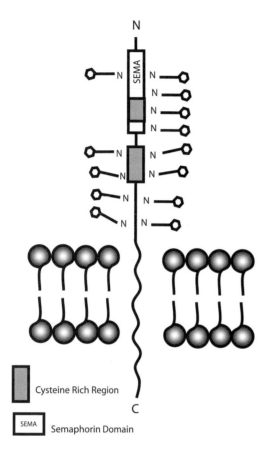

Cysteine Rich Region

SEMA Semaphorin Domain

Molecular Structure

CD232 is a 1568 amino acid transmembrane glycoprotein and a member of the plexin family.

The structure of CD232 is typical of plexins consisting of an extracellular domain containing short cysteine-rich motifs termed Met-related sequences (MRS), glycine- and proline-rich motifs, and a semaphorin domain.

Mol Wt: 200 kDa.

Function

The function of CD232 is unclear. It is the receptor for virally encoded semaphorin (A39R) and semaphorin 7A.

A39R ligation of murine CD232 inhibits integrin-mediated dendritic cell adhesion and chemokine-induced migration in vitro.

$CD232^{-/-}$ mice display normal dendritic cell (DC) development and normal T-cell responses in vitro. However, in vivo migration of $CD232^{-/-}$ DC to lymph nodes and T-cell responses were somewhat reduced compared with wild-type DC.

Ligands

CD232 binds semaphorin 7A (CD108) and the poxvirus semaphorin-like protein A39R.

Expression

CD232 is expressed by monocytes, dendritic cells, and some B cells and neuronal cells.

Gene Name   Entrez Gene#

PLXNC1   10154

Selected Monoclonal Antibodies

M460 (Spriggs; Seattle).

CD233

Other Names

Band 3, AE1, anionexchanger 1, Diego blood group antigen.

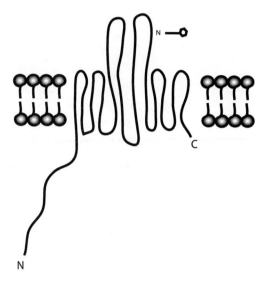

Molecular Structure

CD233 is an integral membrane protein that belongs to the anion exchanger family.

It comprises two structurally and functionally distinct domains.

The N-terminal domain is located in the cytoplasm and has attachment sites for several red cell proteins, including band 4.2, glyceraldehyde 3-phosphate dehydrogenase, hemoglobin, and ankyrin, a component of the red cell cytoskeleton.

The C-terminal domain contains 12–14 transmembrane regions and mediates the stilbene disulphonate-sensitive anion exchange transport.

The C-terminal cytoplasmic tail binds carbonic anhydrase II.

CD233 forms tetramers in the presence of ankyrin; otherwise, it is dimeric.

A single N-linked glycosylation site occurs at Asn 642.

A truncated form of CD233 arising from the use of an alternative promoter in exon 3 is expressed in the kidney.

CD233 is highly polymorphic.

Mol Wt: Reduced, 95–110 kDa; unreduced, 95–110 kDa.

Function

The N-terminal cytoplasmic domain of CD233 links the erythrocyte membrane to the underlying spectrin/actin-cytoskeleton. This assists in maintenance of the integrity of the erythrocyte.

The C-terminal membrane domain mediates exchange of most monovalent anions, but chloride and bicarbonate anions are the predominant substrates. This enables erythrocytes to transport carbon dioxide from the tissues to the lungs.

High anion transport activity and optimal surface expression of CD233 requires the presence of CD235a.

CD233 is involved in clearance of aging and damaged erythrocytes by mediating their recognition by macrophages.

Children with South East Asian ovalocytosis have very rigid red blood cells due to a heterozygous deletion of CD233 and are less susceptible to infection with *Plasmodium falciparum*.

The truncated isoform expressed in the kidney is responsible for transporting bicarbonate out of the cell and into the blood in exchange for plasma chloride. This function plays a part in maintaining whole-body pH homeostasis.

The Diego blood group system comprises 18 blood group antigens all derived from polymorphism in the CD233 gene. Incompatibility of the two most prevalent Diego antigens is a common cause of hemolytic disease of the newborn among indigenous Americans.

CD233 knockout mice have high mortality and severe hemolytic anemia due to unstable erythrocytes. A similar phenotype occurs in band 3 null cattle.

Expression

CD233 is very strongly expressed on erythrocytes (over 1 million copies per cell).

Expression of the truncated form occurs on the basolateral membrane α-intercalated cells of the distal tubules and collecting ducts of the kidney.

Gene Name	Entrez Gene#
SLC4A1	6521

Selected Monoclonal Antibodies

55 (von dem Borne; Amsterdam); BRIC71, BRIC90 (Spring; Bristol); naM127-3A11 (Blanchard; Nantes).

CD234

Other Names

DARC, Fy-glycoprotein, Duffy blood group antigen.

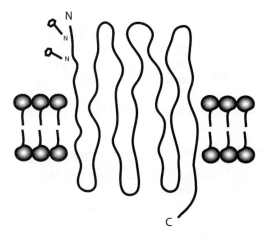

Molecular Structure

CD234 is a 7-transmembrane domain acidic glycoprotein of the chemokine receptor superfamily.

The protein has two N-linked glycosylation sites on the extracellular amino terminal domain and four conserved Cys residues (at the N-terminus, and the first, second, and third extracellular loops) that are paired to form disulfides that help to stabilize the protein.

Mol Wt: Predicted, 36 kDa.

Function

The Duffy antigen binds several chemokines of both the CC and the CXC families with high affinity. Its physiological role might be to act as an intracellular sink to modulate the level of these proinflammatory molecules.

Plasmodium vivax and *Plasmodium knowlesi* use CD234 to bind and enter erythrocytes. Some individuals, usually African or African Americans, carry a mutation in the FY gene that causes a T to C substitution in the promoter region. This substitution disrupts binding of the h-GATA-1 erythroid factor and prevents expression of CD234 in erythroid cells but not in nonerythroid cells. The absence of CD234 renders the red cells resistant to infection with *P. vivax* and *P. knowlesi*.

CD234 knockout mice are healthy and display no developmental abnormalities but lack CXC and CC chemokine binding activity. When challenged with LPS, a significant increase in inflammatory infiltrates is seen in both the lung and the liver of CD234 null mice compared with wild-type mice. However, when toxic doses of LPS were given, a decrease in inflammatory infiltrates was found in the lungs and peritoneal cavity. Other aseptic antigens induced different responses.

Ligands

CD234 is a binding protein for some chemokines, including IL-8, MGSA, RANTES, and MCP-1, and is the human receptor for the malarial parasites *Plasmodium vivax* and *Plasmodium knowlesi*.

Expression

CD234 is expressed by erythrocytes, capillary endothelial cells, Purkinje cells of the cerebellum, and epithelial cells of the kidney collecting duct, lung, and thyroid.

Gene Name   Entrez Gene#

DARC   2532

Selected Monoclonal Antibodies

64-4A8, CBC-512 (Uchikawa; Tokyo); NaM185-2C3 (Blanchard; Nantes).

CD235a, CD235b

Other Names

CD235a: Glycophorin A, PAS-2, sialoglycoprotein A, MN sialoglycoprotein.

CD235b: Glycophorin B, PAS-3, sialoglycoprotein δ, ss-active sialoglycoprotein.

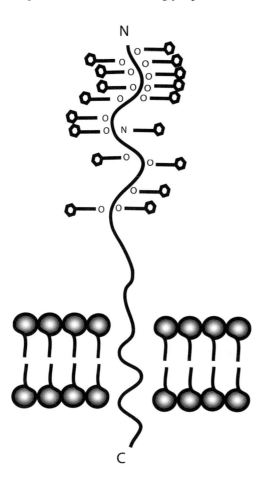

Molecular Structure

CD235a is a type I membrane protein of 131 amino acids that forms α-helical dimers in lipid bilayers.

The CD235a gene (GPA) and the gene encoding Glycophorin B (GPB) are located in tandem on chromosome 4 and are highly homologous and prone to deletions, gene conversions, and crossovers.

The N-terminal extracellular region of CD235a consists of 72 amino acids and has 15 O-glycosylation sites and 1 N-glycosylation site.

The C-terminal cytoplasmic region consists of 36 amino acids.

The 23 amino acid transmembrane domain mediates the noncovalent dimerization of the protein not only within the cell membrane but also in artificial bilayers, in the presence of several detergents and SDS-PAGE conditions.

Mol Wt: Dimer, 65.7 kDa; Monomer, 28–31 kDa.

CD235b is a highly glycosylated type I membrane protein and belongs to the glycophorin A family.

The N-terminal extracellular domain consists of 72 amino acids and has 11 O-linked glycosylation sites. The transmembrane region has 22 residues, and the C-terminal cytoplasmic domain consists of 10 amino acids.

Mol Wt: 20 kDa.

Function

CD235a is the major glycoprotein of the erythrocyte cell membrane, present at 1 million copies per cell.

It is thought to prevent cell agglutination.

The absence of CD235 in humans is not associated with pathology. However, the absence of CD235a alters the structure and anion transport properties of CD233. Anion transport was lower in cells lacking CD235a, and optimal surface expression of CD233 requires CD235a and vice versa.

CD235a carries the M/N blood group antigens.

It is used as by *Plasmodium falciparum* merozoites to attach to erythrocytes as part of a sialic acid-dependent invasion process.

CD235b is a minor sialoglycoprotein of the erythrocyte cell membrane, which carries S/s blood group antigens.

Ligands

CD235a binds CD170, influenza virus, and the erythrocyte binding antigen (EBA-175) of *Plasmodium falciparum*.

Expression

CD235a is expressed by hematopoietic stem cells and is present on all erythroid cells.

CD235b is present on erythrocytes.

Applications

CD235a is a useful marker to study the developmental biology of hematopoietic progenitor cells.

Glycophorin A (GPA) somatic-cell-mutation assay is used to assess mutation events at the GPA M/N locus in bone marrow stem cells.

Gene Name	Entrez Gene#
GYPA	2993
GYPB	2994

Selected Monoclonal Antibodies

11E4B-7-6 (van Agthoven; Marseille); AME-1 (van der Schoot; Amsterdam); BRIC 127, BRIC 163, BRIC256, (Spring; Bristol); HI264 (De-Cheng Shen; China); NaM10-6G4, NaM13-4E4 (Blanchard; Nantes); P.Mac7/4E9 (Blancher; Toulouse). The following react with CD235a and b: HIR2 (DeCheng Shen; China); 14D5D3F7H8, 18D2B1 (Chin; New Jersey); OSK29 (Yamaono; Osaka).

CD236, CD236R

Other Names

Glycophorin C/D (CD236), glycophorin C (CD236R), Gerbich blood group antigen.

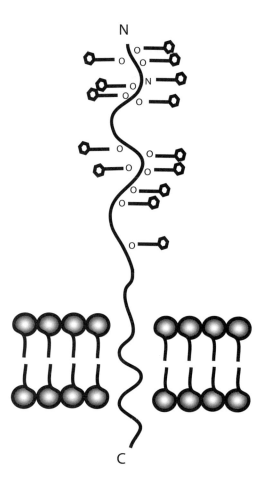

Molecular Structure

CD236 is a type III membrane sialoglycoprotein and glycophorin but bears little homology with the major erythrocyte glycophorins A and B (CD235a and b).

The protein has an extracellular domain of 57 amino acids and contains 14 O-linked and 1 N-linked glycosylation sites.

The transmembrane region consists of 24 residues, and the intracellular portion of 47 amino acids contains the band 4.1 binding region between residues 61 and 77.

Glycophorin D is a truncated form of glycophorin C arising from the use of an alternative translation initiation site at codon 30. As a result, glycophorin D lacks the first 21 N-terminal amino acids, has fewer glycosylation sites, and lacks the N-terminal oligosaccharide chain.

Mol Wt: Glycophorin C, 40 kDa; glycophorin D, 30 kDa.

Function

Together with membrane protein p55, CD236 is linked to the cytoskeletal protein band 4.1. This interaction assists in maintaining the mechanical stability and deformability of erythrocytes.

CD236 acts a receptor for *Plasmodium falciparum* merozoites.

The CD236 gene, GYPC, encodes the Gerbich (Ge) blood group antigens. Naturally occurring anti-Ge antibodies have been found but are not clinically significant. However antibodies to Ge antigens have been associated with transfusion reactions and mild hemolytic disease of the newborn.

Individuals with the Leach phenotype are devoid of CD236 due to a deletion in GYPC gene and have erythrocytes that are elliptocytic and less deformable. Furthermore, these individuals are less susceptible to infection with *Plasmodium falciparum*. No pathology is associated with this phenotype.

The Yussef (Yus) phenotype is due to a 57 base pair deletion in exon 2 of GYPC.

The rare Webb (Wb) antigen arises from a base substitution at nucleotide 23, which results in insertion of an asparagine residue instead of a serine during protein synthesis and loss of a glycosylation site.

Similarly, the Duch (Dh) antigen is the result of a C to T transition at nucleotide 40 and the replacement of leucine by phenylalanine.

Ahonen (Ana) is a rare blood group antigen found only on glycophorin D positive cells.

Ligands

P. falciparum erythrocyte binding protein 2 (PfEBP-2) binds CD236.

Expression

Glycophorin C and glycophorin D are both present on erythrocytes numbering about 135,000 copies/cell and 50,000 copies/cell, respectively. Both glycophorins are detectable in a broad range of other tissues (including kidney, breast, thymus, and adult liver) although at lower levels and with different glycosylation.

Gene Name	Entrez Gene#
GYPC	2995

Selected Monoclonal Antibodies

BGRL 100, BRAC1 (Spring; Bristol); NaM19-3C4 (Blanchard; Nantes). (these antibodies react with Glycophorin C and D.)

Antibodies specific for C are BRIC10, BRAC48, BRIC4 (Spring; Bristol); NaM10-7G11 (Blanchard; Nantes); RB8 (Ikeda; Sapporo).

CD238

Other Names

Kell blood group antigen.

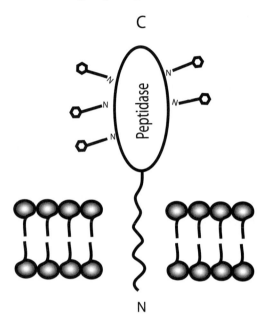

Molecular Structure

CD238 is a type II transmembrane glyco-protein and is classified as a member of the small neprilysin (M13) family of zinc metalloproteases, which includes CD10.

The 722 amino acid protein has an extra-cellular domain of 665 residues with 5 N-linked glycosylation sites.

The signal-anchor transmembrane region consists of 20 amino acids, and the intracellular portion of the protein has 47 amino acids.

There are between 4000 and 18,000 mol-ecules per erythrocyte.

CD238 shows a high level of polymor-phism, which results in at least 22 Kell blood group antigens, some of which have distinct racial prevalence.

Kell antigens are linked by a single disul-phide bond to the XK-protein (32–37 kDa), which traverses the cell membrane 10 times.

Mol Wt: Reduced, 93 kDa; unreduced, 115–200 kDa.

Function

CD238 acts as a zinc endopeptidase that cleaves a large intermediate precursor of endothelin-3 (big endothelin-3) to its bioactive form. One biological function of Endothelin-3 is as a potent vasoconstrictor.

Kell antibodies can suppress outgrowth of BFU-E as well as CFU-GM and CFU-Meg from purified CD34$^+$ cells. This is consistent with clinical findings in alloim-munized pregnancies where the anemia found in the fetus or neonate is due to the suppression of erythropoeisis as well as to antibody-induced hemolysis.

The McLeod phenotype is characterized by loss of the XK-protein and resultant decreased expression of CD238 and is asso-ciated with late onset muscular dystrophy. Erthrocytes from individuals with the McLeod phenotype have a unique mor-phology and are known as ancanthocytes.

CD238 null individuals are found at very low frequency in all populations and are healthy, which implies alternative pathways exist for endothelin-3 activation. KEL null erthryocytes have normal morphology.

Expression

CD238 is expressed on erythroid cells, testis, and at low levels in brain, heart, and skeletal muscle.

Gene Name	Entrez Gene#
KEL	3792

Selected Monoclonal Antibodies

BRIC 107, BRIC 18, BRIC 68, BRIC 203 (Spring; Bristol); 64-3C7, CBC-117 (Uchikawa; Tokyo); NaM18-5A11 (Blanchard; Nantes); RB16, Fuj30 (Ikeda; Sapporo). (Note: Some of these antibodies detect polymorphisms.)

CD239

Other Names

B-CAM, lutheran glycoprotein.

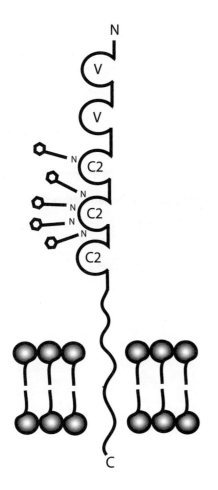

Molecular Structure

CD239 is a type I transmembrane glyco-protein and is a member of the Ig gene superfamily.

CD239 is a carrier of the Lutheran blood group, which comprises at least 18 antigens.

The processed protein consists of 597 amino acids.

The extracellular region comprises 516 residues arranged into 2 N-terminal V-type Ig-like domains followed by 3 C2-type Ig-like domains and has 5 potential N-linked glycosylation sites.

The transmembrane span consists of 21 residues.

The 60 amino acid cytoplasmic region contains a membrane proximal RK motif for spectrin binding in erythrocytes as well as a dileucine motif that is responsible for basolateral targeting of the Lu isoform of CD239 in epithelial cells.

CD239 is phosphorylated at Ser 596, 598, and 621 by glycogen synthase kinase 3 β, casein kinase II, and PKA, respectively.

Mutation of Ser 621 abolishes PKA phosphorylation and impairs binding of CD239 to laminin.

Alternative RNA splicing of intron 13 gives rise to two isoforms that differ in the length of the cytoplasmic tail. The Lu(v13) isoform is the shorter form, which lacks 40 C-terminal amino acids including potential phosphorylation sites and the SH3-binding site. Lu(v13) is identical to the basal cell adhesion molecule (B-CAM).

Mol Wt: Lu isoform, 85 kDa; Lu(v13)/ B-CAM, 78 kDa.

Function

CD239 isoforms are adhesion molecules and appear to mediate intracellular signaling in certain disease states. Lu and B-CAM bind erythroid spectrin. This association with the red cell skeleton is not considered to have structural significance because of the relatively low density of CD239 molecules in the erythrocyte membrane and may have more to do with signaling.

CD239 is over-expressed in sickle cells, and PKA-mediated phosphorylation of the Lu isoform plays a critical role in laminin binding. This may contribute to the vaso-occlusion that occurs in sickle cell disease by allowing sickle cells to bind laminin on endothelial cells under flow conditions.

Normal epidermis expresses CD239 weakly if at all, but strong expression is induced in malignant basal cells and squamous cells, particularly at the basal surface of tumor nests. Laminin expression is upregulated around the tumor nests, potentially enabling progression of epithelial cell tumors.

Ligands

CD239 binds the α5-chain of laminin 10/11.

Expression

CD239 is expressed by erythrocytes and by the basal layer of epithelia and vascular endothelium and is over-expressed by sickle cells. It has wide tissue distribution, with the highest expression occurring in the pancreas and the lowest in brain tissues.

Expression of CD239 is upregulated after malignant transformation of some cell types, including basal and squamous cells and ovarian carcinomas.

Applications

CD239 is a marker of malignant transformation in basal and squamous cell carcinomas and is over-expressed in ovarian carcinomas.

Gene Name	Entrez Gene#
LU	4059

Selected Monoclonal Antibodies

BRIC 221, BRIC 224 (Spring; Bristol); LU-4F2 (Telen; Durham, NC).

CD240CE

Other Names

Rh blood group system, Rh30CE.

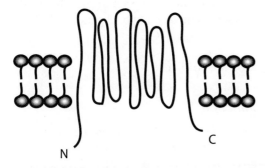

Molecular Structure

CD240CE is a member of the Rh blood group system that incorporates 49 well-defined antigens (see CD240D, CD24DCE, and CD241).

There are 100–200,000 copies per cell.

It is a non-glycosylated protein consisting of 417 amino acids with 12 transmembrane helical domains and 6 cysteine residues, of which 3 are palmitoylated.

The N and C termini are cytoplasmic.

The RHCE gene encodes the Cc and Ee antigens and is closely linked to and shares a high level of homology with RHD, which encodes the RhD antigens (CD240D).

CD240CE and CD240D proteins differ by between 34 and 37 amino acids depending on the CcEe phenotype.

The E (Rh3) and e (Rh5) phenotypes arise from a single amino acid substitution at position 226 in the fourth extracellular loop; Pro226 corresponds to E (Rh3) and Ala226 to e (Rh5).

Similarly the basis of C (Rh2) and c (Rh4) phenotype is a result of a single amino acid substitution at position 102 in the second extracellular loop; Ser 103 corresponds to C (Rh2) and Pro103 to c (Rh4).

Mol Wt: 30 kDa.

Function

CD240CE is closely associated in the erythrocyte membrane with the Rh-associated glycoprotein (RhAG), CD242 (ICAM-4, LW), CD47, and glycophorin B (CD235b).

The core of the Rh complex is thought to consist of two Rh subunits and two RhAG (CD241) subunits to which CD47, CD235b, and LW associate noncovalently.

The function of this large complex is unclear, but there is evidence to suggest CD240D assists in maintaining the mechanical properties of the erythrocyte by association with ankyrin-R of the red cell skeleton.

Expression

CD240CE is expressed by mature erythrocytes and erythroid progenitors at the CFU-E stage.

Gene Name	Entrez Gene#
RHCE	6006

Selected Monoclonal Antibodies

703-7, CBC-107, HIR021 (Uchikawa; Tokyo); Cyn2-4D5 (Blancher; Toulouse).

CD240D

Other Names

RhD, RH1, Rh30D, Rhesus blood group antigen.

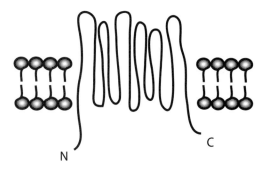

Molecular Structure

CD240D is a member of the Rh blood group system which incorporates 49 well-defined antigens (see CD240CE, CD24DCE, and CD241).

It is a non-glycosylated protein consisting of 417 amino acids with 12 transmembrane helical domains and 5 cysteine residues. Two of these cysteines are intracellular and palmitoylated.

There are 100–200,000 copies per cell.

The N and C termini are cytoplasmic.

The RHD gene encodes the D antigen, which consists of at least 30 epitopes.

RHD is closely linked to and shares a high level of homology with RHCE, which encodes the C/c and E/e antigens (see CD240CE).

CD240D and CD240CE proteins differ by between 34 and 37 amino acids depending on the CcEe phenotype.

Partial D phenotypes arise from missense mutations in RHD encoding single amino acid substitutions or when sections of RHD are replaced with the equivalent region from RHCE.

In Caucasians, the D-negative phenotype is almost always the result of homozygosity for a deletion of the entire RHD gene. In Africans, the D-negative phenotype can be due to deletion of RHD, the presence of an RHD pseudogene (RHDψ), or the presence of a hybrid gene RHD-CE-Ds (see CD240DCE).

Mol Wt: 30 kDa.

Function

CD240D is closely associated in the erythrocyte membrane with the Rh-associated glycoprotein (RhAG), CD242 (ICAM-4, LW), CD47, and glycophorin B (CD235b).

The core of the Rh complex is thought to consist of two Rh subunits and two RhAG (CD241) subunits, to which CD47, CD235b, and LW associate noncovalently.

The function of this large complex is unclear, but there is evidence to suggest CD240D assists in maintaining the mechanical properties of the erythrocyte by association with ankyrin-R of the red cell skeleton.

CD240D is the most immunogenic and clinically important antigen of the Rh system. In the Caucasian population, the major antigenic polymorphism of the Rh system is almost always associated with the presence or absence of the RHD gene (12–18% of Caucasians; 5% of black Africans are D-negative; and almost 100% of people from the Far East are D-positive).

Expression

CD240D is expressed by mature erythrocytes and erythroid progenitors at the CFU-E stage.

Applications

The RhD phenotype of an individual has implications in alloimmune transfusion reactions and hemolytic disease of the newborn.

Gene Name **Entrez Gene#**

RHD   6007

Selected Monoclonal Antibodies

AB5, BRAD3, BRAD5, (Spring; Bristol); HMR49 (Ikeda; Sapporo).

CD240DCE

Other Names

Rh30D/CE.

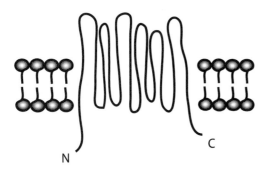

Molecular Structure

CD240DCE is a member of the Rh blood group system, which incorporates 49 well-defined antigens (see CD240CE and CD240D).

It is a non-glycosylated protein consisting of 417 amino acids with 12 transmembrane helical domains.

CD240DCE is the product of a hybrid gene RHD-CE-D that is created when a portion of the RHD gene ranging from one exon to several exons has been replaced by the equivalent region of RHCE. This results in a hybrid protein that stably exists in the red cell membrane but lacks many D epitopes.

RHD-CE-D genes often give rise to partial D phenotypes as well as to the D-negative RHD-CE-Ds gene.

Mol Wt: 30 kDa.

Function

CD240DCE is closely associated in the erythrocyte membrane with the Rh-associated glycoprotein (RhAG), CD242 (ICAM-4, LW), CD47, and glycophorin B (CD235b).

The core of the Rh complex is thought to consist of two Rh subunits and two RhAG (CD241) subunits, to which CD47, CD235b, and LW associate noncovalently.

The function of this large complex is unclear, but there is evidence to suggest CD240DCE assists in maintaining the mechanical properties of the erythrocyte by association with ankyrin-R of the red cell skeleton.

Expression

CD240DCE is expressed by mature erythrocytes and erythroid progenitors at the CFU-E stage.

Gene Name	Entrez Gene#
CD240D	See CD240CE

Selected Monoclonal Antibodies

BRIC 69 (Spring; Bristol).

CD241

Other Names

RhAg, Rh50, Rh associated antigen.

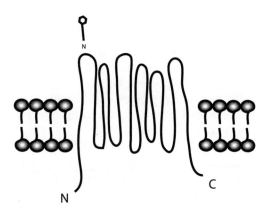

Molecular Structure

CD241 is a glycoprotein and a member of the Rh blood group system. It has 32.9% and 38.5% identity with CD240CE and CD240D, respectively, and a similar secondary structure with 12 transmembrane helical domains.

RHAG has a different chromosomal location to RHD and RHCE and displays very little allelic diversity.

It has a single N-glycosylation site at Asn37. The N-glycan carries ABH and Li antigens.

CD241 is not palmitoylated like CD240CE and CD240D but is phosphorylated.

Erythrocytes carry between 100 and 200,000 copies of CD241 per cell.

The C terminus is cytoplasmic and interacts with the erythrocyte cytoskeleton.

Mol Wt: 50 kDa.

Function

Formation of a complex with CD241 is essential for expression of Rh blood group antigens.

The core of the Rh complex is thought to consist of two Rh subunits and two CD241 subunits, to which CD47, glycophorin B (CD235b), and CD242 (LW, ICAM-4) associate noncovalently.

CD241 and Rh antigens C-terminal cytoplasmic domains bind ankyrin-R, thereby linking the complex with the actin-spectrin-based red cell skeleton.

Recently it has been shown that CD241 functions as an ammonium transporter, facilitating the movement of CH_3NH_2 and NH_3 across the erythrocyte membrane.

The very rare Rh-null phenotype is the result of inactivation of the RHAG gene. The absence of CD241 prevents expression of all Rh antigens. Rh-null individuals have chronic hemolytic anemia of varying severity, increased osmotic fragility, abnormal cation transport and cell morphology (stomato-spherocytosis), and membrane phospholipid organization.

Expression

CD241 is expressed by erythroid progenitors from the BFU-E stage to mature cells.

Gene Name	Entrez Gene#
RHAG	6005

Selected Monoclonal Antibodies

LA20.20, LA18.18, LA23.40 (van der Schoot; Amsterdam).

CD242

Other Names

ICAM 4, LW blood group, Landsteiner–Wiener blood group antigen.

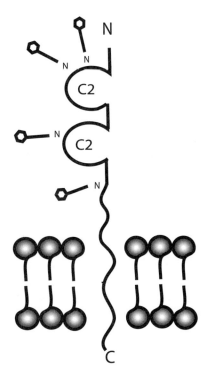

Molecular Structure

CD242 is a type I transmembrane glyco-protein of the Ig gene superfamily that has similarity in structure and sequence to the intracellular adhesion molecules (ICAMs).

The mature protein consists of 249 amino acids, of which 218 residues are extracellular, 21 amino acids span the membrane, and 10 amino acids are intracellular.

The extracellular domain contains two C2-type Ig-like domains and has four potential N-linked glycosylation sites.

The Landsteiner–Wiener antigens arise from a single amino acid variation at posi-tion 100. Gln100 corresponds to LW(A), and Arg100 corresponds to LW(B).

Mol Wt: 42 kDa.

Function

CD242 carries the antigens of the Land-steiner–Wiener blood group system.

It is an adhesion molecule that plays a role in the interaction between red blood cells and macrophages, neutrophils, and platelets and may be involved in differen-tiation of erythroblasts.

CD242 may promote sickle cell adhe-sion to endothelium and potentiate episodes of vaso-occlusion in sickle cell disease.

Ligands

CD242 binds LFA-1 (CD11a/CD18), Mac-1 (CD11b/CD18), β1 and β5 integrins, platelet fibrinogen receptor, and endothe-lial cell vitronectin receptor.

Expression

CD242 is expressed by erythroid progeni-tors from the BFU-E stage to mature cells.

Applications

LW antigens may be depressed in preg-nancy and some malignancies.

Expression of CD242 is elevated in sickle cells.

Gene Name	Entrez Gene#
ICAM4	3386

Selected Monoclonal Antibodies

BS 56, BS87 (Sonneborn; Germany).

CD243

Other Names

MDR-1 (multi-drug resistance protein 1), P-glycoprotein, pgp 170.

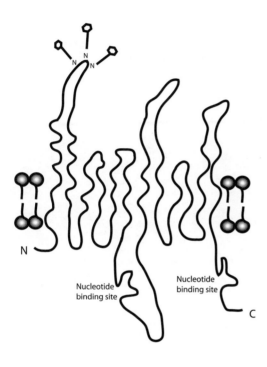

Molecular Structure

CD243 is a glycoprotein that spans the membrane 12 times and is a member of the multi-drug resistance (MDR) subfamily within the ABC family of ATP-binding transport proteins.

The mature protein consists of 1280 amino acids and 12 transmembrane domains, of which 2 are type 1 ABC transmembrane domains, 2 ABC transporter domains, 2 ATP binding sites at amino acid 434 and 1077, and 3 potential N-linked glycosylation sites.

The N and C termini are cytoplasmic.

Several variants have been found that are the result of single amino acid substitutions.

Mol Wt: 170 kDa.

Function

CD243 is an ATP-dependent efflux transporter capable of effluxing a variety of structurally and pharmacologically unrelated neutral and positively charged hydrophobic compounds that are potentially toxic to the cell.

CD243 is expressed at blood-tissue barriers, including the blood-brain barrier, blood-testis barrier, blood-placenta barrier, and blood-ocular barrier. At these sites, CD243 acts to prevent accumulation of harmful substances by effluxing them out of the cell.

Expression of CD243 is high in the intestine, particularly in the ileum and colon, which suggests CD243 limits availability of orally administered drugs.

A multi-drug resistant phenotype can occur in primary and recurrent tumors and is most often related to the upregulated expression of CD243.

Single nucleotide polymorphisms can affect CD243 transport capabilities. For example, patients with resistant epilepsy are likely to have the C3435T polymorphism, and PET (positron emission tomography) imaging showed lower delivery of an anti-epilepsy drug to the brain than in other genotypes.

Expression

CD243 is expressed by endothelial and epithelial cells of many tissues.

It is expressed at low levels in hemopoietic cells, including bone marrow stem cells.

Expression of CD243 can be markedly elevated in various malignancies, including breast and ovarian carcinomas.

Applications

CD243 is a useful marker in evaluating potential drug resistance of tumors and is a prognostic indicator for various tumors.

Selected Monoclonal Antibodies

U1C2 (van Agthoven; Marseille).

Gene Name	Entrez Gene#
ABCB1	5243

CD244

Other Names

2B4.

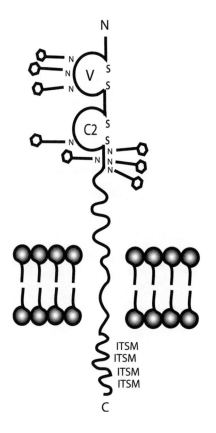

Molecular Structure

CD244 is a type I transmembrane glyco-protein and a member of the CD150 (SLAM) subfamily of the CD2 receptor family within the Ig gene superfamily (see also CD2, CD48, CD58, CD84, CD150, and CD229).

The unprocessed precursor consists of 370 amino acid residues. After cleavage of the 21-residue signal peptide, the mature protein consists of a 208 amino acid extracellular region, 21-residue transmembrane domain, and 120 amino acid cytoplasmic domain.

The extracellular region contains an N-termimal V-set Ig-like domain followed by one C2-set Ig-like domain and has eight potential N-glycosylation sites.

The cytoplasmic region contains four novel tyrosine-based motifs known as tyrosine-based switch motifs (ITSMs; TxYxxV/I) capable of binding several SH2-domain containing proteins, including both activating and inhibitory signaling molecules.

Mol Wt: 70 kDa.

Function

CD244 plays a role in non-MHC restricted cytotoxic activity of NK cells and acts as a costimulatory ligand for both NK cells and T cells in vitro.

During CD244-CD48 mediated homotypic interaction of T cells and NK cells or NK–T-cell interactions, CD244 signaling is proposed to induce optimal activation of T cells and NK cells.

However, interaction of CD244 on NK cells with other CD48$^+$ target cells such as tumor cells can lead to inhibition of NK-cell effector functions.

CD244 knockout mice are phenotypically normal but have an increased capacity to clear CD48$^+$ tumor cells in vivo. Consistent with this finding are the results of cytotoxicity assays performed with CD244$^{-/-}$ splenic NK cells, which demonstrated enhanced killing of CD48$^+$ target cells. These findings are consistent with CD244 acting as an inhibitory receptor.

Ligands

CD244 binds CD48 with high affinity.

Expression

CD244 is expressed by all NK cells, a subset of CD8$^+$ T cells with memory/effector phenotype, skin γ/δ T cells, basophils, and monocytes.

Gene Name	Entrez Gene#
CD244	51744

Selected Monoclonal Antibodies

158 (Colonna; Basle); C1.7.1 (van Agthoven; Marseille); PP35 (Moretta; Genoa).

CD245

Other Names

p220/240, DY12, DY35.

Molecular Structure

CD245 is a transmembrane protein of unknown structure.

Mol Wt: 220–250 kDa.

Function

CD245 is involved in signal transduction and costimulation of T and NK cells.

Weak phosphatase activity was detected in immunoprecipitates from an NK cell line but not from peripheral blood lymphocytes (PBLs).

MAb-cross-linking of CD245 augments proliferation of PBL in the presence of suboptimal concentrations of anti-CD2 mitogenic mAbs.

Anti-CD3-induced T-cell proliferation is unaltered in the presence of anti-CD245.

Expression

CD245 is expressed by all resting peripheral blood lymphocytes (PBLs), monocytes, granulocytes, platelets, and NK cells.

High level expression of CD245 occurs in monocytes and IL-2-dependent T-cell lines but is weak on T cells, thymocytes, granulocytes, and platelets.

Expression of CD245 has been reported on Ewing sarcoma, osteosarcoma cell lines, and weakly on a rhabdomyosarcoma cell line.

Gene Name	Entrez Gene#
	Nonassigned

Selected Monoclonal Antibodies

DY12 (Boumsell; Paris); DY35 (Bensussan; Paris).

CD246

Other Names

Anaplastic lymphoma kinase (ALK).

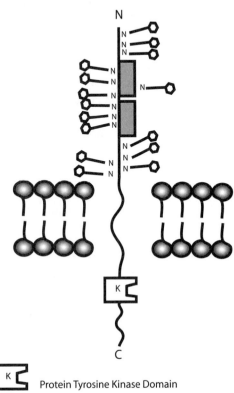

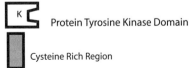

K ⊏ Protein Tyrosine Kinase Domain

▨ Cysteine Rich Region

Molecular Structure

CD246 is a receptor protein–tyrosine kinase. and is a member of the insulin receptor subfamily.

It bears significant homology with leukocyte tyrosine kinase (LTK)

The protein consists of a 1030-residue extracellular region of which the first 20 amino acids represent a putative signal peptide.

The extracellular region has 16 potential N-glycosylation sites and 26 cysteine residues in clusters between amino acids 425–487 and 987–1021.

The transmembrane span consists of 28 amino acids.

The intracellular portion comprises a juxtamembrane region of 64 residues, a 254 amino acid tyrosine kinase domain, and a 244 amino acid carboxyl tail.

The juxtamembrane region contains potential binding site for SH2 domain containing proteins also present in other members of the insulin receptor subfamily and shown to mediate interaction of receptor tyrosine kinases with substrates such as IRS-1.

The tyrosine kinase domain has paired tyrosine residues that are characteristic of autophosphorylation sites of the insulin receptor family.

There are several other potential SH2 and PTB binding sites in the carboxyl tail.

Mol Wt: 200 kDa.

Function

As a receptor tyrosine kinase, CD246 is predicted to play a role in signal transduction via the mitogen-activated protein kinase (MAPK) pathway.

The expression pattern of CD246 suggests it is involved in the normal development and function of the nervous system.

CD246 knockout mice are phenotypically normal, which indicates CD246 is nonessential at least in mice. Interestingly drosophila lacking CD246 do not develop normal gut musculature.

Chromosomal translocations affecting ALK result in the production of a variety of fusion proteins, the most common of which is nucleophosmin (NPM)-ALK. Eighty percent of all ALCLs (anaplastic large cell lymphomas) express NPM-ALK.

The protein fused with CD246 determines the subcellular localization of the fusion protein. Additionally, most fusion proteins have an oligomerization domain resulting in oligomerization of the fusion protein and constitutive activation.

Ligands

Pleiotrophin (PTN) and midkine (MK) are putative ligands for CD246.

Expression

CD246 expression occurs principally in perinatal neural cells. In particular, CD246 is highly expressed in the dienchephalon, midbrain, and ventral half of the spinal chord. It is also expressed in the trigeminal, sympathetic, and enteric ganglia.

After birth, expression decreases but is still detectable in the thalamus, olfactory bulb, and mesenchephalon.

CD246 fusion proteins arising from chromosomal translocation are found in ALCLs and in inflammatory myofibroblastic tumor (IMT). CD246 expression has been reported in peripheral nerve sheath tumors and leiomyosarcoma.

Applications

CD246 is a marker used in the diagnosis of ALCLs and is a potential prognostic indicator in cases of IMT and ALCL.

Gene Name	Entrez Gene#
ALK	238

Selected Monoclonal Antibodies

ALK-1 (Pulford; Oxford); ALKc (van Agthoven; Marseille).

CD247

Other Names

T-cell receptor ζ-chain, CD3 ζ.

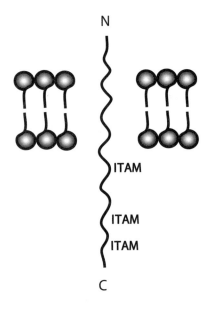

Molecular Structure

CD247 is a type I transmembrane protein that forms disulphide-linked homodimers or heterodimers of its two isoforms CD3ζ and CD3η.

A 21-residue signal peptide is cleaved to produce a mature protein of 143 amino acids.

The extracellular domain consists of only nine residues and has no glycosylation sites.

The 21 amino acid transmembrane region is followed by a cytoplasmic domain that contains 3 immunoreceptor tyrosine-based activation motifs (ITAMs).

CD247 dimers form part of the T-cell receptor (TCR)–CD3 complex in T cells. This complex consists of T-cell receptor α/β or γ/δ heterodimers associated with three distinct dimers: CD3γ/ε, CD3δ/ε, and CD3ζ/ζ (CD247).

Each of these dimers associates with a specific basic residue in the TCR trans-membrane (TM) region. Assembly of the CD247 dimer into the complex requires the interaction of aspartic acid residues in the CD247 TM with an arginine in the TM of TCRα or TCRδ.

Mol Wt: 16 kDa.

Function

CD247 forms a dimeric transmembrane signaling molecule that is associated with the TCR–CD3 complex and is essential for the activation of T cells.

TCR ligation results in phosphorylation of the ITAM motifs of CD247 by tyrosine kinases Lck and Fyn. After phosphorylation, Syk family kinases ZAP-70 and Syk are recruited and activated, ultimately leading to NKκB activation and translocation to the nucleus and T-cell activation.

T-cell activation is self-limiting, and downregulation of TCR triggering involves loss of CD247 probably via internalization and degradation of TCR chains including CD247.

Chronic antigenic stimulation via TCRs can result in prolonged or permanent downregulation of CD247 expression. This has been observed in patients with cancer, leprosy, AIDS, and autoimmune diseases such as SLE in which there are circulating immune complexes.

Ligation of CD43 in T cells and NK cells can also lead to CD247 phosphorylation and recruitment to the CD43 signaling pathway.

CD2 and CD16 (FcγRIII) can associate with CD247 in NK cells.

Expression

CD247 is expressed by all T cells and CD3⁻CD56⁺ CD16⁺ NK cells.

Applications

Expression of CD247 is decreased in CD4$^+$ and CD8$^+$ T cells of some patients with cancer and correlates with poor prognosis and survival.

Selected Monoclonal Antibodies

2H2D9 (van Agthoven; Marseille).

Gene Name	Entrez Gene#
CD3Z	919

CD248

Other Names

TEM1, endosialin, CD164 sialomucin-like protein (CD164L1).

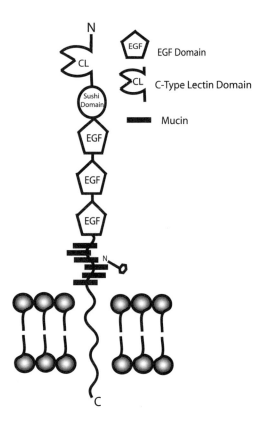

Molecular Structure

CD248 is a type 1 membrane protein and c-type lectin-like protein of 757 amino acids.

The protein is composed of a signal peptide and five globular extracellular domains (which include a C-type lectin domain, a domain with similarity to the Sushi/ccp/scr pattern, and three EGF repeats), a mucin-like region, a transmembrane region, and a short intracellular domain.

CD248 is heavily O-glycosylated with sialylated oligosaccharides.

The N-terminal 360 amino acids of CD248 show homology with thrombomodulin and complement receptor C1qRp.

Mol Wt: 175 kDa.

Function

The structural protein similarities between thrombomodulin (CD141) and CD93 and CD248 suggest a possible role for C248 in cell–cell interactions, particularly during tumor angiogenesis and metastasis.

However, the exact function(s) of CD248 has yet to be elucidated.

Expression

CD248 is considered to be a tumor endothelial cell marker that is also expressed by fibroblast-like cells near the meninges and α-smooth muscle cells in some vessels.

A recent study has suggested CD248 is not expressed by tumor endothelial cells and is only expressed by stromal fibroblasts and a subset of pericytes associated with tumor vessels.

Applications

Expression of CD248 correlates with high tumor grade and aggressive progression of tumors.

Gene Name	Entrez Gene#
CD248	57124

Selected Monoclonal Antibodies

B1/473.16 (Isacke; London).

CD249

Other Names

Aminopeptidase A, glutamyl aminopeptidase.

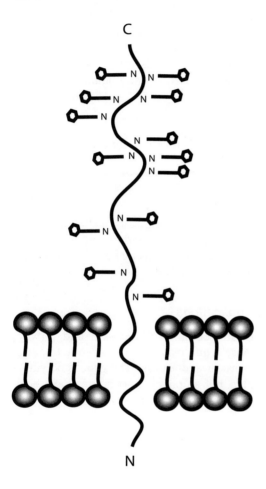

Molecular Structure

CD249 is a type II membrane protein and a member of the M1 peptidase family.

The protein consists of an N-terminal cytoplasmic domain of 18 amino acids, a 21-residue type II signal anchor transmembrane region, and a 918 amino acid extracellular domain.

There are 13 N-linked glycosylation sites.

CD249 forms disulphide-linked homodimers, and each subunit binds one zinc ion.

Mol Wt: 160 kDa.

Function

CD249 is an ectoenzyme that catalyses the release of N-terminal glutamate (and to a lesser extent aspartate) from a peptide.

It plays a role in the renin–angiotensin catabolic pathway and is involved in the formation of brain angiotensin III, which has a stimulatory effect on the central nervous system control of blood pressure.

It plays a regulatory role in angiogenesis.

A possible role for CD249 in regulating B-cell growth and development has been suggested. However, CD249 knockout mice are phenotypically normal and show no abnormality in T- and B-cell development and response to antigen.

The deficient mice do fail to produce the expected angiogenic reaction to hypoxia or growth factors.

Expression

CD249 is expressed by endothelial and epithelial cells, in a variety of tissues, particularly renal proximal tubule cells and the glomerulus of nephrons.

Applications

CD249 is a potential therapeutic target in the treatment of hypertension and prevention of tumor angiogenesis.

Gene Name	Entrez Gene#
ENPEP	2028

Selected Monoclonal Antibodies

2D3 (BD Biosciences; San Diego).

CD252

Other Names

OX40L (OX 40 ligand); TNSF4 (TNF superfamily member 4), CD134 ligand (CD134L).

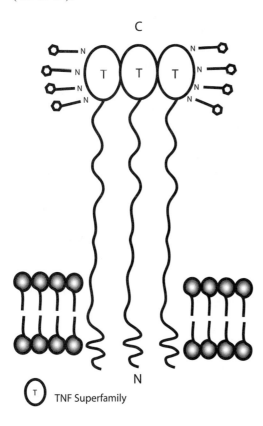

T) TNF Superfamily

Molecular Structure

Type II transmembrane glycoprotein member of the TNF superfamily. By analogy with other TNFSF family members, CD252 probably forms a homotrimer.

183aa long, with four potential N-glycosylation sites.

Mol Wt: Predicted, 21 kDa, Observed, 34 kDa.

Function

Membrane-expressed cytokine that can act as a costimulator through interaction with its ligand on T cells. OX40/OX40 ligand interaction appears to favor Th2 responses.

OX40 on T cells can adhere to OX40 ligand on vascular endothelium.

Ligands

OX40 (TNF receptor superfamily number 4, TNFRSF4).

Expression

Antigen-presenting cells, including B cells and dendritic cells, and endothelium.

Induced in T cells by the HLTLV-1 transcriptional activator p40tax.

Applications

Expressed in psoriatic skin and airways muscle, and may be a therapeutic target in psoriasis and asthma. The gene is polymorphic, but so far no associations have been reported with disease severity.

Gene Name	Entrez Gene#
TNFSF4	7292

Selected Monoclonal Antibodies

SICD134L-1, SICD134L-3, SICD134L-4, SICD134L-5, SICD134L-6 (Zhang; Suzhou).

CD253

Other Names

TRAIL, APO-2 ligand, TNF-like-2 (TL2), TNFSF10.

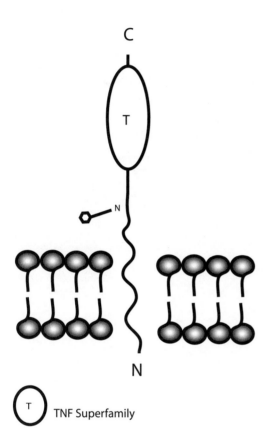

T TNF Superfamily

Molecular Structure

Type II transmembrane glycoprotein member of the TNF family, containing 281 amino acids and with a predicted Mol Wt of 32.5 kDa.

The N-terminal cytoplasmic domain is 17 residues long, whereas the membrane-spanning region consists of 21 hydrophobic residues. The extracellular domain shares significant homology with that of other TNF family members such as FasL (28% identity) and TNF-α (23% identity). The extracellular domain is shed as a 19-kDa protein that forms dimers and trimers of Mol Wt 48 kDa and 66 kDa; TRAIL is also released in a vesicle-associated form.

Splice variants lacking exon 3 (TRAIL β) or exons 2 and 3 (Trail γ) are also expressed.

Function

The principal activity of TRAIL seems to be to induce apoptosis, but the physiological function may be more complex. The multiplicity of receptors is unusual. Gene-knockout studies suggest that TRAIL plays a role in tumor surveillance by immune cells. Blocking of TRAIL with antibody suggests that TRAIL mediates interferon-γ-dependent NK-cell function, including killing of tumor cells and virus-infected cells.

A specific immunological function attributed to TRAIL is the control of CD8 T-cell memory by CD4 cells.

Both splice variants (lacking exons 3 or 2 and 3) have lost their pro-apoptotic activity.

Ligands

TRAIL binds to five related receptors: TRAIL-R1 (death receptor 4, DR4), TRAIL-R2 (DR5), TRAIL-R3 (decoy receptor 1, DcR1), TRAIL-R4 (DcR2), and Osteoprotegerin (OPG), all members of the TNF receptor family.

Expression

TRAIL is expressed widely in lymphoid (spleen, thymus, gut-associated lymphoid tissue) and non-lymphoid (lung, prostate, kidney) tissues. It is expressed by activated

T cells, NK cells, monocytes, and dendritic cells.

Gene Name

TNFSF10

Entrez Gene#

8743

Selected Monoclonal Antibodies

B-S23, B-T24 (Diaclone; Besancon); FMU-TRAIL1 (Jin; Xian).

CD254

Other Names

TRANCE, TNFSF11, RANK ligand (RANKL, hRANKL2).

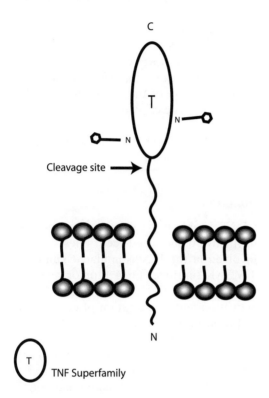

TNF Superfamily

Molecular Structure

Type II transmembrane glycoprotein member of the TNF family, containing 317 amino acids and with a predicted Mol Wt of 34.5 kDa. Predicted to form a homotrimer in the membrane.

Three splice variants, one of them lacking membrane insertion region, as well as a soluble form produced by proteolysis.

Function

Principal factor stimulating osteoclast activation and differentiation. Survival factor for dendritic cells, and plays a role in T-dependent immune responses. May be involved in regulation of apoptosis.

Knockout mice lack osteoclasts and show severe osteoporosis, as well as defective lymphocyte differentiation.

Ligands

Binds RANK (TNFRSF11A) and Osteoprotegerin (TNFRSF11B).

Expression

Expression induced on T cells by activation. Expressed in secondary lymphoid tissue (particularly lymph nodes, less strongly in spleen) and at lower levels in bone marrow, brain, and other tissues.

Applications

Role in bone and immune system suggest that this molecule may be a potential diagnostic and therapeutic target.

Gene Name	Entrez Gene#
TNFSF11	8600

Selected Monoclonal Antibodies

70513 (R&D Systems; Minneapolis).

(CD255)

Other Names

TWEAK, Tumor necrosis factor ligand superfamily member 12, TNF-related weak inducer of apoptosis, APO3 ligand.

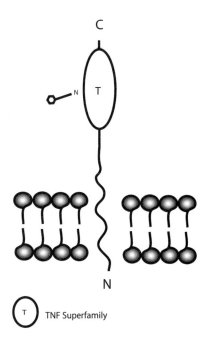

T TNF Superfamily

Molecular Structure

CD255 is a type II transmembrane protein that belongs to a subfamily of the tumor necrosis factor (TNF) superfamily, which includes BAFF, APRIL (CD256), EDA, and TWE-PRIL.

The membrane-bound form consists of 249 amino acids.

The N-terminal cytoplasmic tail consists of 21 residues and a putative serine phosphorylation site.

A signal anchor of 21 hydrophobic amino acids spans the membrane.

The C-terminal extracellular region consists of 207 amino acids and the receptor-binding subdomain predicted to be a β-pleated sheet structure, a single N-linked glycosylation site (position 139), and a proteolytic cleavage site (residue 90–93).

The transmembrane domain is linked to the receptor binding domain via a stalk region containing a high proportion of basic amino acids.

Ligand binding induces the formation of CD255 homotrimers.

A soluble isoform of CD255 consisting of 156 amino acids comprising the receptor-binding portion of the ectodomain results from proteolytic cleavage by furin.

Mol Wt: 18kDa (membrane form), 30–35kDa (soluble).

Function

CD255 is able to weakly induce apoptosis in many tissues and cell lines and is involved in the IFNγ-stimulated killing of TWEAK-sensitive (Fn14$^+$) tumor cells.

In contrast, CD255 can induce NFκB activation and proliferation of endothelial cells and promotes angiogenesis including neovascularization of tumors.

CD255 induces pro-inflammatory cytokine secretion.

Both the soluble and membrane bound forms are biologically active.

Ligands

CD255 binds FN14 (TWEAK-R, CD266, TNFRSF12A), and APO3 (TNFRSF12).

Expression

CD255 is expressed by IFNγ-stimulated peripheral blood lymphocytes and monocytes, endothelial cells, smooth muscle cells, and fibroblasts.

CD255 is expressed at high levels in the central nervous system (CNS), skeletal muscle, heart, and pancreas. Expression has also been detected in spleen, lymph nodes and thymus, first and third trimester placenta, and various tumor cell lines.

Gene Name	Entrez Gene#
TNFSF12	8742

Selected Monoclonal Antibodies

No antibodies confirmed; CD255 designation reserved for this molecule.

CD256

Other Names

APRIL (a proliferation-inducing ligand), TNFSF13, TALL2.

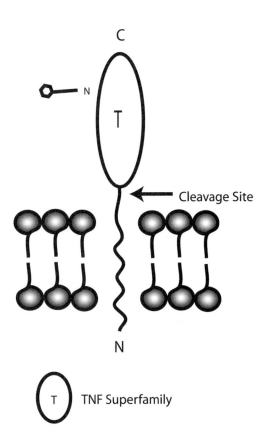

T TNF Superfamily

Molecular Structure

Glycoprotein member of the TNF family, containing 250 amino acids and with a predicted Mol Wt of 27.5 kDa. Predicted to form homotrimers, and can form a heterotrimer with BLyS (CD257).

The N-terminal cytoplasmic domain is 28 residues long, whereas the membrane-spanning region consists of 20 hydrophobic residues. The extracellular domain is 201aa long and shares significant homology with that of other TNF family members, partic-

ularly FasL and TNF-α (both about 20% identical in the extracellular domain).

The extracellular domain is secreted as a result of intracellular proteolysis in the Golgi.

Three splice variants are reported.

Function

CD256 has a role in B-cell development through interaction with BCMA and may additionally induce apoptosis through interaction with other TNFRSF members. May have a role in controlling tumor growth. May also function in the nervous system; acts as a growth factor for glioblastoma cell lines.

Ligands

BCMA (TNFRSF17; CD269) and TACI (TNFRSF13B, CD267).

Expression

CD256 is not generally seen as a membrane protein, because it is secreted after intracellular proteolysis. mRNA expressed in monocyte/macrophages and at high levels by transformed cell lines and some tumors. mRNA expression is downregulated by mitogens.

Soluble protein found at high levels in multiple myeloma. Heterotrimer with BLyS (CD257) found in serum, associated with inflammatory autoimmune disease.

Gene Name	Entrez Gene#
TNFSF13	8741

Selected Monoclonal Antibodies

FMU-APRIL1, FMU-APRIL2, FMU-APRIL3, FMU-APRIL4 (Jin; Xian); Sacha-1 (Murone; Apotech, Epalinges); 172724 (Mortari; R&D Systems, Minneapolis).

CD257

Other Names

BLyS (B lymphocyte stimulator), BAFF, TNFSF13B, TALL1.

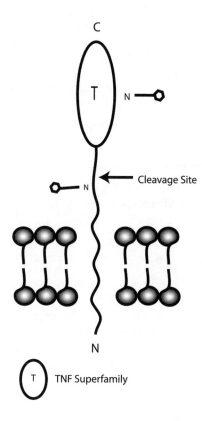

TNF Superfamily

Molecular Structure

Type II transmembrane glycoprotein member of the TNF family, containing 285 amino acids and with a predicted Mol Wt of 31 kDa. Predicted to form homotrimers and can form a heterotrimer with APRIL (CD256).

The N-terminal cytoplasmic domain is 46 residues long, whereas the membrane-spanning region consists of 21 hydrophobic residues. The extracellular domain is 218 αα long, includes 2 sites for N-glycosylation, and shares significant homology with that of other TNF family members, particularly APRIL (33% identical).

The extracellular domain is shed as a result of proteolysis in the extracellular stalk region.

Three splice variants are reported.

Function

Primarily a B-cell survival, activation, and differentiation factor. Confers resistance to apoptosis on some B-cell tumors, including CLL.

Also involved as a costimulator in T–B-cell interactions.

Ligands

BCMA (TNFRSF17; CD269) and TACI (TNFRSF13B, CD267) and BAFFR (TNFRSF13C, CD268).

Expression

Expressed by B lymphocytes and monocyte/macrophages, and at lower levels in non-lymphoid tissues such as placenta, lung, and heart. Upregulated by interferon γ.

Serum soluble BLyS is elevated in patients with autoimmune inflammatory conditions and in multiple myeloma.

Applications

The critical role of BLyS in B-cell survival and activation, including its role in B-cell tumor survival, has made it a target for therapeutic applications.

Soluble BLyS retains the ability to activate cells, unlike many TNF family members, which are active only in membrane-expressed form.

Gene Name   Entrez Gene#

TNFSF13B   10673

Selected Monoclonal Antibodies

FMU-Blys1, FMU-Blys2 (Jin; Xian); Buffy-1 (Murone; Apotech, Epalinges); 137314 (Mortari; R&D Systems, Minneapolis).

CD258

Other Names

LIGHT, TNFSF14.

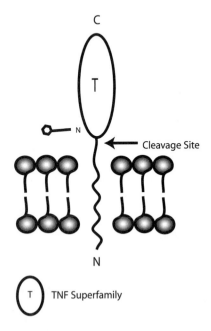

Molecular Structure

Type II transmembrane glycoprotein member of the TNF family. The protein contains 240 residues and has an apparent Mol Wt of 29kDa. The N-terminal cytosolic domain consists of 37 residues, whereas the membrane-spanning sequence is 22-residues long. The 181-residue extracellular domain of LIGHT carries a single N-glycosylation site and shows homology with other TNF members, particularly LTb (34% identity), Fas ligand (31%), and 4-1BBL(29%).

LIGHT is also found as a soluble molecule.

Function

Redundancy in function and receptor binding in the TNF family makes it difficult to work out the physiological function of each member. LIGHT can trigger apoptosis as well as cell activation, by signaling through TRAF3.

LIGHT can act as a costimulator for T-cell proliferation and cytokine secretion, preferentially TH1 cytokines.

LIGHT induces activation of DCs, indicated by upregulation of costimulatory and adhesion molecules and increased antigen presentation.

LIGHT also appears to function in thymic repertoire selection and in aspects of the inflammatory response.

Ligands

LIGHT binds two receptors, both members of the TNF receptor family, HVEM/TR2, and LTbR.

Expression

LIGHT is expressed at low levels in resting blood and tissue leukocytes and is upregulated on activation. It is also expressed in dendritic cells derived by in vitro culture, but not by DCs isolated fresh from blood. Most cancer cell lines do not express LIGHT.

Applications

Research reagents.

Gene Name	Entrez Gene#
TNFSF14	8740

Selected Monoclonal Antibodies

FMU-Light1, FMU-Light2, FMU-Light3, FMU-Light4 (Jin; Xian); 115520 (Mortari; R&D Systems; Minneapolis).

CD261

Other Names

TRAIL-R1, DR4 (death receptor 4), TNFRSF10A.

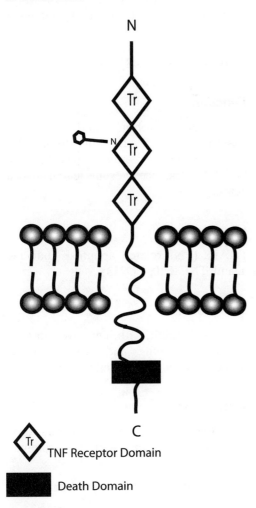

Tr TNF Receptor Domain

■ Death Domain

Molecular Structure

Type I transmembrane protein member of the tumor necrosis factor receptor (TNFR) family, 468 residues long, including a 23-aa signal sequence.

The 216-aa extracellular region contains 3 TNFR cysteine repeats and 1 potential N-glycosylation site.

The 23-residue membrane-spanning domain is followed by a 206-residue cytoplasmic sequence that contains 1 death domain

Predicted Mol Wt: 50 kDa.

Function

On interaction with its ligand, CD261, the adaptor molecule FADD binds to the DR4 death domain, and recruits caspase-8, which initiates a sequence of events leading to cell death.

Ligands

TRAIL (TNF-related apoptosis inducing ligand, TNFSF10, CD253).

Expression

Expressed widely, with high levels in lymphoid tissue and gut tissue.

Applications

A polymorphism in CD261 has been associated with risk of bladder cancer.

Gene Name	Entrez Gene#
TNFRSF10A	8797

Selected Monoclonal Antibodies

B-K32, B-N28, B-N36, B-S26, B-S32, B-T35, (Diaclone; Besancon); FMU-DcR4 (Jin; Xian).

CD262

Other Names

TRAIL-R2, DR5 (death receptor 5), TNFRSF10B.

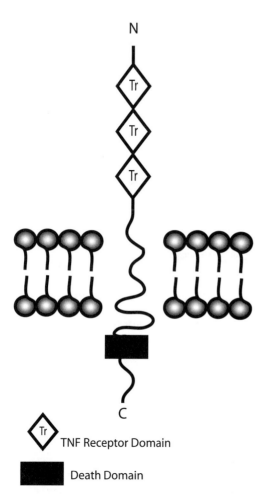

Tr — TNF Receptor Domain

■ Death Domain

Molecular Structure

Type I transmembrane protein member of the tumor necrosis factor receptor (TNFR) family, 440 residues long after removal of the 55aa signal sequence.

Forms a homotrimeric complex.

The 155-residue extracellular domain contains 3 TNFR-cysteine repeats and lacks N-glycosylation sites.

The 21-aa membrane-spanning sequence is followed by the cytoplasmic region, which is 209 residues in length and contains 1 death domain.

Predicted Mol Wt: 48 kDa.

Function

On interaction with its ligand, CD253, the adaptor molecule FADD binds to the DR5 death domain and recruits caspase-8, which initiates a sequence of events leading to cell death.

Ligands

TRAIL (TNF-related apoptosis inducing ligand, TNFSF10, CD253).

Expression

Expressed widely, with high levels in lymphoid tissue, lung, and prostate tissue. Induced by tumor suppressor p53.

Applications

Defective function of CD262 apears to be associated with head and neck carcinoma.

Gene Name	Entrez Gene#
TNFRSF10B	8795

Selected Monoclonal Antibodies

B-B42, B-D37, B-K29, B-L27, B-N32, B-T28 (Diaclone; Besancon); FMU-DcR5.1, FMU-DcR5.2 (Jin; Xian).

CD263

Other Names

TRAIL-R3, TNF-R superfamily-member 10C (TNFRSF10C), DcR1, LIT, TRID.

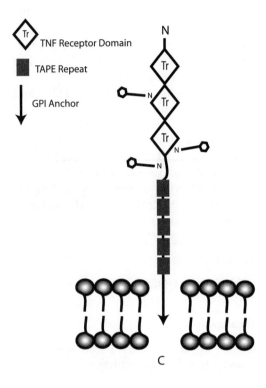

Molecular Structure

CD263 is a glycophosphatidylinositol (GPI)-anchored membrane receptor protein and is a member of the tumor necrosis factor-receptor (TNF-R) superfamily.

The protein has a 23 amino acid signal sequence (N-terminal, and a 23-aa propeptide at the C terminus), which is removed in the mature form, leaving 190-aa mature protein.

The mature protein contains 3 TNFR-Cys repeats, 5 tandem TAPE repeats, and 3 potential N-linked glycosylation sites.

Mol Wt: 65 kDa.

Function

CD263 is a membrane receptor for CD253 (TRAIL) and is thought to act as a decoy receptor, which inhibits TRAIL-induced apoptosis by competing for binding with other TRAIL receptors.

Unlike the TRAIL receptors TRAIL-R1 (CD261) and TRAIL-R2 (CD262), CD263 lacks a death domain and cannot transmit apoptotic signal to the cell upon TRAIL binding.

Normal tissues that express CD263 and CD264 are resistant to TRAIL-induced apoptosis even in the presence of apoptotic signaling receptors CD261 and CD262.

The role of CD263 in malignant tissues is unclear, and various studies reveal conflicting results as to its importance in the control of TRAIL-mediated cell death in tumors.

Ligands

CD263 binds CD253 (TRAIL).

Expression

CD263 is expressed by T and B lymphocytes, NK cells, macrophages, monocytes, and granulocytes.

Expression is also found in hepatocytes and bile duct epithelium, neurons in the brain, germ and Leydig cells, spleen, skeletal muscle, placenta, lung, and heart.

Gene Name	Entrez Gene#
TNFRSF10C	8794

Selected Monoclonal Antibodies

B-D40 (Diaclone; Besancon).

CD264

Other Names

TRAIL-R4, TNF-R superfamily member 10D (TNFRSF10D), TRUNDD, DcR2.

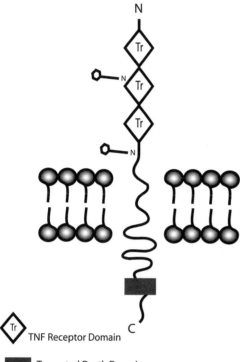

◇ Tr TNF Receptor Domain

▬ Truncated Death Domain

Molecular Structure

CD264 is a type 1 membrane protein and a member of the tumor necrosis factor-receptor (TNF-R) superfamily.

The 331 amino acid protein consists of a 21 residue signal sequence, 156 amino acid extracellular region containing 3 TNFR-Cys repeats and 2 potential N-linked glycosylation sites, a 21-residue transmembrane domain, and a 154 amino acid cytoplasmic region containing a nonfunctional, truncated death domain.

Mol Wt: 35 kDa.

Function

CD264 is a membrane receptor for CD253 (TRAIL) and is thought to act as a decoy receptor by competing for binding with other TRAIL receptors and inhibiting TRAIL-induced apoptosis.

Unlike the TRAIL receptors TRAIL-R1 (CD261) and TRAIL-R2 (CD262), CD264 lacks a functional death domain and cannot transmit an apoptotic signal to the cell upon TRAIL binding.

Normal tissues that express CD263 and CD264 are resistant to TRAIL-induced apoptosis even in the presence of apoptotic signaling receptors CD261 and CD262.

The role of CD264 in malignant tissues is unclear, and various studies have produced conflicting results as to its importance in the control of TRAIL-mediated cell death in tumors.

Ligands

CD264 binds CD253 (TRAIL).

Expression

CD264 is expressed by T and B lymphocytes, NK cells, macrophages, monocytes, and granulocytes.

Expression of CD264 is detectable in fetal kidney, lung and liver and in adult testis, ovary, placenta, prostate, colon, small intestine, pancreas, kidney, lung, and heart.

Gene Name	Entrez Gene#
TNFRSF10D	8793

Selected Monoclonal Antibodies

B-T32, B-R36 (Diaclone; Besancon).

CD265

Other Names

RANK, TNFRSF11A, TRANCER, EOF, FEO, OFE, ODFR, PDB2.

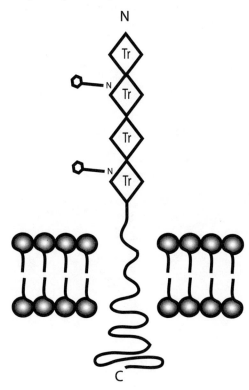

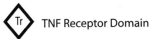 TNF Receptor Domain

Molecular Structure

CD265 is a type 1 membrane protein and a member of the tumor necrosis factor receptor (TNFR) superfamily.

It shares 40% homology with CD40 and associates at the cell surface as a trimer. It is unknown whether trimerization requires ligand binding.

The precursor protein is predicted to have a 21-residue signal peptide, and the mature form consists of 587 amino acids.

The 183 amino acid extracellular domain contains 4 TNFR-Cys repeats and 2 potential N-glycosylation sites.

The transmembrane domain and cytoplasmic domains, are predicted to consist of 21 and 383 residues respectively.

Tumor necrosis factor receptor-associated factors (TRAFs) 1, 2, 3, and 5 interact with CD265 in a membrane distal region of the intracellular tail.

TRAF6 binds to a distinct membrane-proximal Pro-X-Glu-X-X-(aromatic/acid residue) motif of the cytoplasmic domain.

Mol Wt: 97 kDa.

Function

CD265 is the functional receptor for TRANCE (CD254), and together these proteins are required for osteoclast differentiation and activation and bone homeostasis. The CD265/CD254 interaction activates the bone resorption function of osteoclasts.

Signaling by CD265 is mediated by TRAF1, 2, 3, 5, and 6. TRAF6 is the most important adaptor for signaling.

CD265 expression is inducible in dendritic cells (DCs) during maturation and upon ligation by TRANCE activates anti-apoptotic signaling to prolong DC survival.

Immature $CD34^+$ DCs express both CD265 and are capable of autocrine survival signaling.

CD264/CD254 interaction plays a role in the induction of T-cell tolerance.

$CD265^{-/-}$ mice, $CD254^{-/-}$ mice, and $TRAF6^{-/-}$ mice are almost phenotypically identical displaying partially defective JNK activation and complete absence of NFκB activation. These mice are severely osteopetrotic, fail to have tooth eruption, and hematopoiesis is diverted to the liver and spleen. Furthermore, they lack all or almost all lymph nodes, which indicates a critical role for CD265/CD254 signaling in lymph node development.

CD265-mediated signaling is also critical for mammary gland development during pregnancy as $CD254^{-/-}$ mice produce insufficient milk to feed their pups due to the absence of growth and expansion of ductal and alveolar epithelium within mammary glands.

Ligands

CD265 binds TRANCE (CD254).

Expression

CD265 is broadly expressed in human tissues.

It is expressed by all hemopoietic cells with the exception of stem cells and erythrocytes.

Applications

Variants of CD265 are responsible for bone remodeling disorders such as familial Paget's disease of bone (PDB2) and familial expansile osteolysis (FEO), which are characterized by increased osteoclast activity.

Gene Name	Entrez Gene#
TNFRSF11A	8792

Selected Monoclonal Antibodies

80704 (R&D Systems, Minneapolis).

CD266

Other Names

TWEAK-R, TNFRSF12A, Fn14, FN14, TWEAKR.

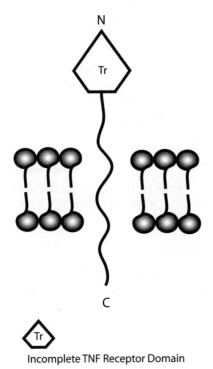

Incomplete TNF Receptor Domain

Molecular Structure

CD266 is a type 1 membrane protein and is the smallest member of the tumor necrosis factor receptor (TNFR) superfamily.

This receptor is leucine-rich (17%) and has eight cysteines but does not have any asparagines or tyrosines.

The immature protein has a 27-residue N-terminal signal peptide that is cleaved to form the 102 amino acid mature protein.

The 53-residue extracellular region contains an incomplete TNFR-Cys domain.

A 21 amino acid transmembrane region is followed by a 29-residue cytoplasmic tail containing a TRAF-binding site flanked by two threonines. TRAF1, TRAF2, TRAF3, and TRAF5 are known to bind this site.

The cytoplasmic threonines are the only potential phosphorylation sites.

Mol Wt: 14 kDa.

Function

CD266-signaling appears to mediate the TWEAK-induced proliferation and migration of endothelial cells and the pro-inflammatory activity of TWEAK.

There is no evidence that CD266 is involved in the apoptotic properties of TWEAK.

TWEAK and CD266 are co-expressed in several cell types and tissues enabling autocrine signaling. Expression of CD266 is upregulated in response to physical damage and certain cytokines, and this would be expected to enhance TWEAK-mediated effects.

Ligands

CD266 binds a tumor necrosis factor-like weak inducer of apoptosis (TWEAK).

Expression

CD266 mRNA expression has been detected in a variety of adult tissues with high levels found in the heart, kidney, lung, placenta and cultured aorta, vascular endothelial cells, and smooth muscle cells.

Normal liver and brain express low levels of CD266, whereas significantly higher levels are found in liver and brain tumors. Similarly over-expression of CD266 has been observed in pancreatic tumors.

Gene Name	Entrez Gene#
TNFRSF12A	51330

Selected Monoclonal Antibodies

ITEM-1 (BD Biosciences; San Diego).

CD267

Other Names

TACI, TNFRSF13B.

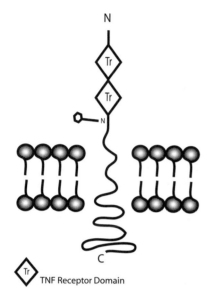

TNF Receptor Domain

Molecular Structure

CD267 is a type III membrane protein and a member of the tumor necrosis factor receptor (TNFR) superfamily.

The protein consists of an extracellular domain of 165 amino acids, which contains 2 TNFR-Cys repeats and 1 potential N-linked glycosylation site; a 21 amino acid transmembrane signal anchor; and a 107 amino acid cytoplasmic domain.

Alternative RNA splicing gives rise to two isoforms. The shorter variant lacks one TNFR-Cys repeat but has been shown to retain its ligand binding capability.

Mol Wt: 32 kDa.

Function

CD267-deficient mice have normal B-cell development; however, B-cell homeostasis and tolerance is impaired, resulting in autoimmunity and the development of lym-phomas. Furthermore, specific activation of CD267 in a human B-cell line induced apoptosis. These findings suggest CD267 is a negative regulator of B-cell activation.

T-independent type 2 response is almost abolished in CD267$^{-/-}$ mice, indicating CD267 provides an essential costimulatory signal for T-independent humoral responses.

Mutations in CD267 are associated with common variable immunodeficiency and IgA deficiency in humans. However, in contrast to CD267$^{-/-}$ mice, lymphoproliferation and autoimmunity are not common features of CD267 deficiency in humans.

Ligands

CD267 binds TALL1 (BAFF, BlyS, CD257) and TALL2 (APRIL, CD256) with high affinity.

Expression

CD267 is expressed by B cells (predominantly CD27$^+$ memory B cells). There are conflicting reports as to whether activated T cells express CD267.

Expression of CD267 has been detected on multiple myeloma cells and B-cell chronic lymphocytic leukemia (B-CLL).

Applications

Agonistic antibody to CD267 is a potential therapeutic agent in the treatment of B-cell lymphoproliferative disorders.

CD267 (TACI)-Ig is being trialed as a decoy receptor for BAFF in the treatment of B-cell malignancies and autoimmune disorders.

Gene Name	Entrez Gene#
TNFRSF13B	23495

Selected Monoclonal Antibodies

165604 (R&D Systems; Minneapolis); FMU-TACI2 (Jin; Xian), 1A1(Mackay; Sydney).

CD268

Other Names

BAFF Receptor, BR3.

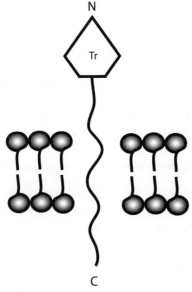

Tr ▷ Incomplete TNF Receptor Domain

Molecular Structure

Type III transmembrane protein member of the tumor necrosis factor receptor (TNFR) family, 172 residues long. The extracellular region contains one N-glycosylation site in the murine molecule, which is absent from the human sequence. Four cysteines are found in the extracellular sequence, fewer than in typical TNFR family members, which contain six or more cysteines.

Splice variants are seen in human and mouse. The human and mouse molecules show 56% identity, including the C-terminal 25aa stretch in the cytoplasmic domain that shows complete identity.

Function

The physiological function of CD268 is not yet clear. It is one of three receptors that bind BAFF, the others being BCMA and TACI. BAFF knockout mice indicate that BAFF is required for the survival of mature B cells, but which receptor is responsible is not clear. Although BAFF-R knockout mice have not yet been analyzed, a naturally occurring mutation in the BAFF R intracellular domain in A/WySnJ mice is associated with apparently normal B-cell precursors but fewer mature B cells. B cells from these mice do not respond to BAFF, whereas mice lacking the other two receptors have normal numbers of mature B cells, indicating it is CD268 that mediates the effects of BAFF on mature B-cell survival.

Ligands

CD268 is one of several receptors that bind the TNF family member BAFF (CD257).

Expression

Expressed in lymphoid tissue and circulating blood leukocytes. Expressed on resting B cells and CD4-positive T cells but down-regulated on activation.

Applications

The role of BAFF in B-cell survival and activation make BAFF R a potential diagnostic reagent. Elevated levels of BAFF are associated with autoimmune diseases, and BAFF or its receptors are thus potential targets for therapy of autoimmune disease. Experimental administration of a CD268-Fc fusion suppresses antibody responses. BAFF-R may also be involved in survival of B-cell malignancies.

Gene Name	Entrez Gene#
TNFRSF13C	115650

Selected Monoclonal Antibodies

FMU-BAFFR1 (Jin; Xian); 11C1 (Mackay; Sydney).

CD269

Other Names

BCMA, BCM, TNFRSF17.

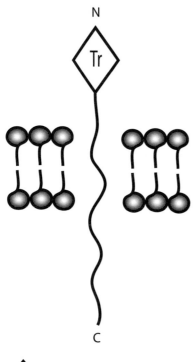

 TNF Receptor Domain

Molecular Structure

CD269 is a type III membrane protein and a member of the tumor necrosis factor receptor (TNFR) superfamily.

The protein consists of a 54 amino acid extracellular domain, 23 amino acid signal anchor, and 107 amino acid cytoplasmic domain.

The extracellular domain has 1 TNFR-Cys repeat.

TRAFs 1, 2, 3, 5, and 6 associate with the cytoplasmic domain.

Mol Wt: 27 kDa.

Function

CD269 is essential for the survival of long-lived bone marrow plasma cells.

CD269-mediated signaling activates NKκB and JNK.

CD269$^{-/-}$ mice have normal serum Ig levels and normal antibody responses but reduced numbers of long-lived bone marrow plasma cells compared with wild-type mice.

A chromosomal aberration of CD269 found in a form of T-cell acute lymphoblastic leukemia (T-ALL) involves a translocation with IL-2 gene.

Ligands

CD269 binds TALL1 (BAFF, BlyS, CD257) with low affinity and TALL2 (APRIL, CD256) with high affinity.

Expression

CD269 is expressed by plasma cells, plasmablasts, and tonsillar germinal center (GC) B cells.

CD269 has low surface density and most remains intracellular where it is associated with peri-nuclear Golgi-like structures.

Applications

CD269 is a potential therapeutic target for the selective elimination of plasma cells in the treatment of antibody-mediated autoimmunity.

Gene Name	Entrez Gene#
TNFRSF17	608

Selected Monoclonal Antibodies

FMU-BCMA1 (Jin; Xian); Vicky-1 (Murone; Apotech, Epalinges).

(CD270)

Other Names

LIGHT-R, HVEM (herpes virus entry mediator).

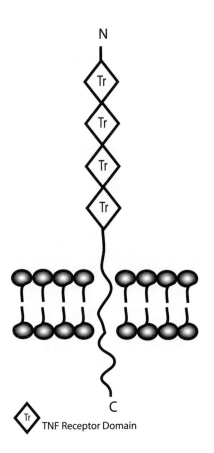

N

Tr

Tr

Tr

Tr

C

Tr TNF Receptor Domain

Molecular Structure

CD270 is a type I transmembrane protein and a member of the TNFR-TNF superfamily.

The unprocessed precursor consists of 283 amino acids and has a signal peptide of 38 amino acids.

The extracellular domain of CD270 consists of 4 cysteine-rich repeat (TNFR-Cys) domains, CRD1-4.

The binding site for LIGHT (CD258) maps to CRD2 and CRD3 and is known as the "DARC" site.

CRD1 contains the distinct but overlapping binding sites for BTLA and herpes virus glycoprotein D (gD).

gD contacts CRD2 as well as CRD1 but on the opposite side to the LIGHT binding site.

Ligand binding induces CD270 trimerization.

Mol Wt: ca. 30 kDa.

Function

LIGHT/LIGHT-R (CD258/CD270) interaction on T cells provides a costimulatory signal via CD270 signaling.

LIGHT/LIGHT-R (CD258/CD270) signaling is implicated in macrophage- and macrophage-derived foam cell-mediated development of atherosclerotic lesions.

Ligation of CD270 with a monoclonal antibody stimulates in an IFNγ-dependent manner the secretion of TNFα and the angiogenic factor IL-8 by the THP-1 monocytic cell line. Furthermore, the THP-1 monocytes produced interstitial collagenase (MMP-1), interstitial collagenase-3 (MMP-13), and gelatinase B (MMP-9). Similarly, CD270 expression correlated with expression of the matrix metalloproteases in foam cell-rich regions of human atherosclerotic lesions.

In contrast to the positive signaling when bound to LIGHT, binding of CD270 to BTLA (CD272) does not trigger CD270 but does provide an inhibitory signal to T cells via BTLA.

Ligands

CD270 binds LIGHT (CD258), BTLA (CD272), LTa3, and glycoprotein D (gD) of Herpes simplex viruses HSV-1 and HSV-2.

Expression

CD270 is expressed on resting T cells, monocytes, and immature dendritic cells. T-cell activation and LIGHT (CD258) binding both downregulate CD270 expression.

Gene Name	Entrez Gene#
TNFRSF14	8764

Selected Monoclonal Antibodies

No antibodies assigned, but CD270 reserved for the LIGHT receptor/ TNFRSF14 molecule.

CD271

Other Names

NGFR (p75), TNFRSF16, NTR, LNGFR.

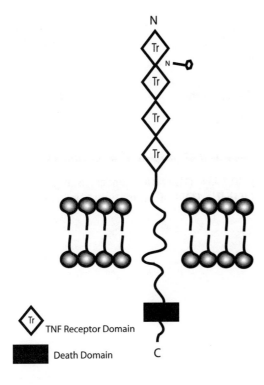

Tr TNF Receptor Domain

Death Domain

Molecular Structure

CD271 is a type 1 membrane protein and a member of the tumor necrosis factor receptor (TNFR) superfamily.

A 28 amino acid signal peptide is cleaved to give a mature protein of 399 amino acids.

The extracellular domain consists of 222 residues and contains 4 TNFR-Cys repeats, a 52 amino acid Serine/threonine-rich region, and 1 potential N-linked glycosylation site.

The transmembrane region consists of 22 amino acids.

The 155-residue cytoplasmic portion of CD271 contains a death domain.

A recently described short isoform (s-p75NTR) retains only the N-terminal TNFR-Cys repeat and does not bind neurotrophin.

The short form is expressed at greatly reduced levels compared with the long form.

Mol Wt: (long form) 75 kDa.

Function

CD271 has diverse and opposing functions due to its capacity to bind a variety of extracellular ligands and associate intracellularly with many different signaling molecules.

CD271 plays a role in cell survival and migration in the vascular system, in tumors such as breast cancer, and in the immune system as well as neurite outgrowth, synaptic transmission, and plasticity.

It is best known as a low affinity neurotrophin receptor, which associates with Trk (tropomyosin-related kinase) receptors to form receptor complexes with high affinity for neurotrophins. Conformational changes imposed by interaction with CD271 modulate the affinity and specificity of Trk receptors for neurotrophins. For example, CD271 restricts TrkA signaling to NGF even though TrkA retains the ability to also bind neurotrophin 3 (NT3). Furthermore, the TrkA-expressing sensory and sympathetic neurons of CD271$^{-/-}$ mice are impaired in their ability to respond to limiting NGF concentrations.

In contrast to the mature neurotrophins, pro-NGF and pro-BDNF bind CD271 (but not Trk receptors) with high affinity and induce apoptosis in cultured neurons.

This finding suggests that the biological role of CD271 may be determined by the local concentrations of pro- and mature neurotrophins.

Mice lacking both CD271 isoforms have a dramatic loss of sensory neurons and Schwann cells and have defective development of major blood vessels compared with mice deficient in the long isoform only. CD271$^{-/-}$ mice have significantly increased numbers of cholinergic neurons, indicating CD271 promotes apoptosis of cholinergic neurons during development.

β-amyloid and aggregated prion protein have both been shown to induce neuronal cell death in vitro and have recently been found to be ligands of CD271.

Ligands

CD271 binds all neurotrophins: NGF, pro-NGF, brain-derived neurotrophic factor (BDNF), pro-BDNF, NT3 and NT4/5, β-amyloid, and aggregated prion protein (CD230).

Expression

CD271 is expressed by neurons, stromal cells, and follicular dendritic cells.

Applications

Analysis of the expression levels of CD271 and NGF may be useful in assessing the prognosis of patients with invasive ductal carcinoma.

Gene Name	Entrez Gene#
NGFR	4804

Selected Monoclonal Antibodies

C40-1457 (BD Biosciences; San Diego); NGFR 5 (DakoCytomation; Glostrup).

CD272

Other Names

BTLA (B and T lymphocyte attenuator).

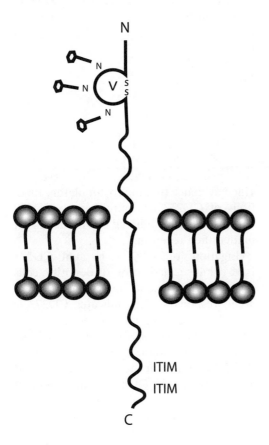

Molecular Structure

CD272 is a type I transmembrane protein and a member of the CD28/B7 family of costimulator molecules within the Ig superfamily.

The precursor protein has a signal sequence of 30 amino acids, and the mature protein consists of 259 amino acids.

The N-terminal extracellular region consists of 127 amino acids and contains a single Ig-like V-type domain and 3 potential N-linked glycosylation sites.

A transmembrane domain of 21 amino acids precedes the C-terminal cytoplasmic tail consisting of 111 residues.

There are 3 tyrosine-based motifs within the cytoplasmic tail that are conserved among mouse, rat, and human CD272 sequences. Two of these motifs are immunoreceptor tyrosine-based inhibitory motifs (ITIMs) and are both required for association with phosphatases SHP-1 and SHP-2.

The third tyrosine-based motif is a Grb-2 recognition consensus.

Mol Wt: 33 kDa (predicted).

Function

CD270 ligation of CD272 induces tyrosine phosphorylation of the CD272 cytoplasmic domain, recruitment of phosphatases SHP-1 and SHP-2, and inhibitory signaling, which results in attenuation of T-cell activation.

CD272 knockout mice have stronger B- and T-cell responses than wild-type mice and increased susceptibility to autoimmunity.

Ligands

CD272 binds CD270 (LIGHT-R, HVEM).

Expression

CD272 is expressed on all mature lymphocytes and developing B and T cells, splenic macrophages, and bone marrow-derived dendritic cells.

Gene Name	Entrez Gene#
BTLA	151888

Selected Monoclonal Antibodies

DTLA9.5 (Olive; Marseille).

CD273

Other Names

B7-DC, PD-L2, PDCD1LG2, PDCG1L2.

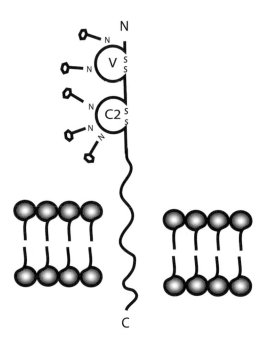

Molecular Structure

CD273 is type I membrane protein and a member of the B7 family of regulatory proteins within the Ig gene superfamily.

The unprocessed protein has a 19 amino acid signal peptide that when cleaved results in a mature protein of 254 amino acids.

The extracellular region consists of 201 residues and contains an N-terminal Ig-like V-type domain followed by an Ig-like C2-type domain and has 5 potential N-linked glycosylation sites.

CD273 has a 21-residue transmembrane span and a cytoplasmic region of 32 amino acids.

Alternative RNA splicing gives rise to three isoforms.

Isoform 2 consists of 183 amino acids and lacks residues 121 to 211 and is not expressed at the cell surface but is associated with the intracellular membrane.

Isoform 3 comprises 182 residues and bears a deletion of residues 183 to 273 and significant amino acid sequence variation between residues 121 and 182 and is probably soluble.

Mol Wt: 25 kDa.

Function

CD273 costimulates the proliferation of T cells, principally $CD4^+$ T cells, and mediates IFNγ production. Several studies have provided evidence that the costimulatory functions of CD273 are unrelated to CD279 binding and are mediated by another as yet unidentified receptor.

Ligation of CD273 by anti-CD273 IgM enhances activation of dendritic cells (DCs) and augments DC stimulation of T-cell responses. This indicates CD273 is capable of signaling into the dendritic cell.

C273 can act as a coinhibitor of the T-cell function when it interacts with PD1 (CD279). A recent study has shown that T-cell-associated CD273 can suppress the proliferation of allo-antigen-specific T cells and IFNγ and IL-2 production via CD279.

Dendritic cells purified from CD273 null mice have a diminished capacity to stimulate T-cell responses to nominal and allogeneic antigens.

Ligands

CD273 binds PD1 (CD279).

Expression

CD273 is expressed by dendritic cells and by activated monocytes and T cells.

CD273 expression is high in the heart, placenta (first trimester), lung, and liver. It is weakly expressed in spleen, lymph nodes, and thymus.

It is highly expressed in primary mediastinal B-cell lymphoma (PMBL) and Hodgkin's lymphoma cell lines.

Applications

CD273 expression is a useful marker to distinguish primary mediastinal B-cell lymphoma from other diffuse large B-cell lymphomas.

Potential exists for CD273 to be a therapeutic target in promoting anti-tumor immunity.

Gene Name	Entrez Gene#
PDCD1LG2	80380

Selected Monoclonal Antibodies

MIH18 (Azuma; San Francisco); PD-L2 (Olive; Marseille).

CD274

Other Names

B7-H1, PD-L1, PDCD1LG1.

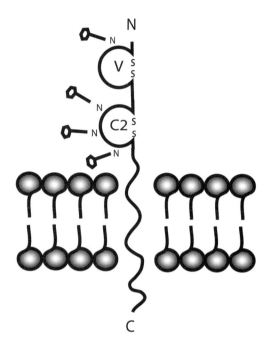

Molecular Structure

CD274 is a type 1 membrane protein and a member of the B7 family of regulatory proteins within the Ig gene superfamily.

An 18 amino acid signal peptide is cleaved to produce a mature protein of 272 amino acids, of which 220 residues are extracellular, 21 residues span the cell membrane, and 31 amino acids are intracellular.

The extracellular sequence contains an N-terminal Ig-like V-type domain followed by an Ig-like C2-type domain, and there are four potential N-linked glycosylation sites.

Variable RNA splicing gives rise to three isoforms: the full length protein and two shorter forms.

The 176-residue isoform 2 lacks amino acids 17–130, and isoform 3 consists of 178 amino acids and lacks residues 179–290.

Mol Wt: 40 kDa.

Function

CD274 can act as both a costimulatory and a coinhibitory molecule for T cells.

Many studies have provided evidence for CD274 having an inhibitory role in regulating T-cell-mediated immune responses, which is similar to the consequences of CD273 binding to CD279.

CD274/CD279 signaling appears to be important in the maintenance of peripheral tolerance and in the prevention of tumor rejection.

Pathogens may exploit CD274 to evade an immune response. For example, the upregulation of CD274 expression by *Shistosoma mansoni* induces T-cell anergy.

Several studies have demonstrated CD274-mediated costimulation of T cells can occur in the absence of CD279, which suggests the existence of alternative receptor(s).

Ligands

CD274 binds PD1 (CD279).

Expression

CD274 is expressed by dendritic cells, activated T cells, and activated monocytes.

It is highly expressed in heart tissue, skeletal muscle, placenta, and lung and weakly expressed in the thymus, spleen, kidney, and liver.

Many tumors, including T-cell lymphomas, carcinomas, melanomas, and glioblastomas express CD274.

Applications

Blockade of CD274 may be a useful tool in cancer immunotherapy.

Gene Name	Entrez Gene#
CD274	29126

Selected Monoclonal Antibodies

1-550, 5-272, 5-496 (Majdic; Vienna); MIH1 (Azuma; San Francisco); SIPD-L1 (2H11) (Zhang; Suzhou); PD-L1.3 (Olive; Marseille).

CD275

Other Names

ICOS ligand (ICOS-L); splice variants hGL50 and B7-homologue 2 (B7-H2) (also known as B7-related protein-1 (B7RP-1) or ligand for ICOS (LICOS).

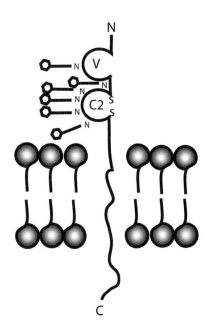

Molecular Structure

A type I transmembrane glycoprotein, homologue of the B7 molecules CD80 and CD86 (with about 25% amino acid identity). The extracellular region consists of one IgV-like and one IgC-like domain. Two splice variants are produced: hGL50 and B7-homologue 2 (B7-H2), also known as B7-related protein-1 (B7RP-1) or ligand for ICOS (LICOS). These variants differ at the C-terminal end of the cytoplasmic sequence.

Function

ICOS-L binds only ICOS and does not bind the ICOS homologues CD28 or CTLA-4 (CD152). Engagement of ICOS on activated T cells by ICOS-L-bearing cells increases cytokine secretion and help for B cells.

ICOS-L knockout mice have not been described. Transgenic mice over-expressing soluble ICOS-L fusion protein showed lymphoid hyperplasia.

The ICOS/ICOS-L interaction appears to be important in the cognate interaction between T cells and antigen presenting cells, and to play a role in pathological situations such as graft rejection and allergy. Most studies have focused on signal transduction through ICOS to the T-cell, but by analogy with the other B7 family members, it is possible that signals are transmitted through ICOS-L to the antigen-presenting cell, endothelial, or B-cell.

Ligands

ICOS (CD278).

Expression

Expressed on B cells, monocytes, macrophages, dendritic cells, and endothelial cells.

Applications

Because of the role of the ICOS/ICOS-L interaction in antigen presentation and pathology such as graft rejection and allergic airway inflammation, the pathway is a target for therapeutic intervention.

Gene Name	Entrez Gene#
ICOSLG	23308

Selected Monoclonal Antibodies

2D3/B7-H2 (San Diego); HIL-131 (Mages; Berlin); SIGL50 (12B11), SIGL50 (11C4) (Zhang; Suzhou); MIH12 (Azuma; San Francisco).

CD276

Other Names

B7-H3 (Long), 4Ig-B7-H3.

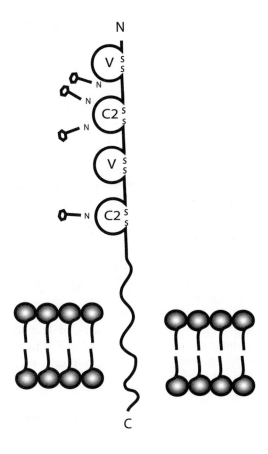

Molecular Structure

CD276 is a type 1 transmembrane protein member of the B7 family of regulatory proteins within the Ig gene superfamily.

Two isoforms are detectable in tissues. The major isoform is the longer form and has four Ig-like domains in the extracellular region arranged as V-type, C-type, V-type, and C-type. The short isoform has 1 V-type and 1 C-type Ig-like domain only.

The long isoform has a short leader peptide of 26 amino acids and a 435 amino acid extracellular region containing the 4 Ig-like domains, a transmembrane region of 31 residues, and a cytoplasmic domain consisting of 42 amino acids.

Mol Wt: 110 kDa (long); 40–45 kDa (short).

Function

CD276 has been described as a costimulatory and coinhibitory ligand. Contradictory results have made the claim of costimulatory functions controversial, and most studies indicate CD276 acts as an inhibitor of T-cell function.

Studies with CD276 null mice provide evidence of inhibitory functions as these mice develop more severe airway inflammation under Th1-polarizing conditions and develop EAE earlier than wild-type mice. Furthermore, antigen presenting cells isolated from CD276 null mice show a twofold increase in alloreactive T-cell proliferation in a MLR response.

CD276 may provide certain tumors with protection against NK cell-mediated killing. Freshly isolated neuroblastoma cells express CD276. MAb-mediated masking of CD276 resulted in enhanced lysis by NK cells.

Expression

CD276 expression is induced upon activation in monocytes, NK cells, dendritic cells, T cells, and B cells.

Applications

Anti-CD276 antibody may be a useful tool for detecting neuroblastoma cells in bone marrow, which is the primary site of neuroblastoma relapse.

Gene Name	Entrez Gene#
CD276	80381

Selected Monoclonal Antibodies

6-311, 7-517, 13-I.241 (Majdic; Vienna).

CD277

Other Names

BT3.1, BTF5.

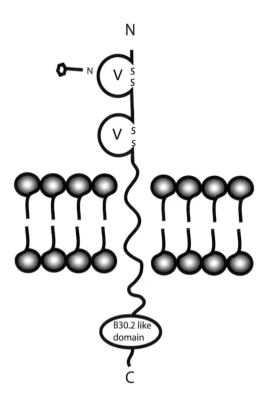

Molecular Structure

CD277 is a type 1 membrane protein and a member of the BT-related subfamily of the B7 family within the Ig superfamily.

The protein has a 29 amino acid signal peptide, and the mature protein consists of 484 residues, of which 225 are extracellular, 17 span the membrane, and 242 comprise the cytoplasmic domain.

The extracellular portion contains two Ig-like V-type domains.

The cytoplasmic region has a B30.2-like domain, which is an approximately 170-residue globular domain.

Mol Wt: 56 kDa.

Function

CD277 is related to the B7 family of proteins, which are regulators of T-cell activation. However, the role of CD277 in the immune response remains to be demonstrated.

Expression

CD277 is expressed by T cells, B cells, NK cells, monocytes, dendritic cells, and a subset of stem cells.

High level mRNA expression of CD277 is found in lymphoid tissues and human umbilical vein endothelial cell (HUVEC), leukemia cell lines, and tumor cell lines derived from breast, ovary, and pancreas.

Gene Name	Entrez Gene#
BTN3A1	11119

Selected Monoclonal Antibodies

19.5 (Olive; Marseille).

CD278

Other Names

ICOS (Inducible Costimulator).

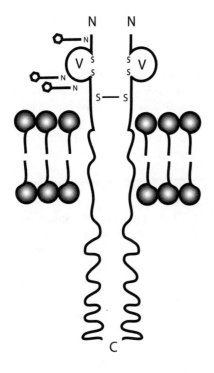

Molecular Structure

Type I transmembrane glycoprotein that forms a disulphide-linked dimer with a molecular weight of 55–60 kDa.

The monomer has a single Ig-V-like domain, a membrane-spanning sequence, and a cytoplasmic tail. The cysteine residue at position 136 forms the disulfide bridge between the chains.

The extracellular sequence contains three potential N-glycosylation sites.

Murine ICOS is 72% identical to human ICOS at the amino acid level.

Function

CD278 (ICOS) provides costimulatory activity for T-cell proliferation, cytokine synthesis, and cognate interaction with B cells. Engagement of ICOS induces secretion of IL-4, IL-5, IL-6, IFNγ, TNFα, and GM-CSF, but not IL-2. CD278 engagement also induces IL-10 secretion and protects T cells from apoptosis.

Knockout mice are generally healthy and have normal T-cell development and numbers, but the T cells show defective T-cell activation and effector function.

ICOS$^{-/-}$ T cells do not make IL-4 and IL-13, resulting in defective Ig class switching. These mice also show impaired germinal center formation.

Blockade of ICOS signaling significantly reduced airway inflammation in a model of allergic airway disease. Anti-CD278 antibody delays graft rejection, apparently by suppressing T-cell activation.

Ligands

Unlike CD28 and CD152 (CTLA-4), ICOS does not bind CD80 and CD86. It provides costimulation to memory T cells by interacting with a different B7 family member, B7H2 (ICOS-L, CD275).

Expression

Expression of ICOS is restricted to activated T cells and is seen on the cell surface 12–48 h after activation. In humans, ICOS is expressed in the thymic medulla and in the T-cell zones of lymph nodes.

Applications

The restricted expression of ICOS on activated cells, together with its role in allergic airway inflammation, EAE, and allograft rejection suggests ICOS as a target for immunotherapy.

Gene Name	Entrez Gene#
ICOS	29851

Selected Monoclonal Antibodies

F44 (Kroczek; Berlin).

CD279

Other Names

PD1, PDC1, hPD-1, SLEB2.

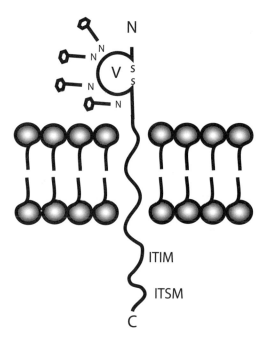

Molecular Structure

CD279 is a type 1 transmembrane protein and belongs to the CD28/CTLA-4 subfamily within the Ig superfamily.

A signal sequence of 20 kDa is cleaved to produce a mature protein of 268 amino acids, of which 150 residues are extracellular, 21 residues span the membrane, and 97 amino acids are intracellular.

The extracellular region has one Ig-like V-type domain and four potential N-linked glycosylation sites.

The intracellular portion of CD279 contains an immunoreceptor tyrosine-based inhibitory motif (ITIM) and an immunoreceptor tyrosine-based switch motif (ITSM). Although both motifs are phosphorylated following CD279 ligation, the ITSM is required for inhibitory activity.

CD279 is monomeric.

A recent study has described four alternatively spliced mRNA variants in addition to the full-length form. One of these isoforms is predicted to be soluble.

Mol Wt: 55 kDa.

Function

Despite being named Programmed Death-1 (PD-1), CD279 has not been shown to induce cell death directly but may do so indirectly.

Cell death may be due in part to CD279-mediated inhibition of cell survival gene bcl-xL expression, downregulation of glucose metabolism, and reduction in Akt activation.

CD279 is an inducible molecule that plays a role in maintaining peripheral self-tolerance and several studies demonstrate that the CD274/CD279 (PD-L1/PD-1) interaction is important in preventing autoimmunity.

CD279-deficient mice develop autoimmune conditions including lupus-like glomerulonephritis and proliferative arthritis in C57BL/6 mice and lethal dilated cardiomyopathy mediated by autoantibodies in BALB/c mice.

Single nucleotide polymorphisms in PDCD1 are associated in humans with susceptibility to systemic lupus erythematosus (SLE) and the presence of nephropathy in SLE, type 1 diabetes, and rheumatoid arthritis.

CD273 ligation of CD279 is associated with inhibition of T-cell proliferation.

Ligands

CD279 binds CD273 (B7-DC) and CD274 (B7-H1).

Expression

CD279 is expressed during thymic development primarily by CD4–CD8- cells and double-negative γ/δ thymocytes and by activated T cells, activated B cells, and activated monocytes. NK-T cells express low levels of CD279.

Applications

SNP (single nucleotide polymorphism) analysis of CD279 may be useful in prognostic evaluation of patients for susceptibility to autoimmune diseases.

Gene Name	Entrez Gene#
PDCD1	5133

Selected Monoclonal Antibodies

J116 (Honjo; Kobe); PD1.3.1 (Live; Marseille).

CD280

Other Names

Endo180, TEM22, MRC2, UPARAP, KIAA0709.

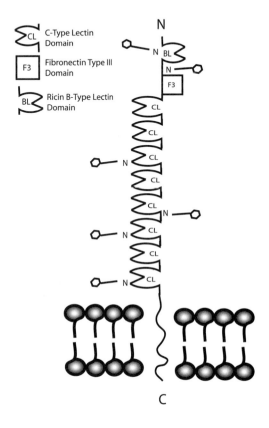

Molecular Structure

CD280 is a type 1 transmembrane protein and an endocytosis receptor of the macrophage mannose receptor (MMR) protein family.

The extracellular portion of CD280 comprises a N-terminal signal sequence followed by 10 extracellular domains: A ricin B-type lectin domain (a cysteine-rich domain with structural similarity to soybean trypsin inhibitor), a fibronectin type II (FnII) domain, and 8 C-type lectin-like domains (CTLD-1 to -8).

Deglycosylation reduces the Mol Wt to 160–170 kDa, indicating that CD280 is N-glycosylated.

The extracellular region is followed by a typical transmembrane region and a short cytoplasmic domain.

Mol Wt: 180 kDa.

Function

CD280 is a constitutively recycled cell-surface adhesion molecule that binds extracellular matrix (ECM) proteins and mediates their uptake and lysosomal degradation.

CD280 expression is not detectable in human breast cancer cells but is present in tumor-associated stromal cells. In a murine model of human ductal mammary adeno-carcinoma, tumor-associated stromal cells were shown to internalize and degrade collagen in a CD280-dependent process. When these tumors were generated in CD280-deficient mice (which are phenotypically normal), collagen turnover was abrogated and the tumors were fibrotic and smaller than the tumors generated in CD280$^{+/+}$ mice.

CD280 forms a complex with urokinase plasminogen activator (uPA) and its receptor (CD87), and this complex may play a role in CD87-dependent cell migration. The addition of uPA to MDA-MB-231 breast cancer cells resulted in clustering of CD280 and CD87 at the leading edge of the polarized cells and increased cell motility. This effect could be abolished by pre-treating the cells with CD280-specific small interfering RNA (siRNA). CD280 expression has been reported at sites of non-neoplastic tissue degenerative diseases, such as osteoarthritis, rheumatoid arthritis, emphysema, and periodontal disease.

Ligands

CD280 binds gelatin, collagen types I, II, IV, and V.

Expression

CD280 is expressed by myeloid progenitors, fibroblasts, a subset of endothelial cells, and a subset of macrophages. It is highly expressed by mesenchymal cells at sites of active tissue remodeling, including during the progression of carcinomas.

Applications

CD280 is a potential therapeutic target in the treatment of carcinomas by limiting ECM degradation and tumor progression.

Gene Name	Entrez Gene#
MRC2	9902

Selected Monoclonal Antibodies

E1/183 (Isacke; London).

CD281

Other Names

TOLL-like receptor 1, TLR1, TIL.

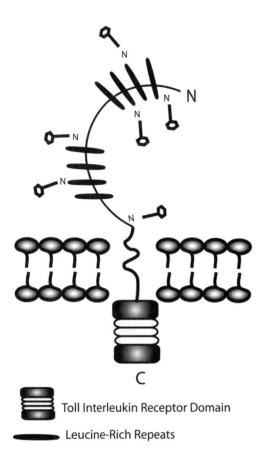

Toll Interleukin Receptor Domain

Leucine-Rich Repeats

Molecular Structure

CD281 is a type 1 transmembrane protein and a member of the CD282 (TLR2) sub-family of the Toll-like receptor (TLR) family (see also CD282–CD291).

The precursor protein has a 24 amino acid signal peptide that when cleaved leaves a mature protein of 762 residues, of which 556 amino acids are extracellular, 21 residues span the membrane, and 185 amino acids are intracellular.

The extracellular region contains eight leucine-rich repeats (LRR) capped at each end by characteristic N-terminal (LRR-NT) and C-terminal (LRR-CT) motifs and six potential N-glycosylation sites.

The LRR are predicted to have a "horseshoe-like" structure and form the ligand binding domain.

The cytoplasmic region contains a toll/IL-1R (TIR) domain.

CD281 forms a heterodimer with CD282 (TLR2).

Mol Wt: 90 kDa.

Function

CD281 is a toll-like receptor and plays a role in innate immunity by recognizing specific pathogen-associated molecular patterns (PAMPs) on pathogens.

PAMP binding of the CD281/CD282 complex triggers intracellular MyD88-dependent signaling pathways and nuclear translocation of NFκB, which ultimately leads to production of pro-inflammatory cytokines to stimulate host defenses and initiate an acquired immune response.

Coexpression of both receptors is required for recognition of ara-lipoarabinomannam, and studies with CD281 and CD282 knockout mice have shown that these receptors cooperate in the recognition of *Borrelia burgdorferi* outer-surface protein A lipoprotein (OspA) as well as mycobacterial 19-kDa lipoprotein and synthetic triacylated lipopeptides.

Ligands

CD281 recognizes *B. burgdorferi* outer-surface protein A lipoprotein (OspA-L), mycobacterial 19-kDa lipoprotein, and tri-acylated lipopeptides.

Expression

CD281 is expressed by monocytes and neutrophils.

CD281 expression is detectable in breast milk.

Gene Name	Entrez Gene#
TLR1	7096

Selected Monoclonal Antibodies

GD2.F4 (e-Bioscience San Diego; Apotech Epalinges).

CD282

Other Names

Toll-like receptor 2, TLR2, TIL4.

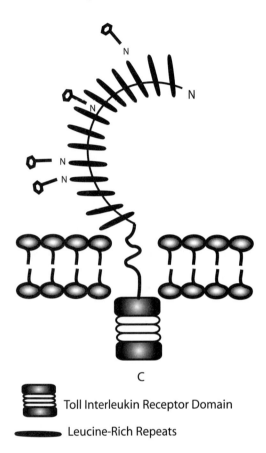

Toll Interleukin Receptor Domain

Leucine-Rich Repeats

Molecular Structure

CD282 is a type 1 transmembrane protein and a member of the Toll-like receptor (TLR) family (see also CD281–CD291).

CD282 forms part of a subfamily of TLRs, which include CD281 (TLR1), TLR6, and TLR10.

CD282 forms heterodimers with CD281 and TLR6.

Cleavage of the 18 amino acid signal peptide results in a mature protein of 766 amino acids, of which 570 residues are extracellular, 21 residues span the membrane, and 175 amino acids are intracellular.

The extracellular domain contains 14 leucine-rich repeats (LRRs) capped at each end by characteristic N-terminal (LRR-NT) and C-terminal (LRR-CT) motifs and has 4 potential N-linked glycosylation sites. Glycosylation of Asn 422 is critical for secretion of the ectodomain.

The LRRs are predicted to have a "horseshoe-like" structure and form the ligand binding domain.

The cytoplasmic region contains a toll/IL-1R (TIR) domain that interacts with the adaptor protein TIR domain-containing adaptor protein (TIRAP).

Mol Wt: 85 kDa.

Function

CD282 functions as a pattern recognition receptor for pathogen-associated molecular patterns (PAMPs) of fungi, protozoan pathogens, and bacteria (particularly peptidoglycan and lipotechoic acids of Gram-negative bacteria).

Ligand binding of CD282 recruits TIRAP and leads to myeloid differentiation primary response gene 88 (MyD88)-dependent signaling resulting in NFκB activation, and pro-inflammatory cytokine production, and it initiates an acquired immune response.

The wide range of bacterial components recognized by CD282 is in part due to its association with CD281 and CD286 (TLR6), which enables discrimination of subtle structural differences between lipopeptides.

Studies of the role of CD282 on T cells suggest CD282 acts as a costimulatory receptor for antigen-specific T-cell development and is involved in maintenance of T-cell memory.

CD282-deficient mice are significantly more susceptible to infection with Gram-positive bacteria than wild-type mice.

Single nucleotide polymorphisms (SNPs) of CD282 have been associated with increased susceptibility to some human infectious diseases, including lepromatous leprosy, tuberculosis, and atopic diseases such as atopic dermatitis and asthma.

Ligands

CD282 recognizes cell membrane components of fungal and protozoan pathogens as well as lipoproteins/lipopeptides of a wide variety of bacteria.

It has been suggested that CD282 binds endogenous heat shock proteins Hsp60, Hsp70, and Gp96. However, these claims are controversial as other studies implicate LPS and LPS-associated protein contamination leading to the observed effects.

Expression

CD282 is expressed by peripheral blood leukocytes, with particularly high expression in monocytes in bone marrow, lymph nodes, and spleen.

Expression of CD282 is detectable in lung, fetal liver, and breast milk and at low levels in other tissues.

Gene Name	Entrez Gene#
TLR2	7097

Selected Monoclonal Antibodies

TL2.1 (Apotech, Epalinges); TL2.3 (eBioscience, San Diego).

CD283

Other Names

Toll-like receptor 3, TLR3.

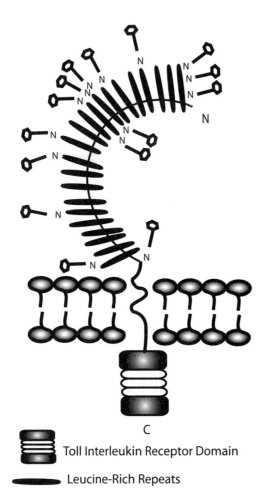

C

⬭⬭⬭ Toll Interleukin Receptor Domain

▬ Leucine-Rich Repeats

Molecular Structure

CD283 is a type 1 transmembrane protein and a member of the toll-like receptor family (see also CD281–CD291).

The unprocessed precursor has a 23-residue signal peptide that is cleaved to give rise to a mature protein of 881 amino acids.

681 residues are extracellular, 21 residues form a transmembrane helix, and 179 amino acids are intracellular.

The ectodomain contains 22 leucine-rich repeats (LRRs) capped at each end by characteristic N-terminal (LRR-NT) and C-terminal (LRR-CT) motifs. The LRRs form a horseshoe-shaped structure, which is the ligand-binding domain. The extensive β-sheet on the protein's concave surface is the site of several modifications including insertions in the LRRs and 11 potential N-linked glycosylation sites.

The cytoplasmic region contains a Toll/IL-1R (TIR) domain that interacts with the adaptor molecule Toll-IL1 receptor-resistance (TIR) domain-containing adaptor inducing IFNβ (TRIF).

Mol Wt: 100 kDa.

Function

CD283 plays a role in the host response to viral infection.

Binding of double-stranded RNA to CD282 recruits the adaptor molecule TRIF, which induces signaling pathways leading via the activation IRF3 and NFκB to pro-inflammatory cytokine and IFN production.

Activation of CD283 also leads to the initiation of a caspase-dependent apoptotic cascade.

A role for CD283 in cross-presentation (presentation in association with MHC class I by cells not infected by the virus) and priming has been suggested for viruses that do not have tropism for dendritic cells. This requires uptake of antigen, for example, by ingestion of infected cells, and TLR3 appears to facilitate this process.

It has been demonstrated that vaccinia virus and Hepatitis C virus (HCV) express proteins that target aspects of the CD283 signaling pathway and efficiently inhibit CD283-induced gene expression.

Ligands

CD283 binds double-stranded RNA.

Expression

CD283 is expressed by fibroblasts, myeloid dendritic cells (monocyte-derived DCs and CD11⁺ blood DCs), microglia, and astrocytes.

Although detectable on the cell surface, most CD283 is located intracellularly and is associated with endosomal compartments.

CD283 expression is detectable in breast milk.

Gene Name	Entrez Gene#
TLR3	7098

Selected Monoclonal Antibodies

TLR3.7 (eBioscience, San Diego).

CD284

Other Names

TOLL-like receptor 4, TLR4.

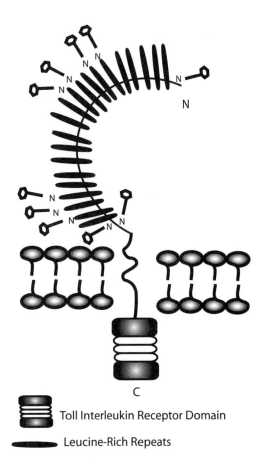

Toll Interleukin Receptor Domain

Leucine-Rich Repeats

Molecular Structure

CD284 is a type 1 transmembrane protein and a member of the Toll-like receptor (TLR) family (see also CD281–CD291).

CD284 forms a complex with the MD2 (Ly96) adaptor protein.

The unprocessed precursor has a 23-residue signal peptide that when cleaved results in an 816 amino acid mature protein.

608 amino acids are extracellular, 21 residues span the membrane, and 187 amino acids are intracellular.

The extracellular domain contains 21 leucine rich repeats (LRRs) capped at each end by characteristic N-terminal (LRR-NT) and C-terminal (LRR-CT) motifs. The LRRs form a horseshoe-shaped structure, which is the ligand-binding domain.

There are 10 potential N-linked glycosylation sites. Glycosylation of Asn-526 and Asn-575 are necessary for the cell surface-expression of CD284 and LPS response. Mutants lacking 2 or more of the other glycosylation sites are unable to interact with LPS.

The intracellular region contains a Toll/IL-1R (TIR) domain that interacts with the adaptor molecules TIR domain-containing adaptor protein (TIRAP) and TRIF-related adaptor molecule (TRAM).

Mol Wt: 85 kDa.

Function

LPS binding of CD284 recruits TIRAP and TRAM, which activate myeloid differentiation primary response gene 88 (MyD88)-dependent and MyD88-independent (TRIF-dependent) signaling pathways, respectively. Activation of both of these pathways is essential for inducing inflammatory cytokine production and favors a Th1 response.

LPS-activated CD284 can induce dendritic cell maturation via TRIF-dependent signaling.

CD284-deficient mice are more susceptible to a number of Gram-negative and Gram-positive bacterial pathogens, respiratory syncytial virus, and the fungal pathogens *Aspergillus fumigatus* and *Candida albicans*. Increased susceptibility was found to be the result of decreased neutrophil recruitment to the site of infection because of defective chemokine production and decreased chemokine receptor expression.

There have been several small studies of the impact of single nucleotide polymorphisms of CD284 on susceptibility to infectious and inflammatory diseases. Larger studies are needed as the generally small numbers of participants and conflicting results make it impossible to draw any conclusions at this time.

Ligands

CD284 binds lipopolysaccharide (LPS) and may be involved in the binding of endogenous ligands such as heat shock proteins Hsp60 and Hsp70 and fibrinogen. However, CD284 binding of endogenous ligands has not been clearly established.

CD284 recognizes the fusion protein of respiratory syncytial virus (RSV) and the fungal pathogens *Aspergillus fumigatus* and *Candida albicans*.

Expression

CD284 is expressed by monocytes, macrophages, granulocytes, dendritic cells, and activated CD4$^+$ T cells.

CD284 expression is detectable in breast milk.

Gene Name	Entrez Gene#
TLR4	7099

Selected Monoclonal Antibodies

HTA125 (Apotech, Epilinges; Serotec, Oxford; eBioscience, San Diego).

(CD285)

Other Names

Toll-like receptor 5, TLR5, TIL3.

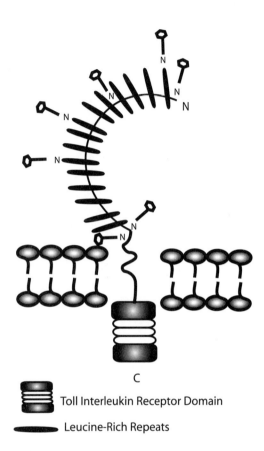

Toll Interleukin Receptor Domain

Leucine-Rich Repeats

Molecular Structure

CD285 is a type 1 transmembrane protein and a member of the Toll-like receptor (TLR) family (see also CD281–CD291).

CD285 forms a subfamily of TLRs based on its genomic structure and amino acid sequence.

Pre-CD285 has a 20 amino acid signal sequence that when cleaved results in a mature protein of 838 amino acids.

The ectodomain consist of 619 amino acids arranged as 15 leucine-rich repeats (LRRs) capped at each end by characteristic N-terminal (LRR-NT) and C-terminal (LRR-CT) motifs. The LRRs form a horseshoe-shaped structure, which is the ligand-binding domain.

There are seven potential N-glycosylation sites.

21 amino acids form the transmembrane domain, and the intracellular region consists of 198 amino acids and contains a 147 amino acid Toll/IL-1R (TIR) domain, which interacts with the adaptor molecule myeloid differentiation primary response gene 88 (MyD88).

Approximately 10% of the population carry a CD290 polymorphism with a stop codon at position 392 (TLR5392STOP), leading to loss of the transmembrane and cytoplasmic domains.

Mol Wt: ca. 120 kDa.

Function

CD285 acts as a receptor for and is activated by bacterial flagellin. Release of pro-inflammatory cytokines and immune cell activation occurs via the MyD88-dependent signaling pathway.

The stop codon polymorphism prevents flagellin-activated signaling and is associated with susceptibility to lung infections by bacterial pathogens such as *Legionella pneumophila* and *Pseudomonas aeruginosa*.

Flagellin/CD285 signaling is implicated in the progression of inflammatory bowel conditions such as colitis, inflammatory bowel disease, and Crohn's disease.

Some bacterial pathogens, including *Helicobacter pylori* and *Campylobacter jejuni*, produce flagellin with specific changes to the CD285 binding site and are thus able to evade detection via CD285.

Ligands

CD285 binds flagellin.

Expression

CD285 is highly expressed in mucosal epithelium as well as peripheral blood leukocytes particularly monocytes. Moderate expression is detectable in CD11c$^+$ immature dendritic cells.

CD285 expression is found also in ovary, prostate, testis, and breast milk.

Gene Name	Entrez Gene#
TLR5	7100

Selected Monoclonal Antibodies

No antibodies assigned, but CD285 reserved for TLR5.

CD286

Other Names

Toll-like receptor 6, TLR6.

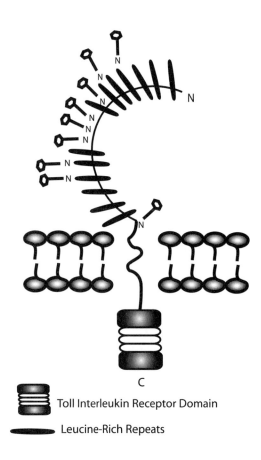

Toll Interleukin Receptor Domain

Leucine-Rich Repeats

Molecular Structure

CD286 is a type 1 transmembrane protein and a member of the Toll-like receptor (TLR) family (see also CD281–D291).

CD286 forms part of a subfamily of TLRs, which includes TLR1 (CD281), TLR2 (CD282), and TLR10 (CD290).

Pre-CD286 has a 31 amino acid signal sequence that when cleaved results in a mature protein of 765 amino acids.

The ectodomain consist of 555 amino acids arranged as 13 leucine-rich repeats (LRRs) capped at each end by characteristic N-terminal (LRR-NT) and C-terminal (LRR-CT) motifs. The LRRs form a horseshoe-shaped structure, which is the ligand-binding domain.

There are nine potential N-linked glycosylation sites.

21 amino acids form the transmembrane domain, and the intracellular region consists of 189 amino acids and contains a 145 amino acid Toll/IL-1R (TIR) domain, which interacts with the adaptor molecule myeloid differentiation primary response gene 88 (MyD88).

CD286 forms heterodimers with CD282.

Mol Wt: ca. 85 kDa.

Function

CD286 is a toll-like receptor and plays a role in innate immunity by recognizing specific pathogen-associated molecular patterns (PAMPs) on pathogens.

CD286 cooperates functionally with CD282 in the recognition of microbial diacyl-lipopeptides.

PAMP binding of CD286/CD282 complex triggers intracellular MyD88-dependent signaling pathways and nuclear translocation of NFκB, which ultimately leads to production of pro-inflammatory cytokines to stimulate host defences and initiate an acquired immune response.

Ligands

CD286/CD282 complex recognizes bacterial diacyl-lipopeptides, including mycoplasmal macrophage-activating lipopeptide-2kDa (MALP-2), soluble TB factor (STF), phenol-soluble modulin (PSM), *B. burgdorferi* outer surface protein A-lipoprotein (OspA-L), and Group B Streptococci heat labile soluble factor (GBS-F).

Expression

CD286 is expressed by monocytes, CD11c⁺ immature dendritic cells, plasmacytoid pre-dendritic cells, and dermal microvessel endothelium.

CD286 expression is detectable in breast milk.

Gene Name	Entrez Gene#
TLR6	10333

Selected Monoclonal Antibodies

HPer6 (eBioscience; San Diego).

(CD287)

Other Names

Toll-like receptor 7, TLR7.

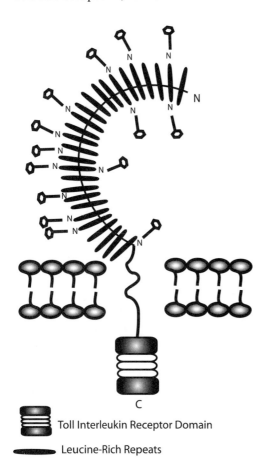

▓ Toll Interleukin Receptor Domain

▬ Leucine-Rich Repeats

Molecular Structure

CD287 is a type 1 transmembrane protein and a member of the Toll-like receptor (TLR) family (see also CD281–CD291).

CD287 forms part of a subfamily of TLRs, which includes TLR8 (CD288) and TLR9 (CD289).

Pre-TLR7 has a 26 amino acid signal sequence that when cleaved results in a mature protein of 1023 amino acids.

The ectodomain consist of 813 amino acids arranged as 27 leucine-rich repeats (LRRs) capped at each end by characteris-tic N-terminal (LRR-NT) and C-terminal (LRR-CT) motifs. The LRRs form a horse-shoe-shaped structure, which is the ligand-binding domain.

There are 14 potential N-linked glycosy-lation sites.

21 amino acids form the transmembrane domain, and the intracellular region consists of 189 amino acids and contains a 148 amino acid Toll/IL-1R (TIR) domain, which interacts with the adaptor molecule myeloid differentiation primary response gene 88 (MyD88).

Function

CD287 acts as a receptor for and is activated by viral single-stranded RNA (ssRNA), which enters the cell via the endosomal pathway. It forms part of the innate defence mechanism against infection by double-stranded (ds) and single-stranded (ss) RNA viruses. The anti-viral response to dsRNA viruses is thought to be in part due to CD287 recognition of de novo synthesized ssRNA that accumulates during viral replication within the cell cytoplasm.

CD287-mediated signaling is MyD88-dependent and leads to the release of pro-inflammatory cytokines, particularly type 1 interferons, and an anti-viral response.

Recent studies have implicated CD287 in the development of an autoimmune response to self-RNA-associated auto-antigens such as nucleoprotein antigens Sm and ribonucleoprotein (RNP). Sm and ribonucleoprotein (RNP) are tightly bound to U-rich small nucleotide (sn) RNAs, which are potential ligands of CD287 (and/or CD288). SnRNA-containing antigen-antibody complexes are able to activate B lymphocytes and dendritic cells via CD287 and/or CD288.

Ligands

CD287 recognizes GU-rich single-stranded RNA.

Expression

CD287 is strongly expressed in predominantly the endosomes of plasmacytoid dendritic cells, B cells, and myeloid dendritic cells.

CD287 expression is detectable in breast milk, brain, placenta, spleen, stomach, small intestine, and lung.

Applications

CD287 agonists such as isatoribine, imiquimod, and resiquimod are thera-peutic agents used to stimulate an anti-viral response in the treatment of HCV infection.

CD287 agonists are currently being assessed as potential adjuvants to vaccines.

Gene Name   Entrez Gene#

TLR7   51284

Selected Monoclonal Antibodies

No antibodies assigned, but CD287 reserved for TLR7.

CD288

Other Names

TLR8, Toll-like receptor 8.

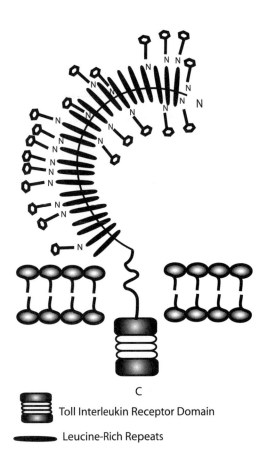

C

Toll Interleukin Receptor Domain

Leucine-Rich Repeats

Molecular Structure

CD288 is a type 1 transmembrane protein and a member of the Toll-like receptor (TLR) family (see also CD281–CD291).

CD288 forms part of a subfamily of TLRs, which includes TLR7 (CD287) and TLR9 (CD289).

Pre-CD288 has a 26 amino acid signal sequence that when cleaved results in a mature protein of 1015 amino acids.

The ectodomain consist of 801 amino acids arranged as 24 leucine-rich repeats (LRRs) capped at each end by characteristic N-terminal (LRR-NT) and C-terminal (LRR-CT) motifs. The LRRs form a horseshoe-shaped structure, which is the ligand-binding domain.

There are 21 potential N-linked glycosylation sites.

21 amino acids form the transmembrane domain, and the intracellular region consists of 193 amino acids and contains a Toll/IL-1R (TIR) domain that interacts with the adaptor molecule myeloid differentiation primary response gene 88 (MyD88).

Mol Wt: 83 kDa.

Function

CD288 is a Toll-like receptor that forms part of the innate defence mechanism against infection by double-stranded (ds) and single-stranded (ss) RNA viruses and its recognition of single-stranded GU-rich RNA. The anti-viral response to dsRNA viruses is thought to be in part due to CD288 recognition of de novo synthesized ssRNA that accumulates during viral replication within the cytoplasm.

Ligation of CD288 triggers the secretion of inflammatory and regulatory cytokines.

Recent studies have implicated CD288 in the development of an autoimmune response to self-RNA-associated autoantigens such as nucleoprotein antigens Sm and ribonucleoprotein (RNP). Sm and ribonucleoprotein (RNP) are tightly bound to U-rich small nucleotide (sn) RNAs, which are potential ligands of CD288 (and /or CD287). SnRNA-containing antigen-antibody complexes are able to activate B lymphocytes and dendritic cells via CD287 and/or CD288.

Ligands

CD288 binds single-stranded GU-rich RNA.

Expression

CD288 is principally found in endosomal or lysosomal compartments of macrophages and subsets of dendritic cells including plasmacytoid dendritic cells.

Gene Name	Entrez Gene#
TLR8	51311

Selected Monoclonal Antibodies

44C143 (Imgenex; San Diego).

CD289

Other Names

TLR9, Toll-like recetor 9.

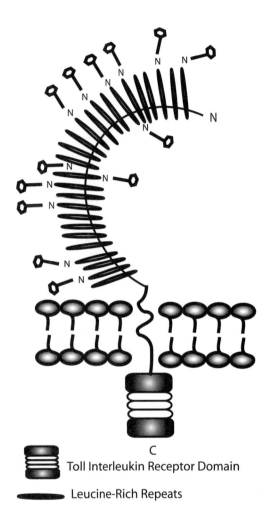

C
Toll Interleukin Receptor Domain

Leucine-Rich Repeats

Molecular Structure

CD289 is a type 1 transmembrane protein and a member of the Toll-like receptor (TLR) family (see also CD281–CD291).

CD289 forms part of a subfamily of TLRs, which includes TLR7 (CD287) and TLR8 (CD288).

Pre-TLR9 has a 25 amino acid signal sequence that when cleaved results in a mature protein of 1007 amino acids.

The ectodomain consist of 1007 amino acids arranged as 26 leucine-rich repeats (LRRs) capped at each end by characteristic N-terminal (LRR-NT) and C-terminal (LRR-CT) motifs. The LRRs form a horseshoe shaped structure, which is the ligand-binding domain.

21 amino acids form the transmembrane domain, and the intracellular region consists of 193 amino acids and contains a Toll/IL-1R (TIR) domain that interacts with the adaptor molecule myeloid differentiation primary response gene 88 (MyD88).

Mol Wt: 115–120 kDa.

Function

CD289 plays a role in the innate immune response, acting as a receptor for unmethylated CpG DNA present in endosomes during bacterial and viral infection.

Activation of CD289 triggers MyD88-dependent signaling and induces high level production of type 1 IFN, particularly IFNα by plasmacytoid and bone marrow derived dendritic cells (DCs), mediates DC maturation, and triggers a Th1-skewed adaptive immune response.

CD289-deficient mice do not produce IFNα in response to challenge with herpesviruses and have impaired DC maturation. Interestingly, control of viral replication was the same in CD289-deficient and wild-type mice challenged with HSV-1, which suggests CD289 is not essential for defence against HSV-1.

Ligands

CD289 binds unmethylated CpG DNA motifs.

Expression

CD289 is expressed at high levels by plasmacytoid dendritic cells and at low levels by other peripheral blood leukocytes.

High level expression is found in the spleen, lymph node, and tonsils.

Gene Name	Entrez Gene#
TLR9	54106

Selected Monoclonal Antibodies

eB72–1665 (eBioscience; San Diego).

CD290

Other Names

TLR10, Toll-like receptor 10.

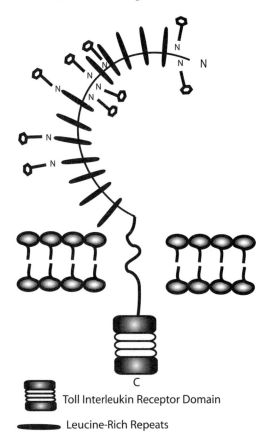

C

≣ Toll Interleukin Receptor Domain

━━ Leucine-Rich Repeats

Molecular Structure

CD290 is a type 1 transmembrane protein and an orphan member of the Toll-like receptor (TLR) family (see also CD281–CD291).

CD290 belongs to the TLR2 subfamily, which includes TLR1, TLR2, and TLR6.

CD290 forms homodimers or heterodimers with CD281 (TLR1) and CD282 (TLR2).

Pre-TLR10 has a 19 amino acid signal sequence that when cleaved results in a mature protein of 792 amino acids.

The ectodomain consist of 557 amino acids arranged as 12 leucine-rich repeats (LRRs) capped at each end by characteristic N-terminal (LRR-NT) and C-terminal (LRR-CT) motifs. The LRRs form a horseshoe-shaped structure, which is the ligand-binding domain.

There are 9 potential N-glycosylation sites.

The transmembrane domain consists of 21 residues, and the intracellular region consists of 214 amino acids and contains a 147 amino acid Toll/IL-1R (TIR) domain, which interacts with the adaptor molecule myeloid differentiation primary response gene 88 (MyD88).

CD290 is highly polymorphic.

Mol Wt: 91–100 kDa.

Function

CD290 is a Toll-like receptor selectively expressed by B lymphocytes.

Study of CD290 function has been hampered by the lack of CD290 expression in mice due to the insertion of retroviral DNA in the TLR10 gene.

Recently a complete TLR10 sequence was detected in the rat genome and low level CD290 expression found in rat plasmacytoid dendritic cells. Therefore it is possible that further study of CD290 function may be continued using a rat model.

A recent study has found a possible link between CD290 polymorphisms and asthma, which suggests a role in the lung.

Expression

CD290 expression is expressed by normal and neoplastic B cells. Pre-B cells express CD290 weakly, and the expression level increases with maturation. The strongest expression of CD290 occurs in activated B cells.

Plasmacytoid dendritic cells and CD1a+ dendritic cells derived from CD34+ precursors resembling Langerhans cells express CD290.

CD290 expression is detectable in lung but is predominantly expressed in immune cell-rich tissues, including spleen, lymph node, thymus, and tonsil.

Gene Name	Entrez Gene#
TLR10	81793

Selected Monoclonal Antibodies

158C114 (Imgenex; San Diego).

(CD291)

Other Names

TLR11, Toll-like receptor 11.

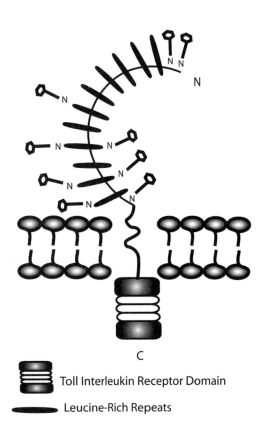

Toll Interleukin Receptor Domain

Leucine-Rich Repeats

Molecular Structure

CD291 is a type 1 transmembrane protein and a member of the Toll-like receptor (TLR) family (see also CD281–CD290).

Unlike the murine TLR11 gene, the human TLR11 gene bears several stop codons and does not encode a full-length protein.

The murine CD290 precursor has a 30 amino acid signal sequence that when cleaved results in a mature protein of 896 amino acids.

The ectodomain consist of 691 amino acids arranged as 11 leucine-rich repeats (LRRs) capped at each end by characteristic N-terminal (LRR-NT) and C-terminal (LRR-CT) motifs. The LRRs form a horseshoe-shaped structure, which is the ligand-binding domain.

There are 9 potential N-glycosylation sites.

The transmembrane domain consists of 21 residues, and the intracellular region consists of 214 amino acids and contains a 184 amino acid Toll/IL-1R (TIR) domain, which interacts with the adaptor molecule myeloid differentiation primary response gene 88 (MyD88).

Mol Wt: 97 kDa.

Function

No role for CD291 has been found in humans, and it is speculated that other TLRs such as TLR5 compensate for the lack of functional CD291.

However, in mice, CD291 recognizes UPEC (uropathogenic *Escherichia coli*) and protects mice from ascending urinary tract infections. Furthermore, CD290 is activated by the protozoan protein profilin and assists in protection against *Toxoplasma gondii* infection and possibly other protozoans such as *Plasmodium* sp.

Ligands

Murine CD291 binds protozoan profilin and recognizes as yet undetermined ligand(s) of human uropathogenic *Escherichia coli* (UPEC).

Expression

Murine CD291 is expressed by macrophages and is strongly expressed by renal and bladder epithelium and weakly expressed by liver epithelium.

Gene Name	Entrez Gene#
TLR11	442887

Selected Monoclonal Antibodies

No antibodies assigned, but CD291 reserved for TLR11.

CD292

Other Names

BMPR1A, ALK-3.

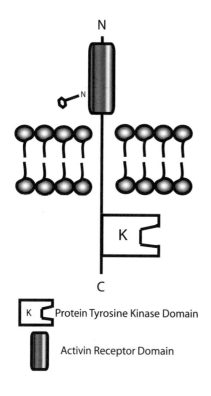

K ⊏ Protein Tyrosine Kinase Domain

Activin Receptor Domain

Molecular Structure

CD292 is a type 1 transmembranc protein and a member of the bone morphogenetic protein (BMP) receptor family of transmembrane serine/threonine kinases within the TGFβ receptor superfamily.

CD292 forms a heterodimer with BMPR II.

A 23 amino acid signal sequence is cleaved to produce a mature protein of 509 amino acids, of which 129 residues are extracellular, 24 residues span the membrane, and 356 amino acids are intracellular.

The extracellular sequence contains an activin receptor domain, whereas the cytoplasmic portion contains a TGFβ-like domain, the protein kinase domain, and 2 ATP-binding sites.

Magnesium or manganese is required as a cofactor for enzymatic activity.

One potential N-glycosylation site is found in the extracellular domain.

Mol Wt: 50–58 kDa.

Function

CD292 plays a role in embryonic development, inducing cell proliferation and differentiation in multiple embryonic tissues.

It forms part of a tetrameric receptor consisting of two CD292 molecules and two BMPRII molecules. Ligand binding activates CD292, which phosphorylates BMPRII enabling activation of SMAD transcriptional regulators.

Bone development and chondrogenesis are regulated by CD292 and CD293, which appear to have overlapping functions.

Studies of CD292-conditional mutant mice have shown that CD292 regulates differentiation and proliferation of hair follicle epithelium and is required for the completion of tooth morphogenesis, the development of atrioventricular valves and annulus fibrosis of the heart, and the development of the spinal cord and skeleton.

Mutations in BMPR1A are associated with Cowden disease, an autosomal dominant cancer syndrome characterized by multiple hamartomas and high risk of breast, thyroid, and endometrial cancers.

Overall, 25–40% of cases of juvenile polyposis syndrome are associated with mutations in BMPR1A.

Ligands

CD292 binds bone morphogenetic protein (BMP)-2 and BMP-4.

Expression

CD292 is expressed by bone progenitor cells, chondrocytes, epithelial cells of epidermis, hair follicles and intestine, and skeletal muscle.

Gene Name	Entrez Gene#
BMPR1A	657

Selected Monoclonal Antibodies

87908 (R&D Systems; Mineappolis).

CDw293

Other Names

BMPR1B, ALK-6.

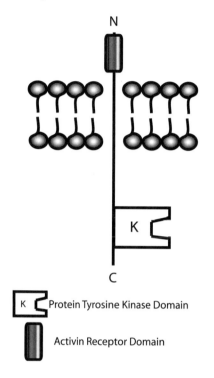

Protein Tyrosine Kinase Domain

Activin Receptor Domain

Molecular Structure

CDw293 is a type 1 transmembrane protein and a member of the bone morphogenetic protein (BMP) receptor family of transmembrane serine/threonine kinases within the TGFβ receptor superfamily.

CD293 forms a heterodimer with BMPR II.

A 13 amino acid signal sequence is cleaved to produce a mature protein of 489 amino acids, of which 113 residues are extracellular, 22 residues span the membrane, and 354 amino acids are intracellular.

The extracellular sequence contains an activin receptor domain, whereas the cyto-plasmic portion contains a TGF β-like domain, the protein kinase domain, and 2 ATP-binding sites.

Magnesium or manganese is required as a cofactor for enzymatic activity.

Mol Wt: 50–58 kDa.

Function

CDw293 plays a role in embryonic development inducing cell proliferation and differentiation in multiple embryonic tissues.

It forms part of a tetrameric receptor consisting of two CDw293 molecules and two BMPRII molecules. Ligand binding activates the CD293/BMPRII complex, which then activates SMAD transcriptional regulators.

Bone development, chondrogenesis, and retinal development are regulated by CD292 and CDw293, which appear to have overlapping functions.

Heterozygous mutations in BMPR1B cause brachydactyly type A2.

Ligands

CDw293 binds bone morphogenetic protein (BMP)-2 and BMP-4.

Expression

CDw293 is expressed by bone progenitor cells, chondrocytes, and in several embryonic tissues.

Gene Name   Entrez Gene#

BMPR1B   658

Selected Monoclonal Antibodies

88614 (R&D Systems, Mineappolis).

CD294

Other Names

CRTH2.

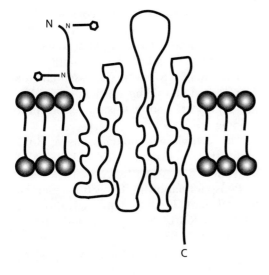

Molecular Structure

CD294 is a G protein-coupled receptor (GPCR) family member, a seven-pass transmembrane protein with an extracellular N terminus. Two potential N-glycosylation sites are found in the N-terminal region. The long cytoplasmic C-terminal region has sites for phosphorylation by protein kinase C.

The protein consists of 395 residues with a calculated Mol Wt of 43 kDa.

The homologous murine protein has a 77% amino acid identity.

Function

CD294 resembles the chemokine receptors and receptors for other chemoattractant stimuli, but its ligand appears to be prostaglandin D2 (PGD2).

PGD2 stimulates various changes in cells expressing CD294, the responses depending on the cell type. In general, the responses can be described as activation. The physiological role of CD294 is not yet clear.

Ligands

Prostaglandin D2.

Expression

CD294 is widely distributed outside the immune system, including gut, heart, and brain. Within the immune system, CD294 shows differential expression and is particularly associated with a subset of T cells that on stimulation produce preferentially IL-4, IL-5, and IL-13, referred to as Th2 cells. It is also expressed by eosinophils and basophils, which, along with Th2 cells, are involved in allergic disease.

Applications

Potentially a marker of TH2 cells.

Gene Name	Entrez Gene#
GPR44	11251

Selected Monoclonal Antibodies

BM16 (Nagata, Saitama; Beckman Coulter, Marseille).

CD295

Other Names

Leptin R, LEPR, OBR, B219.

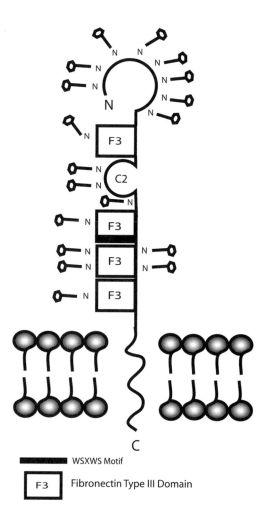

▬▬▬▬▬ WSXWS Motif

| F3 | Fibronectin Type III Domain |

Molecular Structure

CD295 is a type 1 membrane protein and a member of the type 2 subfamily of the type I cytokine receptor family within the Ig gene superfamily.

The CD295 precursor has a 21 amino acid signal sequence that when cleaved results in a mature protein of 1144 residues.

CD295 has an extracellular domain of 818 residues, a transmembrane region of 23 amino acids, and an intracellular domain of 303 amino acids.

Ligand binding induces homodimerization.

The extracellular region consists of an N-terminal fibronectin type III (FnIII) domain followed by an Ig-like domain, 3 FnIII domains, and a WSXWS motif.

The WSXWS motif is essential for correct protein folding, efficient intracellular transport, and cell surface receptor binding.

The cytoplasmic domain has a Box1 motif that is essential for JAK2/STAT3 activation.

Phosphorylation of Tyr 986 is essential for efficient binding and activation of PTPNII, ERK/FOS activation, and interaction with SOCS3, whereas phosphorylation of Tyr1141 is required for STAT3 binding and activation.

Alternative mRNA splicing gives rise to 5 isoforms. The long isoform of CD295 (OB-Rb) is the functional receptor for Leptin. All other isoforms have short cytoplasmic regions (OB-Ra, c, d) or are secreted (OB-Re).

Mol Wt: 130–150 kDa.

Function

CD295 mediates the effects of the multifunctional hormone leptin. CD295 signaling is a critical step in the normal physiology of many cell types regulating food intake and lipid metabolism, immune function, fertility, angiogenesis, and bone formation.

Leptin-induced CD295 signaling in the arcuate nucleus of the hypothalamus modulates neuronal signaling in a negative feedback loop to regulate food intake and energy expenditure. Additionally, CD295 signaling is involved in lipid handling by jejunal epithelium, which when disrupted may contribute to obesity.

Platelets express CD295 and aggregate in the presence of high concentrations of leptin (within the concentration range found circulating in obese people) and ADP. This effect was suggested as a possible link between obesity and cardiovascular disease associated with syndrome X and diabetes.

Näive and memory T-cell proliferation is differentially regulated by leptin-mediated CD295 signaling and promotes the secretion of pro-inflammatory cytokines such as IFN and IL-2 while suppressing regulatory cytokines such as IL-4, thereby favoring a Th1 response.

CD295-deficient mice are obese, infertile, hyperphagic, hypothermic, have increased bone formation and bone density, diabetic, have delayed wound healing, and have impaired T-cell responses.

Similarly ZDF rats lack functional CD295. These rats display defective neovascularization, develop diabetes characterized by reduced glucose-stimulated insulin secretion, increased intracellular triglyceride accumulation, and upregulation of lipogenic enzymes and apoptotic pancreatic β cells.

CD295-deficient humans are morbidly obese, have significant growth retardation and central hypothyroidism with reduced secretion of growth hormone and thyrotropin, and have low T-cell counts and impaired cell-mediated responses. These individuals are predisposed to infectious diseases and are at far greater risk of succumbing to infections in childhood.

Ligands

CD295 binds leptin.

Expression

CD295 is expressed ubiquitously. The OB-Rb isoform is particularly highly expressed in the hypothalamus.

Gene Name	Entrez Gene#
LEPR	3953

Selected Monoclonal Antibodies

52273 (R&D Systems; Mineappolis); JG-8 (Simmons; Melbourne).

CD296

Other Names

ART1.

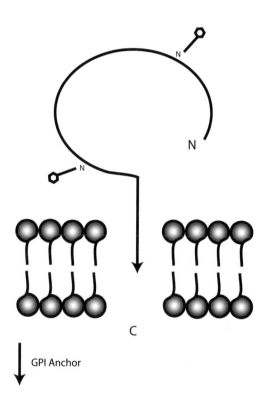

GPI Anchor

Molecular Structure

CD296 is an arginine-specific mono-ADP-ribosyltransferase (ART) anchored to the cell surface via a glycophosphotidylinositol (GPI)-anchor.

The mature protein consists of 273 amino acids and has 2 potential N-glycosylation sites.

The C-terminal half of the CD296 is predicted to be a β-sheet rich region containing the active site. The active site is thought to be formed by the interaction of three regions (I, II, and III).

Regions I and II are defined by a conserved arginine and a consensus Ser-X-Ser motif, respectively, and are involved in stabilizing NAD binding.

Region III contains a catalytic glutamate, which is required for NAD hydrolysis.

The N-terminal portion of CD296 contains α helices and has several regions that influence the transfer of ADP-ribose to an acceptor amino acid or to water.

Mol Wt: 37 kDa.

Function

CD296 catalyzes the transfer of a single ADP-ribose group from NAD onto an arginine of a target protein, thereby reversibly modifying the protein's function.

Substrates of CD296 include integrin α7, defensin-1, CD11a, CD18, as well as ADP-ribosylate guanidine-containing substrates such as agmatine and arginine methyl ester.

CD296 can also ribosylate small soluble proteins such as the basic fibroblast growth factor (FGF-2).

CD296 activity is associated with important cellular events including myocyte differentiation, inflammatory responses, and inhibition of proliferation and cytotoxicity by cytotoxic T cells.

Expression

CD296 is expressed by epithelial cells, a subsct of T cells, heart, and skeletal muscle.

Gene Name	Entrez Gene#
ART1	417

Selected Monoclonal Antibodies

ART1 (Harada; Hiroshima; Koch-Nolte; Hamburg).

CD297

Other Names

ART4, DOK1, DO, Dombrock blood group.

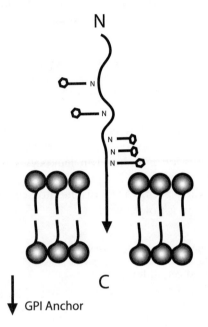

GPI Anchor

Molecular Structure

CD297 is an arginine-specific mono-ADP-ribosyltransferase (ART) anchored to the cell surface via a glycophosphotidylinositol (GPI)-anchor.

29 amino acids are cleaved from the pro-peptide to produce the mature form of CD297.

The protein has a 29 amino acid signal sequence and 5 potential N-linked glycosylation sites.

A single amino acid variation at position 265 is the molecular basis for the Dombrock (Do) blood group system.

Asn 265 is found in the Do(a) antigen, whereas Asp 265 is present in Do(b) antigen.

CD297 carries the Gregory (Gy(a)), Holley (Hy), and Joseph (Jo (a)) antigens.

Mol Wt: 38 kDa.

Function

CD297 catalyzes the transfer of a single ADP-ribose group from NAD onto an arginine of a target protein, thereby reversibly modifying the protein's function.

The Asn265Asp polymorphism occurs within an RGD motif. RGDs are commonly associated with cell–cell interactions involving integrin binding.

Expression

CD297 is expressed by erythrocytes, erythroblasts, and activated monocytes. The expression of CD297 is highest in the spleen but is also detectable in respiratory epithelium.

Expression of CD297 is detectable in the majority of gynecological tumors but not in the equivalent normal tissue.

Applications

DO blood group antigens are useful genetic markers and are sometimes associated with severe hemolytic transfusion reactions due to the presence of anti-Dombrock antibodies in adults.

CD297 is a potential therapeutic target in specific immunotherapy of HLA-A24$^+$ gynecologic cancer patients.

Gene Name	Entrez Gene#
DO	420

Selected Monoclonal Antibodies

MIMA52, MIMA53 (Reid; New York).

CD298

Other Names

Na/K ATPase β3-subunit.

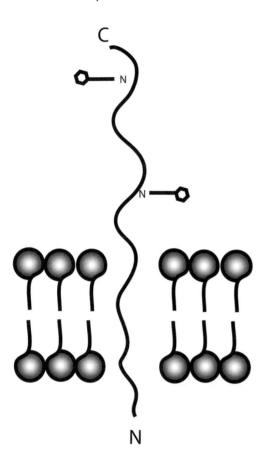

Molecular Structure

The Na/K ATPase consists of three subunits, of which the α subunit is the catalytic component.

CD298, the β-subunit, is a type II transmembrane protein belonging to the Na/K and H/K ATPases β-chain family.

The 35-residue cytoplasmic region is followed by a 21-residue signal/membrane insertion sequence.

The 223-residue extracellular region carries 2 potential N-linked glycosylation sites.

The predicted Mol Wt: is 32 kDa.

Function

The N/K ATPase is a membrane-localized enzyme involved in Na/K transport. Its expression is induced in leukocytes upon activation.

The specific role of the non-catalytic β-chain is not known.

Expression

Found on all leukocytes.

Studies with non-hemopoietic cell lines suggest the protein is also expressed by many other tissues.

Gene Name	Entrez Gene#
ATP1B3	483

Selected Monoclonal Antibodies

P-3E10 (Kasinrerk; Chiang Mai; Thailand).

CD299

Other Names

DC-SIGN2, DC-SIGNR, L-SIGN, CD209L.

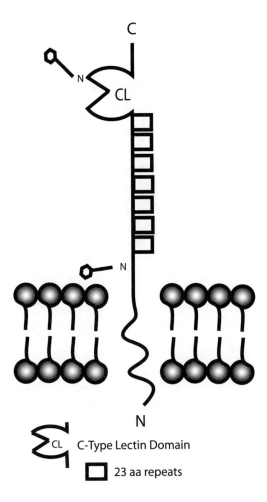

CL — C-Type Lectin Domain

◻ — 23 aa repeats

Molecular Structure

CD299 is a 399 amino acid type II transmembrane protein and a member of the C-type lectin family. It bears a high degree of amino acid sequence homology (77%) to CD209 and has almost certainly arisen as a result of gene duplication.

The 329 amino acid extracellular domain consists of a C-terminal 117-residue C-type lectin domain followed by 7 tandem repeats of a 23 amino acid sequence. The tandem repeats are required for the formation of tetramers.

The protein has 2 potential N-linked glycosylation sites and 6 calcium binding sites.

The 21-residue transmembrane domain is followed by a 43 amino acid intracellular region containing a triacidic cluster and a di-leucine motif, which are potential internalization motifs.

Alternative RNA splicing gives rise to at least 10 isoforms, some of which (isoforms 5, 6, 7, and 10) are potentially secreted.

Further variability arises from polymorphism in the number of tandem repeats that can vary between 3 and 9, although the most common variant has 7 repeats.

Mol Wt: 40.1 kDa.

Function

CD299 is probably a pathogen recognition receptor involved in peripheral immune surveillance in the liver.

Like CD209, CD299 recognizes in a Ca^{2+}-dependent manner high mannose oligosaccharides found on a variety of pathogens such as the gp120 protein of HIV type 1 and appears to mediate endocytosis of pathogens, which are subsequently degraded in lysosomal compartments.

Binding to CD299 is not reversible, which suggests the receptor is not recycled after endocytosis but is degraded within endosomes or lysosomes.

It has been demonstrated in vitro that CD299 can mediate in trans-delivery of HIV-type I, Ebola virus, and Hepatitis C virus to other cellular targets.

Similarly to CD209, CD299 can bind CD50 (ICAM-3), which enables interaction with CD50-expressing T cells. It has yet to be demonstrated whether CD299 induces tolerogenic responses in liver sinusoidal endothelial cells and lymph node endothelial cells.

Ligands

CD299 binds CD50 (ICAM-3) and high mannose moieties of carbohydrate structures of several pathogens such as lentiviruses (including HIV-type I and Ebola virus), human cytomegalovirus, Hepatitis C virus and SARS coronavirus, as well as *Mycobacterium tuberculosis*.

Expression

CD299 is predominantly expressed in liver sinusoidal endothelial cells (LSECs) and by endothelial cells present beneath the subcapsular sinus of lymph nodes, placental endothelium, as well as type II alveolar cells and lung endothelial cells.

Gene Name	Entrez Gene#
CLEC4M	10332

Selected Monoclonal Antibodies

120604 (R&D Systems; Mineappolis).

CD300a, c and e

Other Names

CD300a: CMRF35H, CMRF35H9, IRC1, IRC2, IRP60.

CD300c: CMRF35A, CMRF35A1, CMRF35, LIR.

CD300e: CMRL35L1.

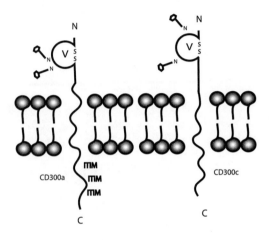

Molecular Structure

CD300a is a type 1 transmembrane protein and a member of the CMRF family within the Ig gene superfamily.

A 17 amino acid signal sequence is cleaved to give a mature protein of 282 amino acids, of which 163 are extracellular, 21 residues span the cell membrane, and 98 amino acids are intracellular.

The extracellular region has 1 Ig-like V-type domain and 2 potential N-linked glycosylation sites. A 45 amino acid membrane proximal region contains several serine and threonine residues that are potentially O-glycosylated. This region is predicted to have a rigid structure.

The Ig-like domain is related to the Ig-binding domains of the Fc receptor for polymeric IgA and IgM.

The cytoplasmic tail contains three putative immunoreceptor tyrosine-based inhibitory motifs (ITIMs) surrounding Tyr233, Tyr256, and Tyr269 and a di-leucine motif (residues 237 and 238).

Tyrosine phosphorylation of ITIMs leads to interaction with protein tyrosine phosphatases SHP-1 and SHP-2.

CD300c is a type 1 transmembrane protein and a member of the CMRF family within the Ig gene superfamily.

The mature protein consists of 204 amino acids following cleavage of a 20 amino acid signal peptide.

The 163 amino acid extracellular portion of CD300c comprises an Ig-like V-type domain, 2 potential N-linked glycosylation sites, and an extended proline-rich membrane proximal region containing several serine and threonine residues, which are potential O-linked glycosylation sites.

The transmembrane domain contains a charged glutamine, which suggests the protein may interact with other molecules in the membrane.

CD300a and c show 80% amino acid identity in the Ig domains but are different in the rest of the molecule. They are encoded by different genes.

CD300e is a type 1 integral membrane protein and a member of the CMRF35 family within the Ig gene superfamily.

Mol Wt: CD330a, 60 kDa; CD300c, 23 kDa (predicted).

Function

CD300a is a receptor that may contribute to the downregulation of cytolytic activity in NK cells.

MAb-cross-linking of CD300a has recently been shown to suppress the effects of IL-5, GM-CSF, and eotaxin on peripheral blood eosinophils in vitro.

Expression

CD300a is expressed by subsets of T cells, B cells, monocytes, mast cells, granulocytes, NK cells, and dendritic cells.

CD300c is broadly expressed by large granular lymphocytes, monocytes, macrophages, granulocytes, and dendritic cells and a proportion of peripheral blood lymphocytes.

CD300e is expressed by monocytes, macrophages, and dendritic cells.

Gene Name	Entrez Gene#
No entry	11314 (a)
	10871 (c)

Selected Monoclonal Antibodies

CMRF35 (Clark; Brisbane) recognizes an epitope shared by CD301 a and e.

CD300e: MMRI-1 (Clark; Brisbane).

CD301

Other Names

MGL, CLECSF14, HMGL, HML2, HML.

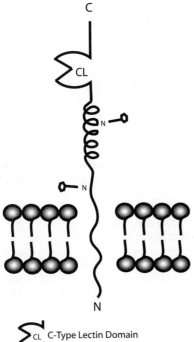

CL C-Type Lectin Domain

Molecular Structure

CD301 is a type II transmembrane glycoprotein and is a member of the type II subfamily of the C-type lectin superfamily.

The 316 amino acid protein comprises an intracellular region of 39 amino acids followed by a 21 amino acid signal anchor transmembrane region and an extracellular region of 256 residues.

The extracellular region contains a C-type lectin domain and 2 potential N-linked glycosylation sites.

Residues 85–176 are predicted to form an α-helical coiled coil. This region is involved in the formation of trimers.

The cytoplasmic domain contains a single endocytosis signaling motif (YENF)

required for interaction with clathrin-coated vesicles.

Alternative mRNA splicing gives rise to 3 isoforms.

Mol Wt: 38 kDa.

Function

CD301 on immature dendritic cells (DCs) is involved in receptor-mediated endocytosis of glycosylated proteins.

CD301 recognizes terminal galactose and N-acetylgalactosamine units, particularly clusters of truncated O-linked carbohydrate chains such as the T and Tn antigens of mucins.

Tn-antigens are expressed by a variety of carcinoma cells, and it has been demonstrated in vitro that murine CD301$^+$ cells can capture tumor cells by interacting with tumor cell carbohydrate epitopes. It is postulated that CD301 might contribute to anti-tumor immunity.

Knockout mice show a deficit in granulation tissue formation.

Ligands

CD301 binds to carbohydrates bearing terminal galactose and N-acetylgalactosamine residues.

Expression

CD301 is expressed by immature dendritic cells and by macrophages.

Applications

CD301 is a marker of immature dendritic cells.

Gene Name	Entrez Gene#
CLECSF14	10462

Selected Monoclonal Antibodies

IB12 (Irimura; Tokyo).

CD302

Other Names

DCL1.

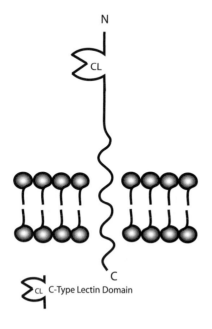

N

CL

C

CL C-Type Lectin Domain

Molecular Structure

CD302 is a type I transmembrane protein with a C-type lectin domain. Limited information is available on structural features. The molecule is structurally related to DEC205 (CD205), and the genes for these molecules are close to each other on the same chromosome.

Reed–Sternberg cells of Hodgkin's lymphoma express a mRNA that is a fusion between DEC205 and CD302.

Mol Wt: 30 kDa.

Function

CD302 functions as an endocytic receptor for glycosylated antigens.

Expression

CD302 is expressed by granulocytes, macrophages, monocytes, and dendritic cells.

Applications

Hodgkin's lymphoma cell lines express a fusion protein encoded by intergenically spliced mRNA for DEC205 and CD302.

Gene Name	Entrez Gene#
CD302	9936

Selected Monoclonal Antibodies

MMRI-20, MMRI-21 (Khan; Brisbane).

CD303

Other Names

BDCA-2, CLECSF11, DLEC, HECL.

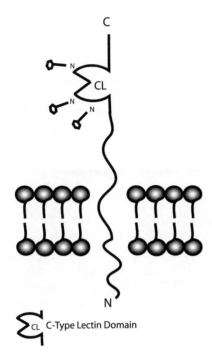

$\sum_{CL}$ C-Type Lectin Domain

Molecular Structure

CD303 is a type II transmembrane protein and a member of the type II subfamily of the C-type lectin superfamily.

The mature CD303 protein consists of an N-terminal cytoplasmic region of 21 amino acids, a transmembrane signal anchor of 23 amino acids, and a C-terminal extracellular region of 169 residue.

The extracellular region contains a single C-type lectin domain and three potential N-linked glycosylation sites.

There are no known signaling motifs in the cytoplasmic domain.

Mol Wt: 38 kDa.

Function

CD303 is a C-type lectin of plasmacytoid dendritic cells (PDC). In vitro studies have found CD303 has a dual function of both capturing and targeting antigen for processing and presentation to T cells and mediating potent inhibition of IFNα/β expression in PDCs.

Triggering of CD303 with mAb activates protein tyrosine kinases, but in the absence of any known cytoplasmic signaling motifs, it remains to be determined whether CD303 interacts with a signaling membrane adaptor molecule.

Expression

CD303 is expressed by plasmacytoid dendritic cells (PDCs).

Applications

CD303 is a specific PDC marker and a potential therapeutic target for the down-regulation of IFNα/β production in patients with systemic lupus erythematosus (SLE).

Gene Name	Entrez Gene#
CLECSF7	170482

Selected Monoclonal Antibodies

AC144, AD5-4B8, AD5-13A11 (Winkels; Miltenyi Biotech, Bergisch Gladbach).

CD304

Other Names

BDCA-4, Neuropilin, Neuropilin-1, VEGF165R.

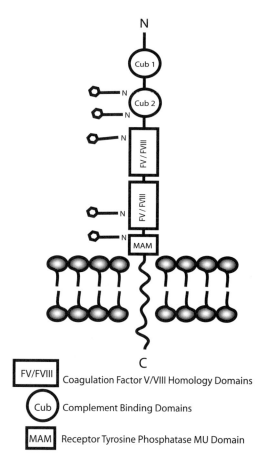

FV/FVIII Coagulation Factor V/VIII Homology Domains

Cub Complement Binding Domains

MAM Receptor Tyrosine Phosphatase MU Domain

Molecular Structure

CD304 is a type I transmembrane glycoprotein.

Removal of a 21 amino acid signal peptide results in a 902 amino acid protein with an extracellular region of 835 amino acids, a transmembrane region of 23 residues, and an intracellular region of 44 amino acids.

The extracellular domain has five potential N-linked glycosylation sites and consists of two N-terminal complement binding (CUB) domains that are predicted to form β barrel structures followed by two coagulation factor V/VIII homology domains and a MAM (meprin, A5, receptor tyrosine phosphatase mu) domain.

Regions within the coagulation factor domains are involved in cell adhesion.

The MAM domain is responsible for dimerization.

Several isoforms arising from alternative mRNA splicing occur including soluble isoforms.

A soluble isoform (sNRP1) consists of the CUB and Factor V/VIII homology domains only.

Mol Wt: 140 kDa; sNRP1: 90 kDa.

Function

CD304 on endothelial cells and tumor cells acts as a receptor for VEGF-A and plays a major role in angiogenesis. Co-expression of VEGFR2 and CD304 significantly enhances VEGF-A-mediated endothelial cell chemotaxis.

Many tumors including breast and prostate carcinomas express CD304, but the corresponding nonmalignant tissues do not. Several studies have shown CD304 is involved in tumor angiogenesis, metastasis, and tumor cell survival.

In contrast, soluble CD304 has anti-angiogenic and anti-tumorigenic activity, probably by binding VEGF-A and inhibiting VEGF-A-induced tyrosine phosphorylation of VEGFR2.

Neuronal CD304 forms a complex with plexin. Semaphorin-3A binding to this complex leads to axonal growth cone collapse and mediates axonal guidance.

CD304–VEGF-A interaction plays a role in neuronal development. A study of the development of facial brachiomotor neurons in the hindbrain of mouse embryos revealed the migration of the cell bodies (somata) of these neurons requires VEGF-A and CD304.

The role of CD304 on plasmacytoid dendritic cells is unclear. There is some suggestion that it may be involved in PDC–T-cell interactions.

Ligands

CD304 is a receptor for semaphorin-3A (sema-3A) and vascular endothelial growth factor-A (VEGF-A, VEGF165).

Expression

CD304 is expressed by endothelial cells, neurons, and several carcinomas.

High level expression of CD304 is found in lineage-, $CD45^{dim}$, and CD11c- $CD123^{bright}$ $CD45RA^+$ $BDCA-1^-$ $BDCA-3^{dim}$ plasmacytoid dendritic cells (PDCs) and at lower levels in $CD34^{dim}$ $CD45RA^{dim}$ $BDCA-2^{dim}$ pre-PDCs and tonsillar $CD3^+$ $CD57^+$ $CXCR5^+$ T cells (TFH cells).

Unlike CD303, CD304 is expressed by PDCs after maturation.

Applications

CD304 is a marker of plasmacytoid dendritic cells.

CD304 over-expression correlates with metastatic disease and poor prognosis for prostate cancer patients.

Gene Name   Entrez Gene#

NRP1   8829

Selected Monoclonal Antibodies

AD5-17F6 (Winkels, Bergisch Gladbach Milteny Biotech).

CD305

Other Names

LAIR1 (Leukocyte-associated Ig-like receptor 1).

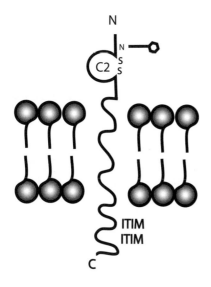

Molecular Structure

Type I transmembrane molecule with a single N terminal extracellular Ig superfamily C2 domain. The cytoplasmic domain carries two inhibitory ITIM motifs.

Several splice variants have been described, with short deletions of either the extracellular or the intracellular regions.

The extracellular domain contains one N-glycosylation site.

Predicted Mol Wt: 31 kDa.

Function

CD305 is an inhibitory molecule; cross-linking LAIR1 results in phosphorylation of the ITIM motifs, leading to inhibition of cellular activation. This inhibitory function has been demonstrated in vitro, with cross-linking by CD305 antibody inhibiting cyto-toxicity by NK or activated T cells.

However, as the ligand for LAIR has not been found, the physiological relevance of this inhibitory function is not known.

Expression

Expressed on the majority of lymphocytes, NK cells, monocytes, and dendritic cells. Among B cells, naive B cells are positive but germinal center cells are negative.

Applications

Research reagents.

Gene Name	Entrez Gene#
LAIR1	3903

Selected Monoclonal Antibodies

FMU-LAIR1.1 (Jin; Xian); 9.1C3 (Ji; Xian); NKTA255 (Poggi; Genoa).

CD306

Other Names

LAIR2 (Leukocyte-associated Ig-like receptor 2).

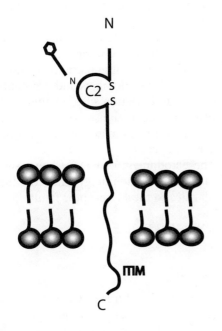

Molecular Structure

LAIR2 consists of 152 amino acids and has a structure similar to LAIR 1, with a single Ig domain and type I orientation (see CD305). Furthermore, the C2 domains of CD305 and CD306 show 84% homology. The proteins are encoded by separate genes. Both proteins contain a single potential N-glycosylation site.

However, the two splice variants that have been identified (LAIR2a and 2b) both lack membrane insertion sequences and cytoplasmic regions, suggesting they are soluble or attached to the membrane indirectly.

Predicted Mol Wt: 16 kDa.

Expression

CD306 is expressed by monocytes.

Gene Name	*Entrez Gene#*
LAIR2	3904

Selected Monoclonal Antibodies

FMU-LAIR2.1, FMU-LAIR2.3 (Jin; Xian).

CD307

Other Names

IRTA2, FcRH5, BXMAS1.

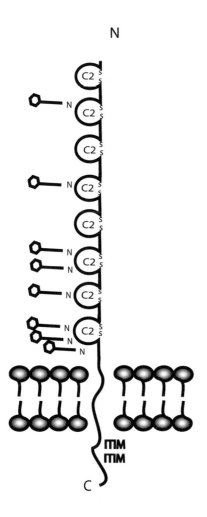

Molecular Structure

CD307 is a type 1 transmembrane glyco-protein and a member of the immunoglo-bulin superfamily receptor translocation associated (IRTA) gene family within the Ig gene superfamily.

CD307 bears significant sequence and structural similarity to Fc receptors.

The gene encoding CD307 is transcribed into three major mRNA isoforms. The predicted proteins share a common signal peptide and six Ig-like domains.

IRTA2a consists of 759 amino acids, has 8 Ig-like domains, followed by 13 unique polar amino acids at its C-terminus, and is secreted.

IRTA2b has six Ig-like domains and is GPI-linked to the membrane.

IRTA2c is a 977 amino acid protein with 8 extracellular Ig domains and 8 potential N-linked glycosylation sites, 23 amino acid transmembrane region, and a 104 amino acid cytoplasmic domain with 2 ITIM consensus sequences.

The ectodomain of CD307 bears significant sequence homology and structural similarities to the Fc receptor family.

Mol Wt: 100 kDa.

Function

The structural features of CD307 isoforms suggest a role in regulating normal B-cell activation. However, the function of this molecule has yet to be demonstrated.

In B-cell malignancies carrying 1q21 abnormalities, CD307 gene expression is often deregulated and is possibly linked to lymphomagenesis.

Ligands

IRTA2c binds heat aggregated human IgG (and presumably antigen complexed IgG) with greater affinity for IgG1 than IgG2 but not monomeric IgG, IgA, IgM, and IgE.

Expression

CD307 is selectively expressed in B lymphocytes, in particular centrocytes of the germinal center light zone and inter-epithelial and inter-follicular B cells.

Applications

CD307 is a B-cell subtype specific marker and is a potential target for immunotherapy in the treatment of B-cell lymphomas (non-Hodgkin's and Burkitt's) and hairy cell leukemia.

Gene Name	Entrez Gene#
FCRL5	83416

Selected Monoclonal Antibodies

F119, F25, F56 (Nagata; Bethesda).

CD308

Other Names

VEGFR1, Flt-1.

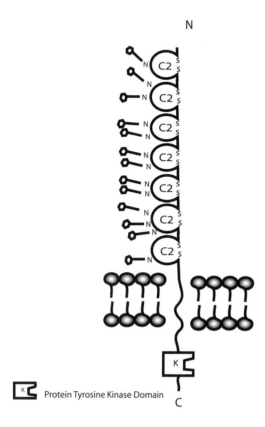

Protein Tyrosine Kinase Domain

Molecular Structure

CD308 is a type I transmembrane glycoprotein member of the CSF-1/PDGF receptor family of type III tyrosine kinase receptors.

CD308, together with VEGFR-2 and VEGFR-3, constitute the flt subfamily of receptors, characterized by seven extracellular Ig-like C2-type domains, a single transmembrane region, and a carboxy-terminal intracellular tyrosine kinase interrupted by a kinase insert sequence.

The precursor has a 26 amino acid signal sequence, and the mature protein consists of 1312 amino acids of which 732 residues are extracellular and form 7 Ig-like C2-type domains.

There are 13 N-linked glycosylation sites in the ectodomain.

The cytoplasmic region consists of 558 residues and contains the 332 amino acid protein kinase domain and 6 phosphotyrosines.

Alternative RNA splicing gives rise to two CD308 isoforms: the membrane bound form (Flt1) and a soluble form (sFlt1).

Mol Wt: Predicted, 152 kDa.

Function

CD308 is an important mediator of stem cell recruitment and mobilization, angiogenesis, and inflammation.

Placental growth factor (PlGF) uses CD308 to stimulate angiogenesis and collateral vessel development to bypass atherosclerotic lesions causing ischemia.

The anti-CD308 monoclonal antibody can suppress angiogenesis in tumors and ischemic retinas, inhibit atherosclerotic plaque formation, inhibit the inflammation and joint destruction associated with autoimmune arthritis, and reduce mobilization of bone-marrow-derived stem cells into the peripheral blood and infiltration of VEGFR-1 expressing leukocytes into tissues.

VEGF-A and PlGF-1 ligation of CD308 induces chemotactic migration of mesenchymal progenitor cells and osteoblasts and stimulates osteoblast proliferation, which suggests CD308 is important in bone formation and remodeling.

CD308-deficient mice die as embryos and have excess endothelial cells in the vasculature. Mice with a defect in the tyrosine kinase domain are viable but display defective monocyte migration in vitro.

Ligands

CD308 binds vascular endothelial growth factor (VEGF), VEGF-B, VEGF-A, and placental growth factor (PlGF).

Expression

CD308 is expressed by most vascular endothelium and by peripheral blood monocytes, osteoblasts, and trophoblasts.

Applications

CD308 is a potential target in the treatment of inflammation and atherosclerotic plaque growth.

Gene Name	Entrez Gene#
FLT1	2321

Selected Monoclonal Antibodies

No antibodies assigned, but CD308 reserved for FLT1.

CD309

Other Names

Vascular endothelial growth factor receptor 2 (VEGFR-2), KDR (human), and Flk-1 (murine).

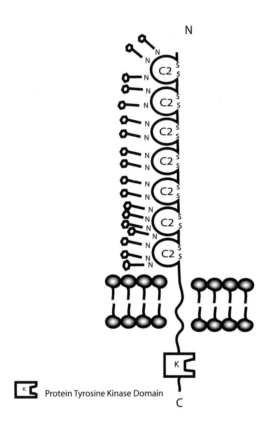

Protein Tyrosine Kinase Domain

Molecular Structure

Type 1 transmembrane glycoprotein member of the CSF-1/PDGF receptor family of type III tyrosine kinase receptors. The glycosylated form has an apparent Mol Wt of 230 kDa. Human and murine homologues are 85% identical in amino acid sequence.

CD309, together with VEGFR-1 and VEGFR-3, constitute the flt subfamily of receptors, characterized by seven extracellular Ig-like C2-type domains, a single transmembrane region, and a carboxy-terminal intracellular tyrosine kinase interrupted by a kinase insert sequence.

The first three extracellular domains are required for ligand binding, whereas the remaining four are involved in receptor dimerisation.

Function

CD309 is involved in regulation of angiogenesis and related functions. Ligand binding leads to receptor dimerization and autophosphorylation, stimulating endothelial cell proliferation and migration, inducing vascular permeability and release of nitrous oxide. Receptor engagement also stimulates expression of proteases required for angiogenesis.

Knockout mice die between embryonic days 8.5 and 9.5 as a result of defects in hematopoiesis and endothelial cell development.

Ligands

Vascular endothelial growth factors (VEGF), including the splice isoforms VEGF121, VEGF145, VEGF165, VEGF189, and VEGF206 (human) or VEGF-A, VEGF-B, VEGF-C, and VEGF-E (murine).

Expression

CD309 is expressed in most embryonic tissues but declines before birth and is expressed at low levels in quiescent adult endothelium. Increased expression in the adult is associated with pathological angiogenesis associated with tumors and diabetic retinopathy.

CD309 is expressed by vascular endothelial cells, megakaryocytes and platelets, retinal progenitors, smooth muscle cells, and pancreatic duct cells.

Expression has been reported on hematopoietic precursors, but this has not been confirmed.

Applications

Because of its role in angiogenesis in tumors and diabetic retinopathy, the KDR signaling pathway is a major therapeutic target. Kinase inhibitors and antibodies designed to inhibit ligand binding are undergoing clinical trials.

Gene Name	Entrez Gene#
KDR	3791

Selected Monoclonal Antibodies

89106 (R&D Systems; Minneapolis).

(CD310)

Other Names

Vascular endothelial growth factor receptor-3, VEGFR3. Flt4.

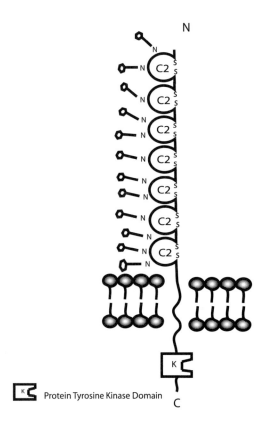

K🗲 Protein Tyrosine Kinase Domain

Molecular Structure

VEGFR3 is a type I transmembrane glycoprotein member of the CSF-1/PDGF receptor family of type III tyrosine kinase receptors.

CD310, together with VEGFR-1 and VEGFR-2, constitute the flt subfamily of receptors, characterized by seven extracellular Ig-like C2-type domains, a single transmembrane region, and a carboxy-terminal intracellular tyrosine kinase interrupted by a kinase insert sequence.

The precursor has a 24 amino acid signal sequence, and the mature protein consists of 1274 amino acids of which 751 residues are extracellular and form 7 Ig-like C2-type domains.

There are 12 N-linked glycosylation sites in the ectodomain.

The cytoplasmic region consists of 501 residues and contains the 329 amino acid protein kinase domain.

Phosphorylation of tyrosine 1063 is essential for CD310 kinase activity.

Phosphotyrosines Y1230/Y1231 and Y1337 all contribute to proliferation, migration, and survival of endothelial cells.

Mol Wt: Predicted, 146 kDa.

Function

CD308 is critical for angiogenesis in embryos and plays a role in angiogenesis and lymphangiogenesis in adults.

Ligand activated CD310 recruits CRKI/II and induces a signal cascade, resulting in activation of c-Jun N-terminal kinase-1/2 (JNK1/2) and signaling for cell survival.

Phosphorylation of tyrosines Y1230 and Y1231 leads to the recruitment of Grb2, which induces activation of AKT and ERK1/2 signaling and ultimately c-JUN expression and pro-survival signaling.

Recent work has shown CD310 and VEGF-C are likely to have a central role in promoting metastasis of tumors to regional lymph nodes.

Primary congenital lymphoedema (Milroy disease) is caused by autosomal dominant mutations in CD310. Onset of lymphoedema can begin at birth and be severe enough to physically impair patients.

Juvenile hemangiomas are related to CD310 mutations and are characterized by benign vascular lesions that expand rapidly in early childhood but spontaneously involute over several years.

Ligands

CD310 binds VEGFR-D and VEGFR-C.

Expression

CD310 is expressed by lymphatic endothelium of normal and malignant tissues. Spindle cells of Kaposi's sarcoma express CD310.

Applications

CD310 is a specific marker of lymphatic endothelium. The expression of CD310 and VEGFD in gastric adenocarcinoma patients correlates with a poor prognosis.

Soluble CD310 decoy receptors are potential therapeutic agents for the prevention of metastasis via the lymphatic system for some tumors such as melanoma and prostate cancer.

Gene Name	Entrez Gene#
FLT4	2324

Selected Monoclonal Antibodies

No antibodies assigned, but CD310 reserved for FLT4.

(CD311)

Other Names

Epidermal growth factor module-containing mucin-like receptor 1, EMR1.

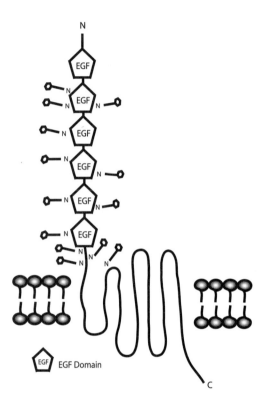

EGF EGF Domain

Molecular Structure

EMR1 is an integral membrane protein belonging to the EGF-TM7 family of cell surface molecules within the LNB-TM7 family of TM7 receptors (see also CD97, CD312, and CD313).

EGF-TM7 family members are characterized by a variable number of N-terminal EGF domains followed by seven membrane-spanning hydrophobic domains that bear homology to the equivalent region in G-protein-coupled peptide hormone receptor family members.

The CD311 precursor comprises 886 amino acids and has a 20 amino acid signal sequence.

The mature protein of 866 residues consists of an N-terminal extracellular region of 579 amino acids followed by 7 transmembrane segments and a C-terminal cytoplasmic tail.

The N-terminal ectodomain contains 6 Ca^{++}-binding EGF-like modules followed by a region of 283 amino acids, of which 27 residues are serines and 25 residues are threonines.

The serine/threonine-rich region is predicted to be heavily O-glycosylated resulting in a rigid stem-like structure. A G-protein-coupled receptor proteolytic site (GPS) motif is located in the stem-like structure; however, it is unknown if CD311 is cleaved into two subunits.

There are 13 potential N-linked glycosylation sites: 8 are found within the EGF domains, 3 in the stem-like structure, and 1 in the first extracellular loop.

There are four potential protein kinase C phosphorylation sites. One is present in the intracellular loop 1 (IC1), another in IC3, and the last two occur within the C-terminal cytoplasmic tail.

A potential casein kinase II phosphorylation site occurs in IC3.

Four isoforms arising from alternative RNA splicing vary in the number of EGF-like domains containing one (EGF4), two (EGF4, 5), three (EGF4, 5, 6), or six (EGF1, 2, 3, 4, 5, 6) EGF domains.

Mol Wt: Predicted, 98 kDa.

Function

The function of CD311 is unknown.

The mouse homologue F4/80 (emr1) has an extra EGF-like domain and has an RGD motif in the extracellular region that the human CD311 protein does not have. The RGD domain may mediate integrin binding and therefore may play a role in cell adhesion.

The expression of F4/80 on tissue macrophages but weak expression in peripheral blood monocytes suggests a role in the terminal differentiation of macrophages.

F4/80 knockout mice are physiologically normal, and no abnormality has as yet been detected.

Expression

CD311 is strongly expressed by peripheral blood monocytes and macrophage cell lines. Weak expression has been detected in solid tumor-derived cell lines.

Applications

CD311 is macrophage-specific marker.

Gene Name	Entrez Gene#
EMR1	2015

Selected Monoclonal Antibodies

No antibodies assigned, but CD311 reserved for EMR1.

CD312

Other Names

Epidermal growth factor module-containing mucin-like receptor 2, EMR2.

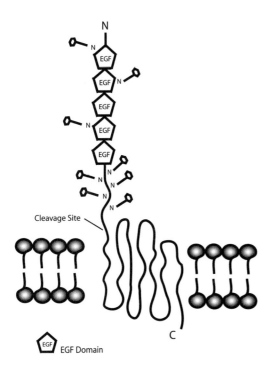

Cleavage Site

C

EGF Domain

Molecular Structure

CD312 is an epidermal growth factor (EGF)-like module-containing mucin-like receptor (EMR) protein and a member of the epidermal growth factor-seven span transmembrane (EGF-TM7) family within the LNB-TM7 family of TM7 receptors (see also CD97, CD311, and CD313).

CD312 shares sequence similarity with CD97, which also binds the glycosaminoglycan (GAG) chondroitin sulphate (CS).

Four isoforms of CD312 have been described, containing two (EGGF1, 2), three (EGF1, 2,5), four (EGF1, 2,3,5), or five (EGF1, 2,3,4,5) EGF domains. Only the largest isoform binds GAGs as it is the fourth EGF domain that interacts with GAGs.

The mature form of the largest CD312 isoform consists of 800 amino acids following cleavage of a 23 amino acid signal sequence.

The protein is post-translationally autocatalytically cleaved at a G-protein-coupled receptor proteolytic site (GPS) motif into two subunits: the α subunit that consists of the N-terminal extracellular EGF-like domains, and a seven-span transmembrane subunit. The two subunits form a heterodimer noncovalently linked via an extended spacer region.

There are eight potential N-linked glycosylation sites.

Mol Wt: 90 kDa.

Function

A recent study suggests CD312 may contribute to the interaction of activated T cells, dendritic cells, and macrophages with B cells, which express the glycosaminoglycan (GAG) chondroitin sulphate.

A recent study found significantly higher expression of CD312 in synovial tissue from rheumatoid arthritis patients than patients with osteoarthritis or reactive arthritis. The majority of CD312+ cells were macrophages and dendritic cells expressing TNFα and costimulatory molecules. CD312 mediated binding of these cells to dermatan sulfate in the synovium.

Ligands

CD312 binds the glycosaminoglycans (GAG) chondroitin sulphate and dermatan sulphate.

Expression

Expression of CD312 is restricted to myeloid cells and activated lymphocytes.

Selected Monoclonal Antibodies

2A1 (Hamann; Amsterdam).

Gene Name	Entrez Gene#
EMR2	30817

(CD313)

Other Names

Epidermal growth factor module-containing mucin-like receptor 3, EMR3.

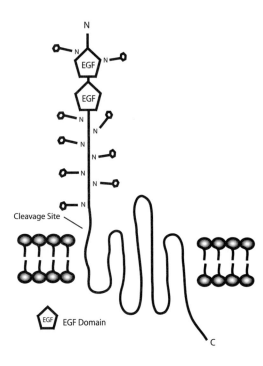

Cleavage Site

EGF EGF Domain

Molecular Structure

CD313 is an epidermal growth factor (EGF)-like module-containing a mucin-like receptor (EMR) protein and a member of the epidermal growth factor-seven span transmembrane (EGF-TM7) family within the LNB-TM7 family of TM7 receptors (see also CD97, CD311, and CD312).

The CD313 precursor comprises 652 amino acids and has a 21 amino acid signal sequence.

The mature protein of 631 residues consists of an N-terminal extracellular region of 336 amino acids followed by 7 transmembrane segments (TM7) and a C-terminal cytoplasmic tail of 50 residues.

The TM7 region has approximately 90% sequence identity to CD312 (EMR2).

The ectodomain contains an N-terminal non-Ca^{++}-binding EGF-like domain followed by a single Ca^{++}-binding EGF-like module. The EGF-like modules are followed by a spacer region of 232 amino acids, which is serine- and threonine-rich and contains a G-protein-coupled receptor proteolytic site (GPS).

The serine/threonine-rich region has the potential to be heavily O-glycosylated, which would make this region a rigid stalk-like structure.

CD313 is predicted to be proteolytically cleaved into two subunits: the α subunit that consists of the N-terminal extracellular EGF-like domains and a seven-span transmembrane subunit. The two subunits form a heterodimer noncovalently linked via the spacer region.

Three isoforms arising from alternative RNA splicing have been described, including a soluble form comprising only the two EGF-like domains.

Function

The function of CD313 is currently unknown.

Ligands

An unidentified ligand for CD313 is expressed by monocyte-derived macrophages and neutrophils.

Expression

Expression of CD313 is highest in neutrophils and weaker in monocytes and macrophages.

CD313 expression is strongest in the spleen, peripheral blood, and lung, and intermediate expression occurs in placenta and bone marrow. Low level expression is found in heart, kidney, liver, pancreas, skeletal muscle, lymph node, thymus, tonsil, and fetal liver. No expression of CD313 is found in the brain.

Gene Name   **Entrez Gene#**

EMR3   84658

Selected Monoclonal Antibodies

No antibodies assigned, but CD313 reserved for EMR3.

CD314

Other Names

NKG2D.

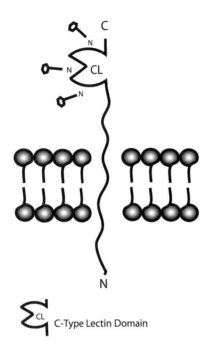

∑CL C-Type Lectin Domain

Molecular Structure

A 42-kDa type II transmembrane glyco-protein member of the C-type lectin family. The extracellular region consists of a single lectin domain linked to a membrane-proximal stalk and contains three potential N-glycosylation sites.

The transmembrane region contains an arginine residue and leads to the 51-aa N-terminal cytoplasmic region.

CD314 exists in the membrane as a disulphide-linked homodimer and requires association with the adaptor molecules DAP10 for membrane expression. DAP10 contains an aspartate residue in the trans-membrane region, which is thought to form a salt bridge to the arginine of CD314.

DAP10 contains a YINM motif, which is phosphorylated to initiate a signal cascade.

Murine NKG2D has an isoform NKG2D-S with a shorter cytoplasmic region, generated by alternative mRNA splicing. This isoform can associate with either DAP10 or DAP12. The latter has an ITAM activation motif.

Function

CD314 recognizes transformed or virus-infected cells expressing CD314 ligands and thereby activates cell-mediated killing.

Ligands

NKG2D binds strongly to at least six ligands in the human, all related to MHC class I. These are MICA and MICB; ULBP-1, -2, and -3; and the RAE-1-like transcript (RAET1E). Mice have orthologs of the ULBP genes but lack MIC genes.

Expression

Constitutively expressed on human NK cells, CD8+ T cells, a minor subset of CD4+ T cells, and most γ/δ T cells.

Mice express NKG2D on NK cells, most γ/δ T cells and a subset of NK1.1 T cells, as well as on activated macrophages.

Applications

CD314 antibodies are used in studies of cytotoxicity particularly in relation to cancer.

Gene Name	Entrez Gene#
KLRK1	22914

Selected Monoclonal Antibodies

149810 (R&D Systems; Mineappolis); ID11 (BD Biosciences; San Diego); ON72 (Beckman Coulter; Marseille).

CD315

Other Names

CD9P1, SMAP6, prostaglandin F2 receptor negative regulator, FPRP, KIAA1436.

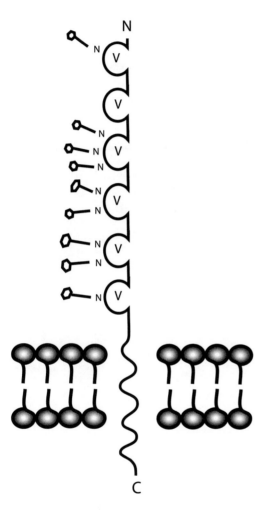

Molecular Structure

CD315 is a type 1 membrane protein and a member of a novel Ig-like protein subfamily known as EWI (glutamine-tryptophan-isoleucine) within the Ig gene superfamily.

Other members of the EWI family include CD101, IgSF3, and CD316 and are characterized by a CxxxEWI motif not found in other Ig proteins, extracellular regions composed exclusively of V-type Ig-like domains, and short cytoplasmic domains. The distal two Ig-like domains have the greatest homology between members of the EWI family.

The CD315 precursor protein has a 25 amino acid signal sequence, which when cleaved results in a mature protein of 854 amino acids.

The 807 amino acid ectodomain comprises 6 V-type Ig-like domains and has 9 potential N-linked glycosylation sites.

The transmembrane region consists of 21 amino acids, and 26 amino acids are intracellular.

A stretch of basic charged amino acids in the cytoplasmic domain may act as binding sites for ERM proteins that are linked to the actin cytoskeleton.

Mol Wt: 135 kDa.

Function

CD315 associates with tetraspanin molecules CD9 and CD81 but not with other tetraspanins.

The rat CD315 molecule was found to reduce the number of PGF-2 α-binding sites on COS cells transfected with the PGF-2 α receptor, and the bovine molecule was found to co-elute from multiple chromatographic procedures with bound tritiated PGF-2 α.

Recent studies have demonstrated CD315 in association with CD81 is involved in regulating cell motility and polarity.

Expression

CD315 is expressed by keratinocytes, a subset of B cells and activated monocytes.

High level expression of CD315 is found in cancer cell lines derived from the colon or fibrosarcoma but not in their normal cell counterparts.

Gene Name	Entrez Gene#
PTGFRN	5738

Selected Monoclonal Antibodies

1F11 (Rubinstein; Paris).

CD316

Other Names

EWI-2, IgSF8, PGRL, CD81P3.

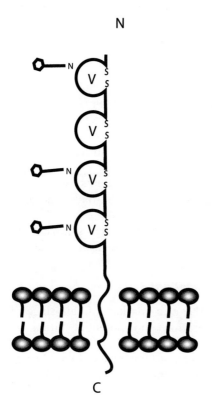

Molecular Structure

CD316 is a type I membrane protein and a member of a novel Ig-like protein subfamily known as EWI (glutamine-tryptophan-isoleucine) within the Ig gene superfamily.

Other members of the EWI family include CD101, IgSF3, and CD315 and are characterized by a CxxxEWI motif not found in other Ig proteins, an extracellular region composed exclusively of V-type Ig-like domains and a short cytoplasmic domain. The distal two Ig-like domains have the greatest homology between members of the EWI family.

The CD316 protein has a 27 amino acid leader peptide, a 556 amino acid extracellular domain, a transmembrane span of 21 amino acids, and a very short cytoplasmic tail.

The extracellular region contains four Ig-like V-type domains and three potential N-linked glycosylation sites.

A stretch of basic amino acids in the cytoplasmic domain may act as binding sites for ERM proteins that are linked to the actin cytoskeleton.

Mol Wt: 63 kDa.

Function

CD316 associates with the tetraspanins CD9 and CD81 and forms stable CD316-CD9 and CD316-CD81 complexes.

The close interaction of CD316 with CD9 and CD81 suggests it participates in the function of CD9 and CD81, including oocyte fertilization, tumor cell metastasis, nervous system development, cell proliferation, myogenesis, and HCV pathogenesis. More recently CD316 in association with CD81 is involved in regulating cell motility and polarity.

Expression

CD316 is expressed by B and T lymphocytes, NK cells, and has been detected in a broad range of tissues.

Gene Name	Entrez Gene#
IGSF8	93185

Selected Monoclonal Antibodies

8A12 (Rubinstein; Paris).

CD317

Other Names

BST2, HM1.24.

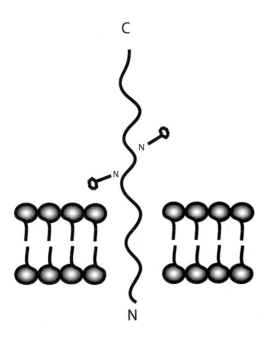

Molecular Structure

CD317 is a type II transmembrane protein.

The protein consists of 180 amino acids, of which the N-terminal 20 residues are cytoplasmic, 28 residues form the signal anchor, and 132 amino acids are extracellular.

The ectodomain has two potential N-linked glycosylation sites.

Mol Wt: 29–33 kDa.

Function

The function of CD317 is unclear at present, but a role for CD317 in the interaction between lymphocytes and bone stromal cells has been suggested.

CD317 is potentially involved in pre-B-cell growth.

Expression

CD317 is expressed by mature Ig-secreting B lymphocytes (plasma cells and lympho-plasmacytoid cells) and T lymphocytes, bone stromal cells, monocytes, NK cells, and dendritic cells and neoplastic plasma cell derived from bone marrow or peripheral blood of patients with multiple myeloma or Waldenstrom's macroglobulinaemia.

CD317 is expressed by synovial cell lines and at high levels by myeloma cell lines.

Applications

CD317 is a marker of late-stage B-cell maturation and potential target in the immunotherapy of patients with multiple myeloma. A humanized mAb is being evaluated as a therapeutic agent in this context.

Gene Name	Entrez Gene#
BST2	684

Selected Monoclonal Antibodies

HM1.24, RS38E, Y129 (Koishihara; Shizuoka).

CD318

Other Names

CDCP-1, SIMA135.

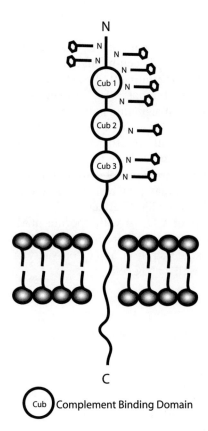

Cub | Complement Binding Domain

Molecular Structure

CD318 is a type I transmembrane protein that contains three complement binding (CUB) domains and nine glycosylation sites in the extracellular domain.

CD318 is expressed as a 140 kDa membrane glycoprotein (gp140) that is cleaved by trypsin to an 80 kDa form (gp80). Plasmin also converts gp140 to gp80.

The cytoplasmic domain has a short hexalysine stretch and five potential tyrosine phosphorylation sites.

Mol Wt: 140 kDa.

Function

CD318 plays a role in early hematopoiesis.

MAb against CD318 was used to stimulate CD34$^+$ bone marrow cells, and this resulted in a two-fold increase in the formation of erythroid colony forming units (CFUs).

An in vitro model of wound activation demonstrated prolonged phosphorylation of the gp80 form of CD318 in foreskin keratinocytes. Whether CD318-mediated signaling plays a role in wound repair of the epidermis is being investigated.

Expression

CD318 is expressed by CD34$^+$ CD133$^+$ bone marrow cells, and keratinocytes.

It is over-expressed in human colorectal cancers.

Applications

CD318 is a marker of hematopoietic progenitor cell subsets, in particular, mesenchymal stem/progenitor cells and neural progenitor cells.

It is an independent marker for the diagnosis of myeloid leukemias.

Gene Name	Entrez Gene#
CDCP1	64866

Selected Monoclonal Antibodies

CUB-1, CUB-2 and CUB-4 (Bühring; Tübingen).

CD319

Other Names

CRACC, SLAMF7, 19A, 19A24, CS1.

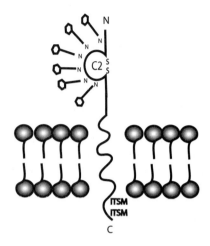

Molecular Structure

CD319 is a type I transmembrane protein and a member of the CD2 family of receptors within the Ig superfamily (see also CD2, CD150, CD224, and CD84).

The protein is predicted to consist of 335 residues with a 22 amino acid signal sequence, 225-residue extracellular region, 23 amino acid transmembrane region, and 85-residue cytoplasmic tail.

The extracellular region contains an Ig-like C2-type domain and has six putative N-linked glycosylation sites.

The intracellular domain has two immunoreceptor tyrosine-based switch motifs (ITSMs).

Two splice variants have been observed in NK cells. The full length or long isoform is the functional molecule. The short isoform lacks the ITSM motifs and does not trigger any signaling pathways.

Mol Wt: 66 kDa.

Function

Unlike other members of the CD2 family, CD319 triggers NK cell-mediated cytotoxicity via the recruitment of extracellular signal-regulated kinases-1/2 instead of a SAP-dependent signaling pathway.

However, although CD319-mediated SAP-independent cytotoxicity occurs in NK cells, two studies have found SAP does associate with the CD319 cytoplasmic tail and therefore may play a signaling role in other CD319-mediated effects.

Ligation of CD319 with specific mAb was shown to induce proliferation, adhesion, cytokine secretion, and cytotoxicity of T cells as well as NK cells.

Ligands

CD319 displays homophilic binding.

Expression

CD319 is expressed by cytotoxic lymphocytes, activated B cells, NK cells, and mature dendritic cells.

Gene Name	Entrez Gene#
SLAMF7	57823

Selected Monoclonal Antibodies

162 (BD Biosciences; San Diego).

CD320

Other Names

8D6.

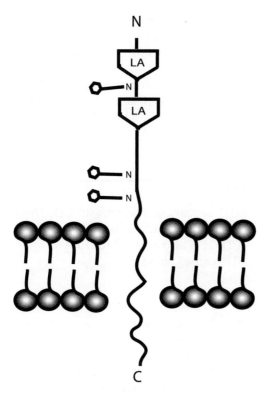

N

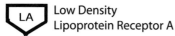

C

LA — Low Density Lipoprotein Receptor A

Molecular Structure

CD320 is a type I transmembrane protein related to the low density lipoprotein receptor (LDL-R) family.

The 282 amino acid protein has an N-terminal signal sequence of 32 amino acids, an extracellular domain of 230 amino acids, a putative transmembrane region of 18 residues, and a short cytoplasmic tail of 32 amino acids.

The extracellular region contains two domains with significant homology to the type A cysteine-rich repeats found in the low density lipoprotein receptor (LDL-R) family. Each domain characteristically has six cysteines with acidic residues separating the fifth and sixth cysteines.

The two domains are separated by an additional cysteine-rich region interrupted by a stretch of four proline residues.

A putative N-glycosylation site is located in the spacer region and two additional sites are present between the second LDL-R type A domain and the transmembrane region.

Mol Wt: 29 kDa (predicted).

Function

CD320 is involved in the follicular dendritic cell (FDC)-mediated proliferation of CD27+ plasma cells in germinal centers.

CD320-specific mAb can partially block proliferation of plasma cells in vitro and in vivo. The mechanisms involved have yet to be determined.

CD320 may play a role in lymphomagenesis as proliferation of a Burkitt's lymphoma cell line occurs in the presence of CD320+ FDC, but the addition of CD320-specific mAb inhibits tumor cell growth.

Expression

CD320 is expressed by follicular dendritic cells.

Applications

CD320 is a potential target of immunotherapy in the treatment of lymphomas.

Gene Name	*Entrez Gene#*
CD320	51293

Selected Monoclonal Antibodies

8D6, 3C8, 4G10, BH2 (Li; San Diego).

CD321

Other Names

JAM-1 (Junctional adhesion molecule-1).

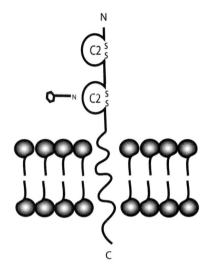

Molecular Structure

A 32–35-kDa type 1 transmembrane glycoprotein with two extracellular Ig superfamily domains.

The membrane-proximal C2 domain carries one potential N-glycosylation site.

A 19aa membrane spanning sequence is followed by a cytoplasmic domain containing two tyrosines and several phosphorylation sites.

X-ray crystallography indicates that CD321 dimerizes, forming a U-shaped dimer. Functional analysis suggests that physiologically dimers form between CD321 molecules on interacting cells, rather than on the same cell.

Function

JAM-1 is an adhesion molecule that is involved in the formation of tight junctions between cells. The exact mechanisms are unknown, and tight junctions are complex regions involving the assembly of several different molecules.

The N-terminal extracellular domain of JAM-1 interacts with the corresponding domain of JAM-1 on the adhering cell and interacts with other tight junction components through binding motifs on the cytoplasmic domain.

CD321 appears to have a role in extravasation of leukocytes, an important process in inflammation and immunity.

CD321 is used as a receptor by reoviruses.

Ligands

CD321 appears to interact with CD321 on interacting cells in forming tight junctions.

CD321 is also a ligand for LFA-1.

Reoviruses bind CD321.

Expression

CD321 is expressed in several tissues, including lung, kidney, and placenta, and on blood leukocytes and platelets. Among leukocytes it is expressed on neutrophils, monocytes, and lymphocytes.

Applications

Currently research reagents, with potential value in immunophenotypic analysis.

Gene Name	Entrez Gene#
F11R	50848

Selected Monoclonal Antibodies

F11 (Naik; Newark).

CD322

Other Names

JAM-2.

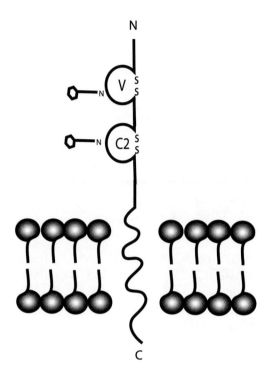

Molecular Structure

CD322 is a type 1 transmembrane protein that is part of a subfamily of junctional adhesion molecules comprising JAM-1 and JAM-3 (VE-JAM) within the Ig super-family.

The precursor protein has a 31 amino acid signal sequence.

The mature protein consists of 279 residues, of which 210 are extracellular, 21 amino acids span the cell membrane, and 48 residues are intracellular.

The extracellular domain contains an N-terminal Ig-like V-type domain followed by an Ig-like C2-type domain.

There are two N-linked glycosylation sites (Asn 104 and Asn192).

The cytoplasmic region has four putative phosphorylation sites. Phosphorylation at Serine 281 appears to be involved in the negative-regulation of CD322 localization to tight junctions.

Mol Wt: 45 kDa.

Function

CD322 associates with JAM-3 and JAM-1 and plays a role in the formation and maintenance of tight junctions and cell polarity of endothelial cells.

The localization of CD322 at tight junctions is regulated by serine phosphorylation and recruits cell polarity protein PAR-3 and another tight junction protein ZO-1.

CD322 may promote the transmigration of human lymphocytes across endothelium by homophilic interaction.

Ligands

CD322 displays homophilic binding and can bind CD323 (JAM-3).

Expression

CD322 is expressed by endothelial cells, monocytes, B cells, and a subset of T cells (probably activated and memory T cells).

It is strongly expressed during embryogenesis and becomes restricted in expression in adult tissues such as the tongue and heart.

Gene Name

Gene Name	Entrez Gene#
JAM2	58494

Selected Monoclonal Antibodies

H36, D22, H31, H33, F24, F26, D33 (Beat; Geneva).

(CD323)

Other Names

JAM-C, JAM-3, VE-JAM, FLJ14529.

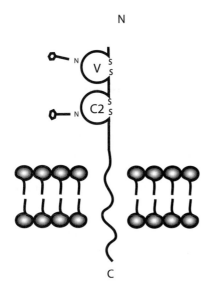

Molecular Structure

CD323 is type I transmembrane protein and is a member of a subfamily of junctional adhesion molecules including JAM-1 (CD321) and JAM-2 (CD322) within the Ig superfamily.

The precursor protein has a 31 amino acid signal sequence that is cleaved to form the mature protein of 279 amino acids.

CD323 has an extracellular domain consisting of 210 amino acids that contains an N-terminal Ig-like V-type domain followed by an Ig-like C2-type domain.

There are two potential N-linked glycosylation sites (Asn104, Asn192) and one potential O-linked glycosylation site (Thr60).

The transmembrane domain consists of 21 amino acids.

The 48 amino acid intracellular domain has 3 potential phosphorylation sites (Tyr 270, 282, 293) and a putative phosphoryla-tion site for casein III kinase (Thr296) or protein kinase C (Ser281). At the C-terminus, there is a potential binding site for PDZ domains.

Mol Wt: 43 kDa.

Function

CD323 localizes to the inter-endothelial tight junctions and plays a role in neutrophil transmigration across endothelial cells via the interaction of CD323 on endothelium with Mac-1 on the surface of neutrophils.

CD323 plays a role in lymphocyte transmigration via homophilic interaction with endothelial cells.

Ligands

CD323 binds Mac-1 (CD11b/CD18) and JAM-2 (CD322) and displays homophilic binding.

Expression

CD323 is expressed by platelets, T cells, and NK cells and is widely expressed by endothelial cells in many tissues with highest expression in placenta, kidney, and brain.

It is expressed by megakaryoblastic cell lines.

Applications

Potential target for anti-inflammatory therapy for inflammatory vascular pathologies.

Gene Name	Entrez Gene#
JAM-3	83700

Selected Monoclonal Antibodies

No antibodies assigned, but CD323 reserved for JAM-3.

CD324

Other Names

E-cadherin, cadherin 1, CDHE, CDH1, uvomorulin, ECAD, Arc1.

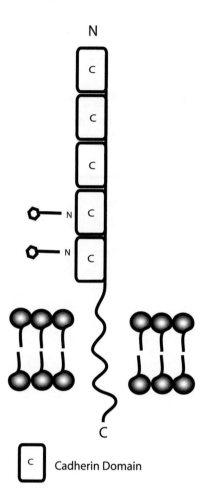

C | Cadherin Domain

Molecular Structure

CD324 is a type I transmembrane protein and a member of the classical cadherin family (which includes N-cadherin (CD325) and P-cadherin).

CD324 forms disulphide-linked homodimers.

The CD324 precursor protein has a 23 amino acid signal sequence and propeptide of 131 amino acids.

The mature protein consists of 728 residues, of which 553 amino acids are extracellular, 24 amino acids form the transmembrane region, and 151 residues are intracellular.

The extracellular domain has five cadherin domains (designated from the N-terminus as EC1–EC5) and two potential N-linked glycosylation sites and binds a single Ca^{2+} ion.

Some studies have identified the EC1 domain as essential for homophilic binding, whereas other studies indicate all five EC1 domains are required.

Tryptophan at position 2 (W2) and the histidine-alanine -valine pocket are essential for the formation adhesive transdimers.

The cytoplasmic domain contains a 14 amino acid stretch, which is serine rich.

Mol Wt: 120 kDa.

Function

CD324 functions as a cell–cell adhesion molecule via calcium-dependent homophilic binding and plays an important role in the intercellular adhesion of epithelial cells. Classical type I cadherins are mostly found in tissues where a high level of cell cohesiveness is required to maintain tissue integrity.

CD324 contributes to cell differentiation and polarity.

It is localized principally in the adherens junctions.

The cytoplasmic domain of CD324 binds β-catenin, which via association with α-catenin and other structural proteins is connected to the actin cytoskeleton.

The connection of CD324 with the actin cytoskeleton is required for normal cell–cell adhesion as mutant CD324 molecules lacking the cytoplasmic domain display weak binding to substrate compared with the wild-type molecule.

CD324 is a suppressor of tumor development and progression, as loss or abnormal function of CD324 is associated with several tumors, including gastric, breast, ovarian, endometrial, and thyroid carcinomas.

CD324 knockout mice embryos die at pre-implantation stage, indicating expression of this cadherin is critical during embryonic development.

Ligands

CD324 displays homophilic binding but has also been found to bind integrin αEβ7 and integrin α2β1.

Expression

CD324 is expressed by non-neural epithelial cells, stem cells, and erythroblasts.

Applications

CD324 expression is downregulated in several carcinomas, and this usually correlates with high grade, tumor progression and a poor prognosis.

Gene Name	Entrez Gene#
CDH1	999

Selected Monoclonal Antibodies

67A4 (Bühring; Tübingen); NCH-38 (Just, DakoCytomation; Glostrup).

CD325

Other Names

N-cadherin, Cadherin 2, NCAD, CDHM, CDH2.

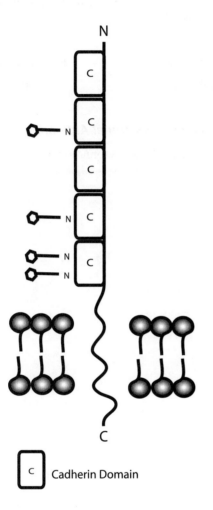

C   Cadherin Domain

Molecular Structure

CD325 is a type I transmembrane protein and a member of the classic cadherin family (which includes E-cadherin (CD324) and P-cadherin).

The precursor protein has a signal sequence of 25 amino acids and a propeptide of 134 residues. The mature protein consists of 740 amino acids, of which 555 residues are extracellular, 21 amino acids form the transmembrane domain, and 157 residues are intracellular.

The extracellular domain has five cadherin domains (designated from the N-terminus as EC1–EC5) and four potential N-linked glycosylation sites and binds a single Ca2+ ion.

Mol Wt: 140 kDa.

Function

CD325 forms a complex with catenins that is linked to the actin cytoskeleton. The CD325-catenin complex plays an important role in synaptic development and the structural and functional plasticity of neurons.

Electrical activity regulates the distribution of CD325 at synapses by mobilizing CD325 and catenins to the synapse.

CD325 is one of the first cadherins recruited to the site of synapse formation, and homophilic interactions across the synaptic gap are thought to stabilize the early synapse. As synapses mature, CD325 accumulates at excitatory but not at inhibitory synapses.

At least two studies have shown antibody to the CD325 extracellular domain can inhibit the induction of long-term potentiation.

CD325 is proteolytically cleaved by presenilin 1 (PS1, a protein implicated in Alzheimer's disease) releasing a peptide N-cad/CTF2. N-cad/CTF2 accumulation in turn downregulates CREB binding protein (CBP)–CREB-mediated transcription. CBP–CREB-mediated transcription is implicated in learning and memory as well as in neurodegenerative disease. Mutations in PS1 found in familial Alzheimer's disease result in decreased cleavage of CD325 and increased CREB-mediated transcription. This suggests CD325 may contribute to memory impairment associated with Alzheimer's disease.

CD325 is expressed on the surface of malignant T cells and was found to modulate adhesion of the T cells to Caco-2 epithelial cells in vitro. This suggests a role for N-cadherin in promoting malignant T-cell adhesion to epithelia as well as their capacity to invade and metastasize to inflammatory sites.

CD325 null mice die as embryos around day 10 of development, indicating that the presence of this cadherin is essential for cmbryonic development.

Ligands

CD325 exhibits homophilic binding.

Expression

CD325 is expressed by neurons, endothelial cells, osteoblasts, and stem cells and is mostly present on cells that do not express CD234 and P-cadherin.

Molt-3 T lymphoblastic leukemia cells express CD325.

Gene Name	Entrez Gene#
CDH2	1000

Selected Monoclonal Antibodies

6G11 (Just; DakoCytomation, Glostrup).

CD326

Other Names

Ep-CAM, EGP40, MIC18, TROP1, EGP, hEGP-2, KSA, M4S1, MK-1, TACSTD1, GA733-2.

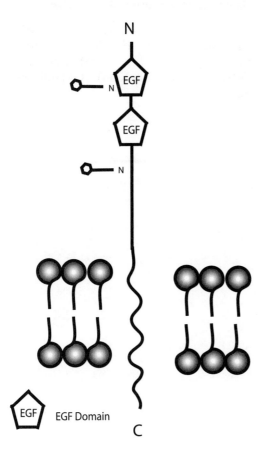

EGF Domain

Molecular Structure

CD326 is a type I transmembrane protein and an adhesion molecule that bears no homology to other known cell adhesion molecules.

The precursor protein has a 21 amino acid signal sequence that is cleaved to give a mature protein of 293 residues.

The extracellular domain consists of 246 amino acids and contains 2 epidermal growth factor (EGF)-like repeats followed by a cysteine-poor stretch of 122 amino acids and 2 putative N-linked glycosylation sites.

The first EGF repeat mediates homophilic binding between CD326 molecules on adjacent cells, whereas the second EGF domain is required for lateral interactions between CD326 molecules to form tetramers.

The transmembrane region consists of 21 amino acids.

The short cytoplasmic domain of 26 residues has 2 binding sites for α-actinin.

Mol Wt: 40 kDa.

Function

CD326 mediates calcium-dependent homotypic cell–cell adhesion with its extracellular domain and is linked to the actin cytoskeleton via its intracellular domain.

CD326-mediated intercellular adhesion is weaker than that mediated by cadherins and is thought to be involved in maintaining cells in position during proliferation.

Expression levels of CD326 correlate inversely with that of E-cadherin (CD324) and cellular differentiation. Hence, CD326 expression declines during cell differentiation and E-cadherin (CD324) expression increases.

A recent study found CD326 to be expressed by intra-epithelial lymphocytes (IELs) in mucosal epithelium, and it has been suggested that CD326-mediated adhesion between IELs and intestinal epithelial cells helps maintain an immunological barrier, which is the first line of defense against mucosal infection.

Ligands

CD326 displays homophilic binding.

Expression

CD326 is expressed by most epithelial cell types with the exception of adult squamous cells of the skin and a few specific epithelial cell types such as hepatocytes.

It is only expressed in neoplasms of epithelial cell origin.

Immature erythroblasts express CD326.

Applications

CD326 is a marker of epithelial cells, and CD326 immunohistochemistry is a means of distinguishing tumors of epithelial and non-epithelial origin.

It is a target of immunotherapy in the treatment of colorectal carcinoma.

Gene Name	Entrez Gene#
TACSTD1	4072

Selected Monoclonal Antibodies

FMU-EpCAM1, FMU-EpCAM2, FMU-EpCAM3, FMU-EpCAM4, FMU-EpCAM6, FMU-EpCAM7, FMU-EpCAM8 (Jin; Xian); 9C4 (Bühring; Tübingen).

CD327

Other Names

Siglec 6, OB-BP1, CD33L, CD33L1, sialic
acid-binding Ig-like lectin 6.

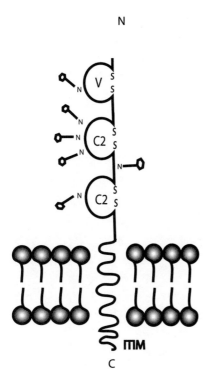

Molecular Structure

CD327 is a type I transmembrane protein
and a sialic acid-binding Ig superfamily
member lectin (Siglecs). Siglecs are a
subset of I-type lectins within the Ig superfamily (see also CD170, CD328, and
CD329).

CD327, Siglec 5, and CD33 form a subgroup of Siglecs that have high overall
amino acid identity to each other and
whose genes are located in close proximity
on chromosome 19.

The mature protein consists of 427
amino acids following cleavage of a signal
peptide of 15 residues.

The 321 amino acid extracellular
domain contains an N-terminal V-type Ig-
like domain followed by 2 C2-type Ig-like
domains and has 6 potential N-linked glycosylation sites.

The transmembrane domain consists of
21 amino acids.

The 85-residue intracellular domain
contains an immunoregulatory tyrosine-
based inhibitory motif (ITIM) and a signaling lymphocyte activating molecule
(SLAM)-like motif that acts as a docking
site for the SLAM-associated protein
(SAP).

Alternative RNA splicing gives rise to
two CD327 isoforms that includes the
membrane-bound form described above
and a soluble form that lacks most of the
intracellular amino acids.

Mol Wt: Predicted, 49 kDa.

Function

As a Siglec-family member, CD327 is
predicted to mediate cell–cell recognition events between specific cell populations in the placenta, spleen, and small
intestine.

The presence of signaling motifs in the
cytoplasmic tail of the membrane-bound
form of CD327 indicates a role in signal
transduction.

The role of CD327 in leptin physiology
is unknown, but it may be important during
embryogenesis given that cyto- and syncytiotrophoblastic cells strongly express
CD327 and leptin.

Ligands

CD327 specifically recognizes Neu5Aca2-
6GalNAca (sialyl-Tn) motifs.

Unrelated to its sialic acid-binding activity, CD327 binds the protein core of leptin
with moderate affinity.

Expression

CD327 is strongly expressed by cyto- and syncytiotrophoblastic cells of placenta and B cells in the spleen and small intestine. Neutrophils express CD327 at low levels.

Gene Name	Entrez Gene#
SIGLEC6	946

Selected Monoclonal Antibodies

E20-1232 (BD Biosciences).

CD328

Other Names

Siglec7, AIRM1, p75, sialic acid-binding Ig-like lectin 7.

N

Molecular Structure

CD328 is a type I transmembrane protein and a sialic acid-binding Ig superfamily member lectin (Siglecs). Siglecs are a subset of I-type lectins within the Ig superfamily (see also CD170, CD327, and CD329).

The CD328 gene is located in chromosome 19 in close proximity to other Siglecs.

The CD328 precursor has an 18 amino acid signal sequence, and the mature protein consists of 449 amino acids, of which 335 are extracellular, 23 residues span the membrane, and 91 amino acids are intracellular.

The extracellular domain contains an N-terminal Ig-like V-type domain followed by two Ig-like C2-type domains and has eight potential N-linked glycosylation sites.

The intracellular domain contains an immunoreceptor tyrosine-based inhibitory motif (ITIM).

Four isoforms arising from alternative RNA splicing have been described.

Mol Wt: 75 kDa.

Function

CD328 mediates sialic acid-dependent cell–cell binding and functions as an inhibitory receptor of NK cells.

Ligand-induced tyrosine phosphorylation of CD328 ITIM leads to recruitment of the cytoplasmic phosphatase SHP-1. SHP-1 blocks signal transduction by dephosphorylating signaling molecules.

CD328 inhibits the differentiation of $CD34^+$ cell precursors toward myelomonocytic cell lineage and the proliferation of leukemic cells in vitro.

CD328 can negatively affect TCR signaling. Ligand binding by CD328 leads to recruitment of SHP-1 and subsequently reduced phosphorylation of Tyr319 on ZAP-70, which plays a critical role in the upregulation of gene transcription after TCR stimulation.

Ligands

CD328 preferentially binds α 2,3- and α 2,6-linked sialic acid but can also bind disialogangliosides such as disialyl Lewis (a) antigen.

Expression

CD328 is predominantly expressed by NK cells but is expressed at lower levels by granulocytes, monocytes, and mainly α/β T cells as well as a small population of C8⁺ memory T cells.

High expression of CD328 is found in the placenta, liver, lung, and spleen.

Gene Name	Entrez Gene#
SIGLEC7	27036

Selected Monoclonal Antibodies

F023-420.2 (BD Biosciences; SanDiego); 6-434, 5-386 (Majdic; Vienna).

CD329

Other Names

Siglec-9, sialic acid-binding Ig-like lectin 9.

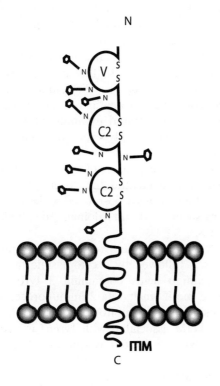

Molecular Structure

CD329 is a type I transmembrane protein and a sialic acid-binding Ig superfamily member lectin (Siglecs). Siglecs are a subset of I-type lectins within the Ig superfamily (see also CD170, CD327, and CD328).

The CD329 gene is located in chromosome 19 in close proximity to other Siglecs.

CD329 shares 84% identity with CD328 at the nucleotide level.

The CD329 precursor has a 17 amino acid signal, and the mature protein consists of 446 amino acids, of which 331 are extracellular, 21 residues span the membrane, and 94 amino acids are intracellular.

The extracellular domain contains an N-terminal Ig-like V-type domain followed by tow Ig-like C2-type domains and has nine potential N-linked glycosylation sites.

The intracellular domain contains a membrane-proximal immunoreceptor tyrosine-based inhibitory motif (ITIM) and a signaling lymphocyte activating molecule (SLAM)-like motif that acts as a docking site for SLAM-associated protein (SAP).

Mol Wt: Predicted, 50.1 kDa.

Function

CD329 can negatively affect TCR signaling. Ligand binding by CD329 leads to recruitment of SHP-1 and subsequently reduced phosphorylation of Tyr319 on ZAP-70, which plays a critical role in the upregulation of gene transcription after TCR stimulation.

A recent study has found CD329 ligation can initiate both apoptotic and non-apoptotic death signaling in neutrophils depending on the pro-inflammatory cytokine environment.

Ligands

CD329 binds $\alpha2,3$- and $\alpha2,6$-linked sialic acids, although the underlying glycan influences the binding avidity. Sialic acids $\alpha2,3$-linked to Galβ1-4GlcNAc are better ligands of CD329 than sialic acids $\alpha2,3$-linked to Galβ1-3GalNAc.

Expression

Intermediate to high levels of CD328 expression are found in monocytes and neutrophils as well as in a minor population of CD16$^+$, CD56$^-$ cells. Weaker expression is detectable in 50% of B cells, NK cells, and CD3$^+\alpha/\beta$ T cells.

Gene Name	Entrez Gene#
SIGLEC9	27180

Selected Monoclonal Antibodies

E10-286 (BD Biosciences; San Diego).

(CD330)

Other Names

Siglec 10, sialic acid-binding Ig-like lectin 10, Siglec-like protein 2.

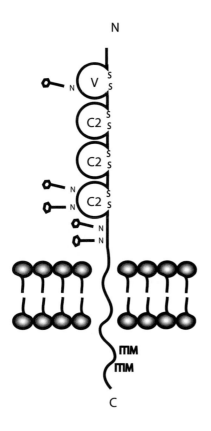

Molecular Structure

CD330 is a type I transmembrane protein and a CD33-related sialic acid-binding immunoglobulin superfamily member lectin (Siglecs). Siglecs are a subset of I-type lectins within the Ig superfamily (see also CD170, CD327, CD328, and CD329).

The CD330 gene maps to the same chromosomal region as other CD33-related Siglecs (chromosome 19q13.3-4).

CD330 is most closely related to Siglec 5, with which it has 69% homology at the amino acid level.

The CD330 precursor has a 16 amino acid signal sequence, and the mature protein consists of 681 amino acids.

The extracellular domain consists of 534 amino acids and contains an N-terminal Ig-like V-type domain followed by 3 Ig-like C2-type domains and has 5 potential N-linked glycosylation sites.

The V-type domain bears a critical arginine residue (Arg120) that interacts with the carboxyl group of sialic acid as well as two conserved aromatic residues (Phe26 and Tyr124) required for interaction with the N-acetyl and glycerol side chains of sialic acid.

The unique pattern of cysteines in the V-type domain and the N-terminal C-2 type domain of CD33-related Siglecs form intra-sheet and interdomain disulphide bonds.

A transmembrane region of 21 amino acids is followed by a cytoplasmic tail of 126 amino acids containing 3 tyrosine-based motifs including 2 immunoreceptor tyrosine-based inhibitory motifs (ITIMs). The ITIM associated with Tyr667 is phosphorylated by Src family kinases Lck, Jak3, and Emt and recruits SHP-1 and to a lesser extent SHP-2.

The motif associated with Tyr691 resembles a signaling lymphocyte activating molecule (SLAM)-like motif that acts as a docking site for SLAM-associated protein (SAP), although SAP binding has yet to be demonstrated.

Alternative RNA splicing gives rise to six isoforms (Long, Sv1, Sv2, Sv3, Sv4, and isoform 6). Isoforms Long, Sv1–Sv4 retain the V-type domain but vary in the number and arrangement of C2-type domains. Isoform Sv2 is a soluble form of CD330.

Mol. Wt: 90–120 kDa

Function

The role of CD330 remains unclear, but based on the structure of the cytoplasmic tail, it is predicted to act as an inhibitory receptor.

Binding assays have demonstrated that the CD330 extracellular domain binds peripheral blood leukocytes.

The expression of CD330 by eosinophils and upregulation of CD330 expression on eosinophils from asthmatics has led to the suggestion that CD330 may modulate eosinophil activity during an allergic reaction.

CD330 expression has been found to be upregulated on some transformed blood cell lines.

Ligands

CD330 preferentially binds α2,6 sialylated glycoconjugates but can also bind α2,3 sialylated glycoconjugates including GT1b ganglioside.

Expression

The CD330 long isoform is strongly expressed by eosinophils, neutrophils, and monocytes in bone marrow, spleen, and spinal chord, whereas the Sv1 isoform is weakly expressed in the same tissues.

The Sv3 isoform is expressed in T and B cells, whereas the Sv4 isoform is restricted to CD56⁻CD16⁺ NK cells.

Isoform Sv2 is the most abundantly expressed isoform and is strongly expressed in lymph node, lung, ovary, and appendix.

Gene Name	Entrez Gene#
SIGLEC10	89790

Selected Monoclonal Antibodies

No antibodies assigned, but CD330 reserved for Siglec-10.

CD331

Other Names

FGFR1, FLT2, FLG.

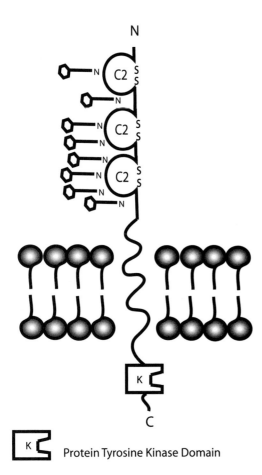

Protein Tyrosine Kinase Domain

Molecular Structure

CD331 is a type I membrane protein and a receptor tyrosine kinase (RTK) of the fibroblast growth factor receptor (FGFR) subfamily within the Ig superfamily (see also CD332, CD333, and CD334).

The precursor has a 21 amino acid signal sequence.

The mature protein consists of 801 amino acids, of which 355 residues are extracellular, 21 amino acids span the membrane, and 425 residues are intracellular.

The extracellular domain contains three Ig-like C2-type domains (D1–D3 or IgI–IgIII), a stretch of residues in the linker connecting D1 and D2 known as the "acid box," a heparin binding site in D2, and eight potential N-linked glycosylation sites.

D2 and D3 form the primary binding pocket for FGF, whereas D1 and the acid box have an autoinhibitory role.

Binding of FGF induces dimerization of CD331 and results in a tetrameric complex. Essential cofactors associated with this complex are cell-surface heparin sulphate proteoglycans.

The cytoplasmic domain has 2 ATP binding sites and a 290 amino acid protein kinase domain that is split by a short insert.

Dimerization promotes autophosphorylation in trans of critical tyrosines in the activation loop that stabilizes the receptor in an active conformation and leads to in cis phosphorylation of tyrosine residues within the TK domain. Autophosphorylation of Tyr653 and Tyr654 is essential for the upregulation of kinase activity.

Intracellular phosphotyrosines serve as binding sites for signal transduction molecules such as SHC, FRS2, and phospholipase Cγ (PLCγ).

Autophosphorylated Tyr766 is the binding site for PLCγ.

Eighteen isoforms arising from alternative RNA splicing have been described. Of most significance is the cell-type specific obligatory splicing that generates two forms of D3 with different FGF binding characteristics (FGFR1b and FGFR1c).

Mol Wt: 130 kDa.

Function

CD331 mediates some pleiotropic responses to fibroblast growth factors (FGF). During development of the embryo, FGF-induced CD331-mediated signaling plays a critical role in morphogenesis by regulating cell proliferation, differentiation, and migration.

In adults, CD331-mediated signaling is involved in tissue repair and wound healing, tumor angiogenesis, and growth.

Disruption of FGFR1 and targeted disruption of the FGFR1c isoform in mice are both embryonically lethal at E9.5-E12, whereas FGFR1b$^{-/-}$ mice are phenotypically normal.

Point mutations in CD331 are responsible for Pfeiffer syndrome, which is characterized by craniosynostosis syndrome (premature fusion of cranial sutures) and broad thumbs and toes.

Somatic mutations of FGFR1 cause autosomal dominant Kallmann syndrome (KAL2), in which the olfactory bulb fails to develop.

Alterations in CD331 expression or translocation and fusion of FGFR1 with other genes are associated with a variety of malignancies.

Five different fusion partners for FGFR1 have been found in association with 8p11 myeloproliferative syndrome (EMS). EMS is characterized by eosinophilia, myeloid hyperplasia, and lymphoblastic lymphoma. The FGFR fusion proteins are constitutive tyrosine kinases that have transforming activity.

Over-expression of CD331 is associated with breast cancer and astrocytomas, whereas abnormal expression of CD331 occurs in prostate cancer and pancreatic adenocarcinoma.

Ligands

CD331 is a high affinity receptor for acidic and basic fibroblast growth factors (FGF). FGFR1b binds FGF1, -2, -3, and -10, and FGFR1c binds FGF1, -2, -4, -5, and -6.

Expression

CD331 is expressed by fibroblasts and epithelial and endothelial cells.

Applications

CD331 is a potential target of tyrosine kinase inhibitors currently under development for use in the treatment of various cancers.

Gene Name	Entrez Gene#
FGFR1	2260

Selected Monoclonal Antibodies

133105 (R&D Systems; Minneapolis).

CD332

Other Names

FGFR2, KGFR, TK14, BEK, KSAM-1.

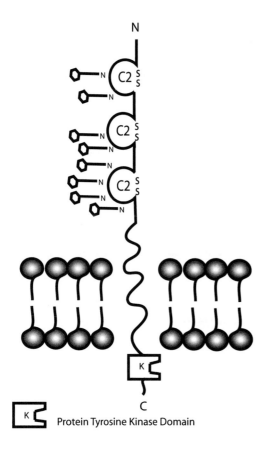

K **[** Protein Tyrosine Kinase Domain

Molecular Structure

CD332 is a type I membrane protein and a receptor tyrosine kinase (RTK) of the fibroblast growth factor receptor (FGFR) subfamily within the Ig superfamily (see also CD331, CD333, and CD334).

The precursor has a 21 amino acid signal sequence.

The mature protein consists of 800 amino acids, of which 356 residues are extracellular, 21 amino acids span the membrane, and 423 residues are intracellular.

The extracellular domain contains three Ig-like C2-type domains (D1–D3 or IgI–IgIII), a stretch of residues in the linker connecting D1 and D2 known as the "acid box," a heparin binding site in D2, and eight potential N-linked glycosylation sites.

D2 and D3 form the primary binding pocket for FGF, whereas D1 and the acid box have an autoinhibitory role.

Binding of FGF induces dimerization of CD331 and results in a tetrameric complex. Essential cofactors associated with this complex are cell-surface heparin sulphate proteoglycans.

The cytoplasmic domain has 2 ATP binding sites and a 290 amino acid tyrosine kinase (TK) domain that is split by a short insert.

Dimerization promotes autophosphorylation in trans of critical tyrosines in the activation loop that stabilizes the receptor in an active conformation and leads to in cis phosphorylation of a tyrosine residue within the TK domain.

Intracellular phosphotyrosines serve as binding sites for signal transduction molecules such as SHC, FRS2, and phospholipase Cγ (PLCγ).

Nineteen isoforms arising from alternative RNA splicing have been described, including two soluble forms. Of most significance is the cell-type-specific obligatory splicing that generates two forms of D3 with different FGF binding characteristics (FGFR2b and FGFR2c).

Mol Wt: 115–135 kDa.

Function

CD332 mediates some of the pleiotropic responses to fibroblast growth factors (FGF). During development of the embryo, FGF-induced CD332-mediated signaling plays a critical role in morphogenesis by regulating cell proliferation, differentiation, and migration.

In adults, CD332-mediated signaling is involved in tissue repair and wound healing, tumor angiogenesis, and growth.

Null mutations of FGFR2 in mice are embryonically lethal at E10.5 due to defective cell migration through the primitive streak and a posterior axis defect.

Selective disruption of FGFR2b results in death of the mice immediately after birth and is characterized by defective development of limbs, lungs, anterior pituitary, thyroid, and teeth.

Targeted disruption of FGFR2c leads to viable mice with impaired skull and bone development.

In humans, point mutations in FGFR2 are associated with a variety of human skeletal disorders including Crouzon syndrome, Jackson–Weiss syndrome, Apert syndrome, Beare–Stevenson cutis gyrata, Pfieffer syndrome, and Saethre–Chotzen-like syndrome. Many of these mutations are specific nucleotide substitutions and have been found to be germline mutations of paternal origin.

Downregulation of FGFR2 expression is observed in malignant astrocytomas.

A switch in isoform expression from FGFR2b to FGFR2c has been found to be associated with prostate cancer, and a novel splice site mutation coupled with a point mutation in FGFR2 is linked to gastric cancer.

Ligands

CD332 binds acidic and basic fibroblast growth factors (FGFs) with high affinity. Isoforms FGFR2b and FGFR2c bind FGF1, -3, -7, -10, and -22 and FGF1, -2, -4, -6, -9, -17, and -18, respectively.

Expression

CD332 isoform FGFR2b is exclusively expressed in epithelial cells, whereas FGFR2c is exclusively expressed in mesenchymal cells.

Gene Name   Entrez Gene#
FGFR2   2263

Selected Monoclonal Antibodies

98739, 98725, 98707, 98726 (R&D Systems; Minneapolis).

CD333

Other Names

FGFR3, JTK4.

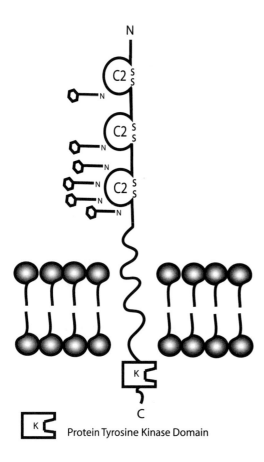

K $\vdash$ Protein Tyrosine Kinase Domain

Molecular Structure

CD333 is a type I membrane protein and a receptor tyrosine kinase (RTK) of the fibroblast growth factor receptor (FGFR) subfamily within the Ig superfamily (see also CD331, CD332, and CD334).

The precursor has a 22 amino acid signal sequence.

The mature protein consists of 784 amino acids, of which 353 residues are extracellular, 21 amino acids span the membrane, and 410 residues are intracellular.

The extracellular domain contains three Ig-like C2-type domains (D1–D3 or IgI–IgIII), a stretch of residues in the linker connecting D1 and D2 known as the "acid box," a heparin binding site in D2, and six potential N-linked glycosylation sites.

D2 and D3 form the primary binding pocket for FGF, whereas D1 and the acid box have an autoinhibitory role

Binding of FGF induces dimerization of CD331 and results in a tetrameric complex. Essential cofactors associated with this complex are cell-surface heparin sulphate proteoglycans.

The cytoplasmic domain has 2 ATP binding sites and a 290 amino acid tyrosine kinase (TK) domain that is split by a short insert.

Dimerization promotes autophosphorylation in trans of critical tyrosines in the activation loop that stabilizes the receptor in an active conformation and leads to in cis phosphorylation of a tyrosine residue within the TK domain.

Intracellular phosphotyrosines serve as binding sites for signal transduction molecules such as SHC, FRS2, and phospholipase Cγ (PLCγ).

Three isoforms arising from alternative RNA splicing have been described. Of most significance is the cell-type specific obligatory splicing that generates two forms of D3 with different FGF binding characteristics (FGFR3b and FGFR3c).

The third isoform, FGFR3 δ 8-10, is secreted.

Mol Wt: 115–135 kDa.

Function

CD333 mediates some pleiotropic responses to fibroblast growth factors (FGF). During development of the embryo, FGF-induced CD333-mediated signaling plays a critical role in the growth and development of the skeleton.

FGFR3 knockout mice are viable but have an inner ear defect and bone overgrowth due to chondrocyte hypertrophy.

FGFR3 mutations in humans are associated with several skeletal disorders including Beare–Stevenson cutis gyrata, Muenke syndrome, Saethre–Chotzen-like syndrome, achondroplasia, severe achondroplasia with developmental delay and acanthosis nigricans, thanatophoric dysplasia types I and II, and hypochondroplasia. Many of these mutations are specific nucleotide substitutions and have been found to be germline mutations of paternal origin.

Abnormal expression of CD333 is linked to a variety of cancers.

Activating mutations in FGFR3 appear to play a central role in the development of papillary bladder tumors. Furthermore, FGFR3 δ8-10 acts as an inhibitor of FGF1-induced cell proliferation of normal uroepithelium. In aggressive bladder carcinomas, the level of FGFR3 δ8-10 expression is significantly reduced.

Constitutively active kinases resulting from the translocation and fusion of FGFR3 with other proteins are associated with multiple myeloma and peripheral T-cell lymphoma.

Other mutations of FGFR3 are found in thyroid carcinoma, cervical carcinoma, and colorectal carcinoma.

Germline mutations of FGFR3 associated with achondroplasia and thanatophoric dysplasia are also associated with 35% of cases of bladder cancer and 25% of cervical cancers.

Ligands

CD333 binds acidic and basic fibroblast growth factors (FGFs) with high affinity. Isoforms FGFR3b and FGFR3c bind FGF1, and -9 and FGF1, -2, -4, -6, -8, -9, -16, -17, -18, and -19, respectively.

Expression

CD333 is expressed by fibroblasts and epithelial cells. Isoform FGFR3b is exclusively expressed in epithelial cells, whereas FGFR3b and FGFR3c are both expressed in fibroblasts.

FGFR3 δ8-10 is the predominant isoform expressed in non-proliferating uroepithelial cells. However, expression of FGFR3 δ8-10 is reduced and FGFR3c is the predominant isoform expressed in aggressive bladder carcinomas.

Gene Name

Gene Name	Entrez Gene#
FGFR3	2261

Selected Monoclonal Antibodies

136334, 136312 (R&D Systems; Minneapolis).

CD334

Other Names

FGFR4, JTK2, TKF.

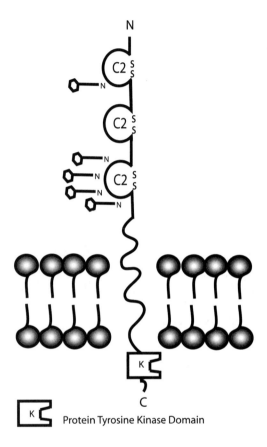

Protein Tyrosine Kinase Domain

Molecular Structure

CD334 is a type I membrane protein and a receptor tyrosine kinase (RTK) of the fibroblast growth factor receptor (FGFR) subfamily within the Ig superfamily (see also CD331, CD332, and CD333).

The precursor has a 21 amino acid signal sequence.

The mature protein consists of 781 amino acids, of which 348 residues are extracellular, 21 amino acids span the membrane, and 412 residues are intracellular.

The extracellular domain contains three Ig-like C2-type domains (D1–D3 or IgI–IgIII), a stretch of residues in the linker connecting D1 and D2 known as the "acid box," a heparin binding site in D2, and five potential N-linked glycosylation sites.

D2 and D3 form the primary binding pocket for FGF, whereas D1 and the acid box have an autoinhibitory role.

Binding of FGF induces dimerization of CD331 and results in a tetrameric complex. Essential cofactors associated with this complex are cell-surface heparin sulphate proteoglycans.

The cytoplasmic domain has 2 ATP binding sites, a 289 amino acid tyrosine kinase (TK) domain that is split by a short insert, and lacks several lysines that are conserved in CD331, CD332, and CD333.

Dimerization promotes autophosphorylation in trans of critical tyrosines in the activation loop that stabilizes the receptor in an active conformation and leads to in cis phosphorylation of a tyrosine residue within the TK domain.

Intracellular phosphotyrosines serve as binding sites for signal transduction molecules such as SHC, FRS2, and phospholipase Cγ (PLCγ).

No cell-type-specific alternative RNA splicing has been observed for CD334.

Mol Wt: 110 kDa.

Function

CD334 mediates some of the pleiotropic responses to fibroblast growth factors (FGF). It plays a role in the differentiation of skeletal muscle cells.

Disruption of CD334 signaling interrupts chick limb muscle formation.

CD334 knockout mice are phenotypically normal but demonstrate defective muscle regeneration.

Bile acid synthesis in mice is regulated by FGF15-induced CD334 signaling in hepatocytes, which represses the CYP7A1 gene (encoding cholesterol 7 α-hydroxylase). CYP7A1 catalyzes the first and rate-limiting step in bile acid synthesis. FGF15 is the murine equivalent of human FGF19.

The Gly388Arg polymorphism in CD334 is associated with breast, colon, prostate cancer, head and neck squamous cell carcinoma, and lung adenocarcinoma.

A recent study has shown that endo-cytosed FGF1 bound to CD334 follows a different intracellular pathway to that of FGF1 bound to CD331, CD332, or CD333. FGF1/CD334 is targeted to the recycling compartment, whereas when other FGFRs bound to ligand are internal-ized, they are mainly sorted to lysosomes for degradation.

Ligands

CD334 is a high affinity receptor for acidic fibroblast growth factors (FGFs) binding FGF1, -2, -4, -6, -8, -9, -16, -17, -18, and -19.

Expression

CD334 is expressed by epithelial cells, fibroblasts, and skeletal muscle cells.

Applications

The expression level of CD334 is a prog-nostic indicator for lung adenocarcinoma, breast, colon, and prostate cancer.

CD334 is a potential therapeutic target of tyrosine kinase inhibitors for the treat-ment of various cancers.

Gene Name	Entrez Gene#
FGFR4	2264

Selected Monoclonal Antibodies

137114 (R&D Systems; Minneapolis), 4FR6D3 (Bühring; Tübingen).

CD335

Other Names

NKp46, NCR1, Ly94.

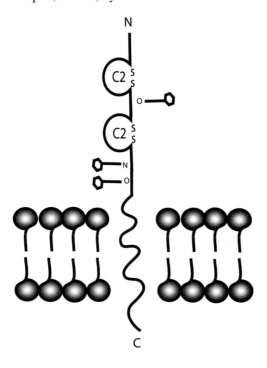

Molecular Structure

CD335 is a type I membrane protein and belongs to the natural cytotoxicity receptor (NCR) family within the Ig superfamily. Other NCR family members are CD336 and CD337.

The precursor protein has a 21 amino acid signal sequence.

The mature protein consists of 283 amino acids, of which 237 residues are extracellular, 21 amino acids span the cell membrane, and 25 amino acids are intracellular.

The extracellular domain has two Ig-like C2-type domains, two O-linked glycosylation sites, and one potential N-linked glycosylation site.

The transmembrane region contains a positively charged arginine that is predicted to associate with the CD3 ζ chain (CD247).

The intracellular domain has no known signaling motifs.

Five RNA splice variants have been characterized. Apart from the full-length molecule, the remaining four variants all lack regions of the extracellular domain with the exception of the membrane proximal Ig-like domain, which is conserved.

Mol Wt: 46 kDa.

Function

CD335 is a major lysis receptor for NK cells and mediates direct lysis of autologous virus-infected cells and tumor cells.

Sialic acid residues on NKp46 are thought to be involved in recognition of viral hemagglutinins.

CD335 lacks any cytoplasmic signaling motifs but associates with the CD3 ζ chain, which bears an immunoreceptor tyrosine-based activation motif (ITAM) and delivers activating signals.

The surface density of CD335, CD336, and CD337 correlates with the magnitude of NK-cell cytolytic activity against target cells.

Variation in the surface density of these molecules occurs within and between individuals.

Prolactin can upregulate CD335 and CD337 expression, and cortisol downregulates expression of both NCRs.

CD335-mediated cytotoxicity of tumor cells is suicidal for NK cells as CD337 engagement with tumor cell ligands leads to upregulation of FasL protein synthesis and release. FasL ligation of Fas on the NK cell surface triggers caspase 3-dependent apoptosis.

Ligands

CD335 binds to influenza virus hemagglutinin (HA) and the HA-neuraminidase of the Sendai virus.

Recent studies have identified heparan-sulphate proteoglycans (HSPGs) on the surface of tumor cells as ligands of CD335.

Expression

CD335 is expressed by resting and activated NK cells.

Applications

CD335 is a specific marker of NK cells.

Gene Name	Entrez Gene#
NCR1	9437

Selected Monoclonal Antibodies

900 (BD Biosciences); B28 (Beckman Coulter); 195314 (R&D Systems; Minneapolis); D2.9A5, 461.G1 (Mandelboim; Jerusalem).

CD336

Other Names

NKp44, NCR2, Ly95.

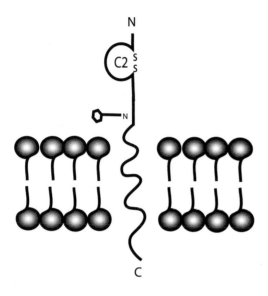

Molecular Structure

CD336 is a type I membrane protein and belongs to the natural cytotoxicity receptor (NCR) family within the Ig superfamily. Other NCR family members are CD335 and CD337.

The precursor protein has a 21 amino acid signal sequence.

The mature protein consists of 255 amino acids, of which 171 residues are extracellular, 21 amino acids span the cell membrane, and 63 amino acids are intracellular.

The extracellular domain has one Ig-like C2-type domain and one potential N-linked glycosylation site.

The intracellular domain has no known signaling motifs.

Mol Wt: 44 kDa.

Function

CD336 is a cytotoxicity-activating receptor that may contribute to the increased efficiency of activated NK cells to mediate lysis of autologous virus-infected cells and tumor cells.

CD336 lacks any cytoplasmic signaling motifs but associates with DAP12/KARAP that bears an immunoreceptor tyrosine-based activation motif (ITAM) and delivers activating signals.

The surface density of CD335, CD336, and CD337 correlates with the magnitude of NK-cell cytolytic activity against target cells.

Variation in the surface density of these molecules occurs within and between individuals.

CD336-mediated cytotoxicity of tumor cells is suicidal for NK cells as CD337 engagement with tumor cell ligands leads to upregulation of FasL protein synthesis and release. FasL ligation of Fas on the NK-cell surface triggers caspase 3-dependent apoptosis.

Ligands

CD336 binds the hemagglutinins of both Influenza and Sendai viruses.

Expression

CD336 is expressed by IL-2 activated NK cells and a minor subset of γ/δ T cells.

Gene Name	Entrez Gene#
NCR2	9436

Selected Monoclonal Antibodies

Z231 (Beckman Coulter; Marseille).

CD337

Other Names

NKp30, NCR3, Ly117, 1C7.

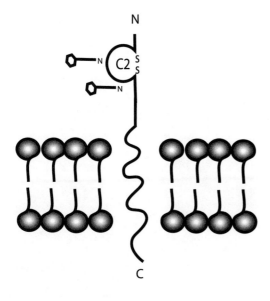

Molecular Structure

CD337 is a type I membrane protein and belongs to the natural cytotoxicity receptor (NCR) family within the Ig superfamily. Other NCR family members are CD335 and CD336.

The precursor protein has an 18 amino acid signal sequence.

The mature protein consists of 183 amino acids, of which 117 residues are extracellular, 21 amino acids span the cell membrane, and 45 amino acids are intracellular.

The extracellular domain has one Ig-like C2-type domain and two potential N-linked glycosylation sites.

The transmembrane region contains a positively charged arginine that is predicted to associate with the CD3 ζ chain (CD247).

The intracellular domain has no known signaling motifs.

Mol Wt: 30 kDa.

Function

CD337 is a cytotoxicity-activating receptor that is partially responsible for NK-cell-mediated lysis of tumor cells but is the main receptor involved in killing immature dendritic cells.

CD337-mediated NK-cell interaction with immature DCs does not always end in DC death. Binding of NK cell CD337 with DC ligands promotes release of TNFα and IFNγ by NK cells, which in turn promotes maturation of DC. This function is controlled by HLA-specific inhibitory NK receptors.

The surface density of CD335, CD336, and CD337 correlates with the magnitude of NK-cell cytolytic activity against target cells.

Variation in the surface density of these molecules occurs within and between individuals.

Prolactin can upregulate CD335 and CD337 expression, and cortisol downregulates expression of both NCRs. Transforming growth factor β (TGFβ) downregulates the surface expression of NKp30 and inhibits NKp30-mediated killing of immature dendritic cells.

CD337-mediated cytotoxicity of tumor cells is suicidal for NK cells as CD337 engagement with tumor cell ligands leads to upregulation of FasL protein synthesis and release. FasL ligation of Fas on the NK cell surface triggers caspase 3-dependent apoptosis.

Ligands

CD337 is reported to bind membrane-associated heparan sulphate proteoglycans on tumor cells. However, a recent study has found heparan sulphate glycosaminoglycans (GAG) are ligands of CD337.

Expression

CD337 is expressed by resting and activated NK cells.

Applications

CD337 is a specific marker of NK cells.

Gene Name

NCR3

Entrez Gene#

259197

Selected Monoclonal Antibodies

Z25 (Beckman Coulter; Marseille); 210845, 210857 (R&D Systems; Montpellier).

CD338

Other Names

ABCG2, BCRP, BCRP1, ABCP, MRX, MXR, MXR1, BMDP. ABC15, EST157481.

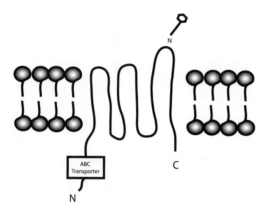

Molecular Structure

CD338 is an integral membrane protein and the second member of the G subfamily of human ATP-binding cassette (ABC) transporter superfamily (hence also known as ABCG2).

The protein consists of 655 amino acids and comprises a 395 amino acid N-terminal intracellular region that contains a nucleotide binding domain followed by a membrane-spanning domain (MSD) with 6 α-helical transmembrane domains.

Three potential N-linked glycosylation sites are located in the extracellular loops of the MSDs.

The C-terminus is cytoplasmic.

CD338 is predicted to form disulphide-linked homodimers or homotetramers.

Alternative RNA splicing gives rise to two isoforms.

Mol Wt: 72 kDa.

Function

CD338 acts as a xenobiotic efflux transport protein that can transport chemotherapeutic drugs, organic anions, and a variety of toxic chemicals across the cell membrane using ATP hydrolysis to drive the efflux process against a concentration gradient.

The normal sites of CD338 expression are tissues involved in absorption, distribution, and elimination of drugs, which indicates a role for CD338 in drug disposition, potentially providing protection against cytotoxic substrates.

Over-expression of CD338 can render cells resistant to several drugs used in chemotherapy such as mitoxantrone, daunorubicin, and doxorubicin.

CD338 is also known as the breast cancer resistance protein; however, it does not appear to be a major contributor to drug resistance in breast cancers.

There have been many studies that indicate that CD338 may contribute to drug resistance in some subgroups of leukemia patients.

Expression of CD338 is upregulated in human glioblastomas and is often found to be elevated in gastric, hepatocellular, endometrial, colon, and small cell lung carcinomas and melanoma.

The function of CD338 in human stem cells is unclear. Studies of CD338$^{-/-}$ mice have shown that CD338 expression not only provides protection against exogenous cytotoxic substrates but also protects against the effects of hypoxia by preventing the intracellular accumulation of heme, which is toxic to mitochondria.

Expression

CD338 is expressed by a subpopulation of hematopoietic stem cells as well as stem cells from a variety of other tissues, including skeletal muscle, liver, heart, and pancreas.

CD338 is strongly expressed in placenta syncytiotrophoblasts, the apical membrane of small intestinal epithelium, the liver canalicular membrane, and the luminal surface of brain microvascular endothelium, particularly in the putamen, substantia nigra, pituitary, and thalamus.

Applications

CD338 can be used as a marker to select for stem cells, potentially enriching for stem cells with greater resistance to cytotoxic substrates and hypoxia.

CD338 inhibitors are used in conjunction with cytotoxic drugs as part of chemotherapy for various cancers.

Gene Name	Entrez Gene#
ABCG2	9429

Selected Monoclonal Antibodies

5D3 (BD Biosciences, San Diego).

CD339

Other Names

Jagged1, JAG1, JAGL1, hJ1.

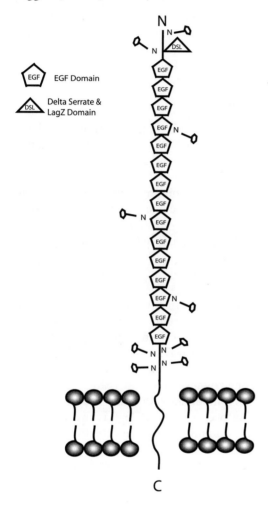

EGF — EGF Domain

DSL — Delta Serrate & LagZ Domain

N — C

Molecular Structure

CD339 is a type 1 transmembrane protein and a member of the jagged ligands family.

The precursor protein has a 22 amino acid signal sequence. The mature CD339 protein consists of 1185 amino acids, of which 1034 are extracellular, 26 residues span the cell membrane, and 125 amino acids are intracellular.

The extracellular region has 1 DSL (Delta, Serrate, and LagZ) domain fol-lowed by 15 EGF-like domains and a jux-tamembrane region that is cysteine rich.

EGF-like domains 4, 5, 6, 7, 10, 11, 14, and 15 bind calcium.

There are nine potential N-linked glyco-sylation sites.

Mol Wt: 150 kDa.

Function

CD339 acts as the ligand for some Notch receptors and is involved in mediating Notch signaling.

It appears to be involved in cell fate decisions during hematopoiesis and during early and late development of the mammalian cardiovascular system.

CD339-mediated signaling inhibits myoblast differentiation and induces fibroblast growth factor-induced angiogenesis (in vitro).

Mutations of JAG1 are responsible for Alagille syndrome (ALGS), an autosomal dominant development disorder that affects the structure of the liver, heart, skeleton, eye, kidney, and other organs.

CD339 mutations are responsible for tetralogy of Fallot (TOF), a congenital disorder of the heart characterized by pulmonary stenosis, ventricular septal defects, dextroposition of the aorta, and hypertrophy of the right ventricle.

Ligands

CD339 binds Notch1, Notch2, and Notch3.

Expression

CD339 is expressed by stromal cells and epithelial cells.

Gene Name	*Entrez Gene#*
JAG1	182

Selected Monoclonal Antibodies

188331 (R&D Systems; Minneapolis).

CD340

Other Names

HER2/neu, ERBB2, p185^{HER2}.

K $\rule{}{}$ Protein Tyrosine Kinase Domain

Molecular Structure

CD340 is a type 1 transmembrane protein, and a member of the ERBB family of receptor tyrosine kinases that includes the human receptors EGFR (ERBB1), ERBB3 (HER3) and ERBB4 (HER4).

The mature protein consists of 1233 aa of which 630 aa are extracellular, 23 aa span the membrane, and 580 aa are intracellular.

Consistent with the extracellular domain (ECD) of other ERBB family members, the ECD of CD340 comprises four domains (I–IV), and domains II and IV are cysteine-rich. However, CD340 does not bind any known ERBB ligand.

There are seven potential N-linked glycosylation sites.

The cytoplasmic region has a protein tyrosine kinase domain.

Alternative splicing results in several transcripts not all of which have been characterized. Allelic variation occurs at amino acids 654 and 655 for isoform a and at amino acids 624 and 625 for isoform b.

Mol Wt: 185 kDa.

Function

Although no direct ligand binding has been observed for CD340, it forms heterodimers with ligand-bound ERBB family members and plexin-B1. Heterodimerization stabilizes ligand binding, and contributes to kinase-mediated activition of MAPK, phospholipase-Cγ and PI-3K signaling pathways. ERBB-heterodimers play a role in a wide range of cellular responses that vary depending on the ligand and the cell type.

CD340 forms a stable complex with plexin-B1 bound by its ligand Sema4D (CD100). CD340-mediated phosphorylation of plexin-B1 is involved in RhoA activation and ultimately in axonal growth cone collapse.

Homodimerization and receptor activation occurs when CD340 is overexpressed as occurs in several cancers. In most cases overexpression is the result of gene amplification and increased promoter activity rather than mutations.

Expression

CD340 is expressed by bone marrow CD271^{+} Mesenchymal stem cells (MSC), subsets of C-ALL blasts and in B-lymphoblastic leukemia.

Several types of epithelial cells express CD340 and overexpression of CD340 is a characteristic of many cancers including neuroblastomas, and carcinomas of the breast, stomach, lung, ovary, colon, and cervix.

Applications

Therapeutic target in the treatment of HER2-positive breast cancer with Trastuzumab (Herceptin).

CD340-overexpression by carcinoma cells correlates with aggressive disease and a poor prognosis.

CD340 is a marker for bone marrow-MSC.

Gene Name   Entrez Gene#

ERBB2   2064

Selected Monoclonal Antibodies

13A1, 24D2, 13D1 (Bühring, Tübingen).

CD344

Other Names

Frizzled-4, Fz-4, hFz-4, FzE4.

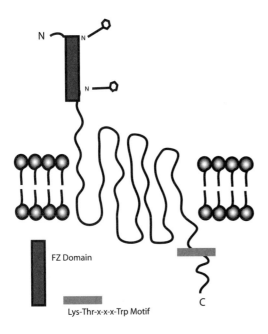

FZ Domain

Lys-Thr-x-x-x-Trp Motif

Molecular Structure

CD344 is a member of the Frizzled family of proteins within the superfamily of G protein-coupled receptors (GPCR). Ten Frizzled genes have been identified in the human genome (see CD349 and CD350).

It is an integral membrane protein of 501 amino acids with a 186-residue extracellular N-terminus containing the cysteine-rich ligand-binding site (FZ domain), seven transmembrane-spanning domains and a 39-residue cytoplasmic C-terminal tail that contains a Lys-Thr-X-X-X-Trp motif. This motif is the binding site for PDZ-domain containing proteins and is essential for activation of the Wnt/β-catenin pathway.

Recent studies have suggested Frizzled proteins may form heterodimers.

Mol Wt: Unprocessed precursor, 59.8 kDa.

Function

Frizzled proteins are essential for the regulation of tissue and cell polarity, embryonic development, regulation of proliferation, and many other processes in developing and adult organisms.

CD344 is a receptor for Wnt proteins and norrie and participates in the activation of the Wnt/β-catenin pathway (canonical Wnt signaling). This process is predicted to involve CD344 coupling to members of Gαi/o family of G proteins.

Patients with familial exudative vitreoretinopathy (FEVR) carry mutations in FZD4. This disease is characterized by a failure of peripheral retinal vascularization leading to retinal degeneration and associated progressive hearing loss indicating CD344 plays a role in retinal angiogenesis.

CD344$^{-/-}$ mice are infertile due to impaired corpora lutea formation and function. They also exhibit vascular defects in the retina, cochlea, and cerebellum, and defects in cell survival in the cerebellum as well as progressive dysfunction and distention of the oesophagus.

Ligands

CD344 binds Wnt proteins and norrin (Norrie disease pseudoglioma homolog).

Expression

CD344 is predominantly expressed in the kidney, lung, brain, and liver. It is also expressed by fetal neuronal progenitor cells and neuronal intestinal cells.

Applications

CD344 is a marker for neuronal stem cells.

Gene Name	Entrez Gene#
FZD4	8322

Selected Monoclonal Antibodies

CH3A4A7 (Bühring, Tübingen).

CD349

Other Names

Fz-9, hFz9, FzE6, Frizzled-9.

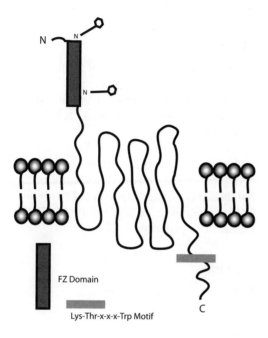

FZ Domain

Lys-Thr-x-x-x-Trp Motif

Molecular Structure

CD349 is a member of the Frizzled family of proteins within the superfamily of G protein-coupled receptors (GPCR). Ten Frizzled genes have been identified in the human genome (see CD344 and CD350).

It is an integral membrane protein of 569 amino acids with a 207-residue extracellular N-terminus containing the cysteine-rich ligand-binding site (FZ domain), seven transmembrane-spanning domains and a 62-residue cytoplasmic C-terminal tail that contains a Lys-Thr-X-X-X-Trp motif. This motif is the binding site for PDZ-domain containing proteins and is essential for activation of the Wnt/β-catenin pathway.

Recent studies have suggested Frizzled proteins may form heterodimers.

Mol Wt: Unprocessed precursor, 64.5 kDa.

Function

Frizzled proteins are essential for the regulation of tissue and cell polarity, embryonic development, regulation of proliferation, and many other processes in developing and adult organisms.

CD349 is a receptor for Wnt proteins and participates in the activation of the Wnt/β-catenin pathway (canonical Wnt signaling). This process is predicted to involve CD349 coupling to members of Gαi/o family of G proteins.

CD349 is important factor in the development of the nervous system and is critical for hippocampal development.

Knockout mice display aberrant B-cell development, and abnormal plasma cell homeostasis. Fzd9$^{-/-}$ mice have pronounced splenomegaly, thymic atrophy and lymphadenopathy with age and accumulation of plasma cells in lymph nodes.

Ligands

CD349 binds Wnt proteins including Wnt-2 and Wnt-7a.

Expression

CD349 is expressed predominantly in adult and fetal brain, testis, eye, skeletal muscle, and kidney. CD349 is also expressed by the parenchymatic cells around large vessels of the placenta, by the CFU-F forming Mesenchymal stem cells (MSC) of bone marrow, and placenta, by neural precursor cells.

Applications

CD349 is a marker for bone marrow and placenta MSC.

Gene Name	Entrez Gene#
FZD9	8326

Selected Monoclonal Antibodies

W3C4E11 (Buhring, Tubingen).

CD350

Other Names

Fz10, hFz10, FzE7, Frizzled-10.

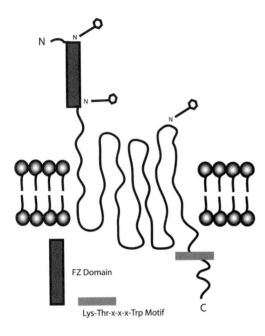

FZ Domain

Lys-Thr-x-x-x-Trp Motif

Molecular Structure

CD350 is a member of the Frizzled family of proteins within the superfamily of G protein-coupled receptors (GPCR). Ten Frizzled genes have been identified in the human genome (see CD344 and CD350).

CD350 is an integral membrane protein of 561 amino acids with a 205-residue extracellular N-terminus containing the cysteine-rich ligand-binding site (FZ domain), seven transmembrane-spanning domains and a 58-residue cytoplasmic C-terminal tail that contains a Lys-Thr-X-X-X-Trp motif. This motif is the binding site for PDZ-domain containing proteins and is essential for activation of the Wnt/β-catenin pathway.

Recent studies have suggested Frizzled proteins may form heterodimers.

Mol Wt: Unprocessed precursor, 65.3 kDa.

Function

Frizzled proteins are essential for the regulation of tissue and cell polarity, embryonic development, regulation of proliferation, and many other processes in developing and adult organisms.

CD350 is a receptor for Wnt proteins and participates in the activation of the Wnt/β-catenin pathway (canonical Wnt signaling). This process is predicted to involve CD350 coupling to members of Gαi/o family of G proteins.

Ligands

CD350 binds Wnt proteins.

Expression

Highest levels of CD350 are expressed in the placenta and fetal kidney, followed by fetal lung and brain.

CD350 is also expressed on syncytiotrophoblasts of placental villi and is highly expressed in the cervical cancer cell line, HeLa S3, and the colon cancer cell line, SW40.

Gene Name	Entrez Gene#
FZD10	11211

Selected Monoclonal Antibodies

1/4C4 (Buhring Tubingen).

Index

ABC15, CD338 molecule, 541
ABCG2, CD338 molecule, 541
ABCP, CD338 molecule, 541
ABC transporter domains, 8
ABO antigens, CD175/175s molecules, 318
Abortion, CD66f molecule expression, 159
AC133, CD133 molecule, 252
Activated leukocyte cell adhesion molecule,
    CD166, 301–302
Activation-induced molecule (AIM), CD69
    molecule, 161
Acute lymphoblastic leukemia (ALL):
    CD7 molecule, 51–52
    CD13 molecule, 63
    CD24 molecule, 79
    CD65/CD65s molecules, 152
    CD96 molecule, 197
    CD153 molecule, 281–282
    CD158 molecule, 291
    CD164 molecule, 299
    CD165 molecule, 300
    CD231 molecule, 383
    CD340 molecule, 544–545
Acute myeloid leukemia (AML):
    CD7 molecule, 51–52
    CD13 molecule and, 63
    CD24 molecule, 79

CD33 molecule, 93
CD64 molecule, 151
CD65/CD65s molecules, 152
CD96 molecule, 197
CD116 molecule, 224
CD123 molecule, 238
CD162/162R molecules, 296
CD168 molecule, 306
CD170 molecule, 309–310
CD318 molecule, 509
AD2, CD165 molecule, 300
ADAM (a disintegrin and metalloproteinase)
    family, 12
basic properties, 12
    ADAM-8, CD156a molecule, 286
    ADAM-10, CD156c molecule, 288
    ADAM-17, CD156b molecule, 287
aDb2 complex, 70
Adenocarcinoma:
    CD227 molecule, 376–377
    CD310 molecule, 497
    CD331 molecule, 529
Adenosine deaminase-binding protein, CD26
    molecule, 81
Adenosine diphosphate (ADP)/adenosine
    triphosphate (ATP), hydrolysis by
    CD39 molecule, 101

ADP-ribosyl cyclase, CD38 molecule, 99
AE1, CD233 molecule, 385
Agammaglobulinemia, CD179b molecule, 391
Ahonen (Ana) blood group antigen, CD236 molecule, 391
AIM, CD69 molecule, 161
AIRM1, CD328 molecule, 523–524
Alagille syndrome (AGS), CD339 molecule, 543
ALCAM, CD166, 301
ALK-3, CD292 molecule, 470
ALK-6, CD293 molecule, 472
Allergic responses and disease:
  CD124 molecule, 240
  CD125 molecule, 242
  CD193 molecule, 334
  CD275 molecule, 440
  CD278 molecule, 443
  CD294 molecule, 473
  CD330 molecule, 526–527
Allograft rejection. *See* Graft rejection
Alloimmune transfusion reactions, CD240CE molecule, 396–397
Alpha-IIb integrin chain, CD41 molecule, 104
Alpha-L integrin chain, CD11a molecule, 56
Alpha-M integrin chain, CD11b molecule, 58
Alpha-X integrin chain, CD11c molecule, 60
Alzheimer's disease:
  CD91 molecule, 189–190
  CD204 molecule, 347–348
  CD228 molecule, 378
  CD325 molecule, 517–518
Amino acid sequences, website sources for, 24, 27–28
Aminopeptidase A, CD249 molecule, 411
Aminopeptidase N (APN), CD13 molecule, 62
β-Amyloid protein, CD271 molecule, 433–434
Anaphylatoxin, CD88 molecule binding, 186
Anaplastic large cell lymphoma (ALCL), CD246 molecule, 406–407
Anaplastic lymphoma kinase (ALK), CD246 molecule, 406–407
Angiogenesis:
  CD105 molecule, 209–210
  CD202b molecule, 344–345
  CD248 molecule, 410
  CD249 molecule, 411
  CD308 molecule, 492–493
  CD309 molecule, 494–495
Angiopoietins, CD202b molecule ligands, 344–345
Angiosarcomas, CD144 molecule, 269

Angiotensin-converting enzyme (ACE), CD143 molecule, 266–267
Anion exchange family, CD233 molecule, 385–386
Anionexchanger 1, CD233 molecule, 385
ANP, CD13 molecule, 62
ANPEP, CD13 molecule, 62
Antibodies, research, diagnosis, and therapy applications, 14–15
Antibody-dependent cellular cytotoxicity (ADCC):
  CD16 molecule, 67–68
  CD32 molecule, 92
Anti-inflammatory therapy:
  CD11a/b molecules, 56–59
  CD121a/b molecules, 233–235
  CD156b molecule, 287
  CD323 molecule, 514
Anti-thrombotic therapy, CD41 molecule, 104–105
Aplastic anemia, CD115 molecule, 222–223
APN, CD13 molecule, 62
APO-1 ligand, CD95 molecule, 195
APO-2 ligand, CD253 molecule, 413
APO-3 ligand, CD255 molecule, 416
Apoptosis:
  CD31 molecule, 89–90
  CD36 molecule, 97
  CD49e molecule, 127
  CD60 molecule, 143
  CD95 molecule, 195
  CD99 molecule, 201–202
  CD110 molecule, 217
  CD134 molecule, 253
  CD174 molecule, 317
  CD178 molecule, 321–322
  CD256 molecule, 418
  CD261 molecule, 421
  CD262 molecule, 422
  CD263 molecule, 423
  CD264 molecule, 424
Apoptosis antigen 1, CD95 molecule, 195
APRIL (a proliferation-inducing ligand), CD256 molecule, 418
APT1, CD95 molecule, 195
Arc1, CD324 molecule, 515–516
Arginine-specific mono-ADP-ribosyltransferase (ART):
  CD296 molecule, 476
  CD297 molecule, 477
ART1, CD296 molecule, 476
ART4, CD297 molecule, 477

Asparagine, glycosylation, 13
Aspergillus fumigatus, CD284 molecule ligand, 444–445
Asthma:
  CD62L molecule, 146–147
  CD62P molecule, 148–149
  CD124 molecule, 240
  CD213α1 molecule, 359–360
  CD252 molecule, 412
  CD282 molecule, 450–451
  CD290 molecule, 466–467
  CD330 molecule, 526–527
Astrocytes, CD15 molecule expression, 66
Atherosclerosis:
  CD36 molecule, 97
  CD40 molecule, 103
  CD68 molecule, 160
  CD91 molecule, 189–190
  CD204 molecule, 347–348
  CD169 molecule, 307–308
  CD270 molecule, 431–432
  CD308 molecule, 492–493
ATP-binding cassette (ABC) transporter superfamily:
  CD243 molecule, 400–402
  CD338 molecule, 541–542
Autoimmune disorders:
  CD5 molecule, 50
  CD7 molecule, 52
  CD26 molecule, 82
  CD30 molecule, 87
  CD40 molecule, 103
  CD122 molecule, 236
  CD150 molecule, 277
  CD152 molecule, 279–280
  CD154 molecule, 283–284
  CD201 molecule, 342–343
  CD226 molecule, 374–375
  CD269 molecule, 430
  CD279 molecule, 444–445

B4, CD19 molecule, 71
B7 regulatory protein family:
  B7–1, CD80 molecule, 173
  B7–2, CD86 molecule, 183
  B7-DC, CD273 molecule, 436
  B7-H1, CD274 molecule, 438
  B7-H2, CD275 molecule, 440
  B7-H3, CD276 molecule, 441
  CD277 molecule, 442
B7-related protein-1 (B7RP-1), CD275 molecule, 440

B29, CD79b molecule, 172
B70, CD86 molecule, 183
B219, CD295 molecule, 474
B220, CD45 molecule, 115
Ba, CDw78 molecule, 170
BA-1, CD24 molecule, 79
BabA adhesin, CD15 molecule, 66
Bacterial diacyl glycerides, CD36 molecule, 97
BAFF, CD 257 molecule, 419
BAFF receptor (BAFFR), CD 268 molecule, 429
Band 3, CD233 molecule, 385
B and T lymphocyte attenuator (BTLA), CD272 molecule, 435
Basigin, CD147 molecule, 273
BB-1, CD80 molecule, 173
B-B4, CD138 molecule, 257
B-CAM, CD239 molecule, 393
B-cell chronic lymphocytic leukemia (B-CLL):
  CD5 molecule, 49–50
  CD6 molecule, 51
  CD70 molecule, 162
  CD79b molecule, 172
  CD267 molecule, 428
B-cell growth factor (BCGF), CD23 molecule signaling, 77–78
B-cell receptor (BCR):
  CD5 molecule, 49–50
  CD19 molecule, 71
  CD20 molecule, 72
  CD21 molecule, 73
  CD22 molecule binding, 75–76
  CD38 molecule, 99
  CD79a molecule, 171
  CD79b molecule, 172
  CD81 molecule, 174
  CD85j molecule, 180–181
  CD179a molecule, 323
  CD179b molecule, 324
B cells:
  CD5 molecule, 49
  CD10 molecule, 55
  CD19 molecule, 71
  CD20 molecule, 72
  CD24 molecule, 79
  CD37 molecule, 98
  CD40 molecule, 102–103
  CD70 molecule, 162
  CD75/CD75s/CDw76 molecules, 168
  CD257 molecule, 419
  CD267 molecule, 428
  CD317 molecule, 508

BCG infection, CD119 molecule, 228

B-CLL. *See* B-cell chronic lymphocytic leukemia

BCM, CD269 molecule, 430

BCM1, CD48 molecule, 121

BCMA, CD269 molecule, 430

BCRP/BCRP1, CD338 molecule, 541–542

BDCA-2, CD303 molecule, 485

BDCA-4, CD304molecule, 486

Beckwith-Wiedemann syndrome, CD221 molecule, 366

BEK, CD332 molecule, 530–531

BEN, CD166, 301

Ber-H2 antigen, CD30 molecule, 87

Bernard-Soulier syndrome, CD42 molecules, 106–111

β-chain, CD131 molecule, 250

Bgp35, CD20 molecule, 72

Bgp95:
  CD19 molecule, 71
  CD180 molecule, 325

Bgp135, CD22 molecule, 75

Bile transport, CD66a molecule, 153–154

Biliary glycoprotein (BCP), CD66a molecule, 153

Birbeck granules (BG), CD207 molecule, 352–353

Bladder cancer, CD261 molecule, 421

BLAST-1, CD48 molecule, 121

Blast-2, CD23 molecule, 77

BLAST alignment, protein sequence similarity comparisons, 27, 29

BL-CAM, CD22 molecule, 75–76

BL-KDD/F12, CD97 molecule, 198–199

BLR1, CD185 molecule, 330

B lymphocyte stimulator (BLyS), CD257 molecule, 419

B lymphocyte surface antigen B1, CD20 molecule, 72

BMDP, CD338 molecule, 541–542

BMPR1A, CD292 molecule, 470

BMPR1B, CDw293 molecule, 472

Bone disorders:
  CD254 molecule, 415
  CD265 molecule, 426

Bone marrow grafts:
  CD11 molecules and, 57
  CD31 molecule, 90
  CD90 molecule, 188

Bone marrow stromal cells, CD157 molecule, 289

Bone morphogenetic protein (BMP) receptor family (BMPR):
  BMPR1A, CD292 molecule, 470–471
  BMPR1B, CDw293 molecule, 472

Bone sialoprotein (Bsp1), CD51/CD61 complex binding, 131

BONZO, CD186 molecule, 331

Borrelia burgdorferi infection:
  CD281 molecule, 488–489
  CD286 molecule, 458–459

BP-3/IF7, CD157 molecule, 289

Bp50, CD40 molecule, 102

BR3, CD268 molecule, 429

Breast cancer:
  CD10 molecule, 55
  CD44 molecule, 114
  CD60b molecule, 143
  CD105 molecule, 106
  CD146 molecule, 271–272
  CD166 molecule, 301–302
  CD168 molecule, 305–306
  CD175/175s molecule, 318
  CD202b molecule, 344–345
  CD227 molecule, 376–377
  CD271 molecule, 433–434
  CD280 molecule, 446–447
  CD331 molecule, 529
  CDw338 molecule, 541–542
  CD340 molecule, 544–545

Breast cancer resistance protein, CD338 molecule, 541–542

Breast milk:
  CD281 molecule, 449
  CD283 molecule, 452–453
  CD286 molecule, 458–459

BST-1, CD157 molecule, 289

BST-2, CD317 molecule, 508

BT3.1, CD277 molecule, 441

BTF5, CD277 molecule, 441

BTLA, CD272 molecule, 435

Burkitt's lymphoma associated antigen (BLA), CD77 molecule, 169

Burkitt's lymphoma receptor 1 (BLR1), CD185 molecule, 330

Burkitt's lymphoma receptor 2 (BLR2), CD197 molecule, 338

BXMAS1, CD307 molecule, 490

BY55, CD160 molecule, 293

C1aR precursors, CD93 molecule, 192

C1qR1, CD93 molecule, 192

C1q receptor precursor, CD93 molecule, 192

C3b. *See also* Complement receptors
  CD35 molecule binding, 95–96
  CD46 molecule, 117–118
C3b/C4b receptor, CD35 molecule, 95–96
C3/C4 convertases:
  CD46 molecule, 117–118
  CD55 molecule binding, 136–137
C3dg:
  CD21 molecule binding, 73
  CD35 molecule binding, 95
C3d receptor, CD21 molecule, 73–74
C4b:
  CD35 molecule binding, 95–96
  CD46 molecule binding, 117–118
C5a/5a (desArg), CD88 molecule, 186
C5a-receptor (C5a-R), CD88 molecule, 186
C8-a, CD59 molecule, 142
C9, CD59 molecule, 142
C33, CD82 molecule, 175
Cadherin domain, 8, 12
Cadherin family:
  CD144 molecule (VE-cadherin/cadherin 5), 268–269
  CD324 molecule (E-cadherin/cadherin 1), 515–516
  CD325 molecule (N-cadherin/cadherin2), 517–518
cADPr hydrolase 2, CD157 molecule, 289
Calcium-dependent lectin superfamily. *See* C-type lectin receptor family
Campath-1, CD52 molecule, 132
Carbohydrate structures, 10
Carcinoembryonic antigen (CEA) family:
  CD66a molecule, 153–154
  CD66b molecule, 155
  CD66c molecule, 156
  CD66d molecule, 157
  CD66e molecule, 158
  CD66f molecule, 159
Carcinoma:
  CD10 molecule, 55
  CD15 molecule, 66
  CD24 molecule, 79
  CD44 molecule, 114
  CD82 molecule, 175
  CD97 molecule, 199
  CD146 molecule, 271–272
  CD175/175s molecules, 318
  CD239 molecules, 393–394
  CD262 molecule, 422
  CD271 molecule, 433–444
  CD274 molecule, 438–439

CD280 molecule, 446–447
CD304 molecule, 487
CD324 molecule, 515–516
CD326 molecule, 519–520
CD340 molecule, 544–545
Cardiotrophin-1 receptor, CD130 molecule and, 249
Cardiovascular disease, CD143 molecule, 266–267
Cartilage link protein family, CD44 molecule, 113–114
CCL receptors. *See* Chemokine, C-C motif receptors (CCR)
CC-CKR1, CD191 molecule, 332
Chemokine, C-C motif receptors (CCR):
  CCR1, CD191 molecule, 332
  CCR2, CD192 molecule, 333
  CCR3, CD193 molecule, 334
  CCR4, CD194 molecule, 335
  CCR5, CD195 molecule, 336
  CCR6, CD196 molecule, 337
  CCR7, CD197 molecule, 338
  CCR8, CDw198 molecule, 339
  CCR9, CDw199 molecule, 340
CD2 family:
  CD2 molecule, 44
  CD5 molecule, 49
  CD45 molecule, 49
  CD48 molecule, 121
  CD58 molecule, 141
  CD150 molecule and, 276–277
CD2R molecule, 44
CD3 complex, 46
CD3-TCR complex, 46
CD3ζ, CD247 molecule, 408–409
CD4⁺CD25⁺ regulatory T cells, 80
CD9P1, CD315 molecule, 505–506
CD11 β subunit, CD18 molecule, 70
CD30 ligand, CD153 molecule, 281–282
CD33L, CD327 molecule, 521–522
CD40 ligand (CD40L), CD154 molecule, 283–284
CD81P3, CD316 molecule, 507
CD95 ligand, CD178 molecule, 321–322
CD128A, CD181 molecule, 326
CD128B, CD182 molecule, 327
CD134 ligand (CD134L), CD252 molecule, 412
CD164 sialomucin-like protein (CD164L1), CD248 molecule binding, 410
CD209L, CD299 molecule, 479
CDCP-1, CD318 molecule, 509
CDH1, CD324 molecule, 515–516

CDH2, CD325 molecule, 517–518
CDHE, CD324 molecule, 515–516
CDHM, CD325 molecule, 517–518
CD-Hub database:
    protein nomenclature on, 19
    Website, 17
CD markers:
    applications of, 14–15
    human leukocyte differentiation antigens
        and, 4
    protein domains, 7–9
    transmembrane helix prediction, 31–32
cDNA libraries, human leukocyte
        differentiation antigens and, 4
CDw149 molecule. *See* CD47
CEA, CD66c molecule, 158
CEA-CAM5, CD66e molecule, 158
Centroblast markers, CD77 molecule, 169
Ceramide dodecasaccharide 4c, CD65/CD65a
        molecule, 152
Ceramide trihexoside (CTH), CD77 molecule,
        169
c-fms, CD115 molecule, 222
CGM1, CD66d molecule, 157
CGM6, CD66b molecule, 155
Chemokine receptors. *See* G-protein-coupled
        receptors (GPCRs)
Chemotaxis:
    CD11b molecule, 58–59
    CD11c molecule, 60–61
    CD47 molecule, 119–120
    CD87 molecule, 184–185
    CD140b molecule, 262–263
    CD185 molecule, 330
    CD192 molecule, 333
    CD196 molecule, 337
    CDw198 molecule, 339
    CDw199 molecule, 340
    CD304 molecule, 486–487
Choline transporter-like family, CD92
        molecule, 191
Chondroitin sulphate binding:
    CD56 molecule, 138–139
    CD97 molecule, 198–199
    CD171 molecule, 311–312
    CD204 molecule, 347–348
    CD206 molecule, 350–351
    CD312 molecule, 500–501
Chronic lymphocytic leukemia (CLL):
    CD5 molecule, 49–50
    CD6 molecule, 51
    CD23 molecule, 77–78

CD63 molecule, 150
CD70 molecule, 162
CD77 molecule, 169
CD79b molecule, 172
CD139 molecule, 259
CD267 molecule, 428
Chronic myeloid leukemia:
    CD109 molecule, 216
    CD177 molecule, 320
    CD318 molecule, 509
CHTL1, CD92 molecule, 191
Ciliary neurotrophic factor, CD130 molecule
        and, 249
Circulating endothelial cells (CECs), CD126
        molecule, 244
c-kit, CD117 molecule, 225
CKR2, CD192 molecule, 333
CKR3, CD193 molecule, 334
CKR5, CD195 molecule, 336
CKR6, CD196 molecule, 337
CKRL1, CDw198 molecule, 339
Class II associated invariant chain peptide
        (CLIP), CD74 molecule, 166–167
Class II-specific chaperone, CD74 molecule,
        166–167
CLECSF11, CD303 molecule, 485
CLECSF14, CD301 molecule, 483
Cluster analysis, human leukocyte
        differentiation antigens and, 4
CMRF family, CD300a/c/e molecules, 481–482
Coagulant activity, CD174 molecule, 317
Coagulation factor III, CD142 molecule, 265
Collagen binding:
    CD26 molecule, 82
    CD29/CD49 complexes, 86, 122–124
    CD36 molecule, 97
    CD49b molecule, 123
    CD138 molecule, 257–258
    CD167a/b molecules, 303–304
    CD204 molecule, 347
    CD280 molecule, 446–447
Common acute lymphoblastic leukemia
        antigen (CALLA), 55
Common β chain, CD131 molecule, 250
Common γ chain, CD132 molecule, 251
Complement binding (CUB) domains:
    CD304 molecule, 486–487
    CD318 molecule, 509
    Structure and function, 8
Complement control protein (CCP) domains:
    CD21 molecule, 73–74
    CD25 molecule, 80

CD35 molecule, 95–96
CD46 molecule, 117–118
CD55 molecule, 136–137
CD62E molecule, 145
CD62L molecule, 146–147
CD62P molecule, 148–149
Complement receptor type 1 (CR1), CD35 molecule, 95
Complement receptor type 2 (CR2), CD21 molecule, 73
Complement receptor type 3 (CR3):
  CD11b molecule, 58
  CD21 molecule, 73
  CD35 molecule, 95
Complement receptor type 4 (CR4):
  CD11c molecule and, 60–61
  CD35 molecule, 95
Congenital amegakaryocytic thrombocytopaenia, CD110 molecule and, 217
Connecting segment-1 (CS-1), CD29/CD49d complex binding, 86, 125–126
Conserved Domain Database (CDD), protein domain conservation on, 27–28, 30
Coronary artery disease, CD146 molecule, 271–272
Coronaviruses:
  CD13 molecule and, 62
  CD299 molecule, 479–480
Cowden disease, CD292 molecule, 470–471
Coxsackie viruses, CD55 molecule, 136–137
CpG DNA motifs, CD289 molecule, 464–465
CRACC, CD319 molecule, 510
Creuzfeldt-Jacob Disease (CJD), CD230 molecule, 382
CRFB4, CD210b molecule, 357
Crk binding, CD140a molecule, 260–261
Crohn's disease:
  CD212 molecule, 358
  humanized anti-CD126 antibody therapy, 358
CRTH2, CD294 molecule, 473
CS1, CD319 molecule, 510
CSF-1/PDGF receptor family:
  CD308 molecule, 492–493
  CD309 molecule, 494–495
  CD310 molecule, 496–497
CSF-1R, CD115 molecule, 222
CSF-3R, CD114 molecule, 221
CTLA-4, CD152 molecule, 279–280

C-type lectin domain, 8, 11–13
C-type lectin receptor family:
  CD69 molecule, 161
  CD72 molecule, 164
  CD94 molecule, 193–194
  CD161 molecule, 294
  CD205 molecule, 349
  CD206 molecule, 350–351
  CD207 molecule, 352–353
  CD209 molecule, 355–356
  CD222 molecule, 367–368
  CD248 molecule, 410
  CD299 molecule, 479–480
  CD301 molecule, 483
  CD302 molecule, 484
  CD303 molecule, 485
  CD314 molecule, 504
CUB domain. *See* Complement binding domains
Cutaneous leukocyte antigen, CD62E molecule binding, 145
CXCR1, CD181 molecule, 326
CXCR2, CD182 molecule, 327
CXCR3, CD183 molecule, 328
CXCR4, CD184 molecule, 329
CXCR5, CD185 molecule, 330
CXCR6, CD186 molecule, 331
Cytokine receptor gene family:
  CD114 molecule, 221
  CD118 molecule, 227
  CD119 molecule, 228
  CD129 molecule, 248
  CD131 molecule, 250
  CD132 molecule, 251
  CD142 molecule, 265
  CD210 molecule, 357
  CD212 molecule, 358
  CD213α1/2 molecules, 359–360
  CD295 molecule, 474–475
Cytokines:
  CD23 molecule, 77–78
  CD40 molecule, 102
  CD44 molecule, 114
  CD69 molecule, 161
  CD100 molecule, 203–204
  CD108 molecule, 215
Cytotoxic T-cell subset:
  CD8 molecule, 53
  CD152 molecule, 279–280
  CD226 molecule, 374–375
Cytotoxic T lymphocyte antigen, CD152 molecule, 279–280

D11, CD163 molecule, 297
DAF, CD55 molecule, 136
DAP-12 homodimers, CD172b molecule, 314
DARC, CD234 molecule, 387
DCL1, CD302 molecule, 484
DC-LAMP, CD208 molecule, 354
DcR1, CD263 molecule, 423
DcR2, CD264 molecule, 424
DC-SIGN, CD209 molecule, 355
DC-SIGN2 / DC-SIGNR, CD299 molecule, 479
Death domain:
  CD91 molecule, 195
  CD120a molecule, 229–230
  CD120b molecule, 231–232
  CD261 molecule, 421
  CD262 molecule, 422
  CD264 molecule, 424
  CD271 molecule, 433–434
  structure and function, 8
  TRAIL receptors, 7
Death receptor 4 (DR4), CD261 molecule, 421
Death receptor 5 (DR5), CD262 molecule, 422
DEC-205, CD205 molecule, 349
Decay accelerating factor, CD55 molecule, 136
Defensins, CD196 molecule, 337
Denatured proteins, CD11b/c molecule binding, 58, 60–61
Dendritic cells:
  CD1e molecule accumulation in, 43
  CD83 molecule, 176
  CD86 molecule, 183
  CD101 molecule, 205
  CD137 molecule, 256
  CD208 molecule, 354
  CD209 molecule, 355–356
  CD301 molecule, 483
Dengue virus, CD209 molecule ligand, 355–356
DEP-1, CD148 molecule, 274
Dermatan sulphate, CD312 molecule, 500–501
DF3 antigen, CD227 molecule, 376
Diabetes mellitus. See Type 1 diabetes; Type 2 diabetes
Diacyl glycerides, CD36 molecule ligands, 97
Diacyl-lipopeptides, CD286 molecule ligands, 458–459
Diego blood group system, CD233 molecule, 385–386
Dipeptidylpeptidase (DPP) IV, CD26 molecule, 81–82

Discoidin domain receptor (DDR) 1/2, CD167a/b molecules, 303–304
Disease association, 32
Disseminated intravascular coagulation, 264
DLEC, CD303 molecule, 485
DM-GRASP, CD166, 301
DNAM-1, CD226 molecule, 374
DO blood group antigens, CD297 molecule, 477
DOK1, CD297 molecule, 477
Dombrock (DO) blood group antigen, CD297 molecule, 477
Donohue syndrome, CD220 molecule, 363–364
Double-stranded RNA receptor, CD283 molecule, 452–453
DPP IV ectoenzyme, CD26 molecule, 81
Dr adhesions, CD55 molecule ligands, 136–137
Drap-27, CD9 molecule, 54
Ductal carcinomas, CD271 molecule, 433–434
Duffy blood group antigen, CD234 molecule, 387
Duch (Dh) antigen, CD236 molecule, 391
DY12, CD245 molecule, 405
DY35, CD245 molecule, 405

E123, CD109 molecule, 216
E2, CD99 molecule, 201
EA1, CD69 molecule, 161
E-ATPDase, CD39 molecule, 101
Ebola virus, CD209 molecule ligand, 355–356
EBV receptor, CD21 molecule, 73
EC3.1.34, CD45 molecule, 115
EC3.4.11.2, CD13 molecule, 62
EC3.4.14.5, CD26 molecule, 81
EC3.6.1.5, CD39 molecule, 101
ECAD, CD324 molecule, 515–516
E-cadherin, CD324 molecule, 515–516
Echoviruses, CD55 molecule binding, 136–137
ECMR-III, CD44 molecule, 113
Ecto-5′-nucleotidase, CD73 molecule, 165
Ecto-apyrase family, CD39 molecule, 101
Ecto-diphosphohydrolase, CD39 molecule, 101
Ectodomains, CD317 molecule, 508
Ectonucleotide pyrophosphatase/ phosphodiesterase (E-NNP) enzymes, CD203c molecule, 346
EGF domain, 8
EGF module-containing mucin-like receptors (EMR):
  EMR1, CD311 molecule, 498–499
  EMR2, CD312 molecule, 500–501
  EMR3, CD313 molecule, 502–503

EGF-TM7 family:
    CD91 molecule, 198–199
    CD311 molecule, 498–499
    CD312 molecule, 500–501
    CD313 molecule, 502–503
EGP/EGP40, CD326 molecule, 519–520
8AE, CD109 molecule, 216
8D6, CD320 molecule, 511
8p11 myeloproliferative syndrome (EMS),
        CD331 molecule, 529
ELAM-1, CD62E molecule, 145
EMBL Ensembl GeneView website:
    gene expression information on, 32–33
    genetic information on, 20–26
    gene variation, 20
    protein structural models on, 28, 30
Embryonic stem (ES) cells, CD118 molecule,
        227
Endo180, CD280 molecule, 446
Endocam, CD31 molecule as, 89
Endoglin, CD105 molecule, 209
Endopeptidases, CD10 molecule, 55
Endosialin, CD248 molecule, 410
Endothelial cell vitronectin receptor, CD242
        molecule, 400
Endothelial protein C receptors (EPCR),
        CD201 molecule, 342–343
E-NPP3, CD203c molecule, 346
Entactin, CD29/CD49c complex binding, 86,
        124
Enteroviruses, CD55 molecule binding,
        136–137
Envelope protein 2 (E2), CD81 molecule,
        174
EOF ligand, CD265 molecule, 425
Eosinophil eotaxin receptor, CD193 molecule,
        334
Eosinophils, CD16 expression on, 67–68
Eotaxin ligands:
    CD193 molecule, 334
    CD195 molecule, 336
Ep-CAM, CD326 molecule, 519–520
Ephrin A2, CD156c molecule and, 288
Epidermal growth factor (EGF):
    CD62P molecule, 148–149
    CD91 molecule, 189–190
    CD97 molecule, 198–199
    CD141 molecule, 264
    CD311 molecule, 498–499
    CD312 molecule, 500–501
    CD313 molecule, 502–503
    CD326 molecule, 519–520

Epidermal growth factor module-containing
        mucin-like receptor 1 (EMR1), CD311
        molecule, 498–499
Epidermal growth factor module-containing
        mucin-like receptor 2 (EMR2), CD312
        molecule, 500–501
Epidermal growth factor module-containing
        mucin-like receptor 3 (EMR3), CD313
        molecule, 502–503
Episialin, CD227 molecule, 376
Epithelial membrane antigen (EMA), CD227
        molecule, 376
Epstein-Barr Induced gene 1 (EBI1), CD197
        molecule, 338
Epstein-Barr virus (EBV):
    CD19 molecule, 71
    CD21 molecule, 73–74
    CD30 molecule, 88
    CD83 molecule, 176
    CDw210 molecule, 357
ERBB receptor tyrosine kinase family, CD340
        molecule, 544–545
ERBB2, CD340 molecule, 544–545
Erythrocyte binding antigen (EBA-175),
        CD235a molecule, 388–389
Erythrocytes, CD240DCE molecule, 398
Erythroid progenitors, CD240DCE molecule,
        398
Erythroid spectrin, CD239 molecules,
        393–394
Erythropoietic cells, CD71 molecule, 163
Escherichia coli ligands:
    CD55 molecule, 136–137
    CD66c molecule, 156
    CD66e molecule, 158
    CD291 molecule, 468–469
E-selectin:
    CD34 molecule, 94
    CD44 molecule, 114
    CD62E molecule, 145
EST157481, CD338 molecule, 541–542
EWI family. *See* Glutamine-tryptophan-
        isoleucine family
Ewing's sarcoma, CD99 molecule,
        201–202
ExPASy, protein sequence information on,
        23–24, 27–28
Experimental allergic encephalomyelitis
        (EAE), CD200 molecule, 341
Extracellular metalloproteinase inducer
        (EMMPRIN), CD147 molecule,
        273

Factor VII/VIIa, CD142 molecule ligand, 265

Factor Xa, CD142 molecule ligand, 265

Familial expansile osteolysis (FEO), CD265 molecule, 426

Familial exudative vitreoretinopathy (FEVR), CD344 molecule, 546

Familial Hibernian fever (FHF), CD120a molecule, 229

Fas, CD95 molecule, 195

Fas ligand, CD178 molecule, 321–322

Fatty acid translocase (FAT), CD36 molecule, 97

Fc-α receptor, CD89 molecule, 187

FcεRI-γ CD16 molecule signaling, 67

FcεRII, CD23 molecule, 77–78

Fcγ receptor family:
  CD89 molecule, 187
  FcγRI, CD64 molecule, 151
  FcγRII, CD32 molecule, 91–92
  FcγRIIIa, CD16a molecule, 67–68
  FcγRIIIb, CD16b molecule, 67–68

FcRH5, CD307 molecule, 490

FCRIIIA, CD16a molecule, 67

FCRIIIB, CD16b molecule, 67

FEO, CD265 molecule, 425

Fetomodulin, CD141 molecule, 264

FGFR. *See* Fibroblast growth factor receptors

Fibrinogen binding:
  CD11/CD18 complexes, 58, 60
  CD41/CD61 complex, 104, 144
  CD51/CD61 complex, 131, 144
  CD54 molecule, 134
  CD284 molecule, 444–445

Fibroblast activation protein (FAP), CD26 molecule, 82

Fibroblast growth factor receptors (FGFR):
  CD138 molecule, 257–258
  FGFR1, CD331 molecule, 528–529
  FGFR2, CD332 molecule, 530–531
  FGFR3, CD333 molecule, 532–533
  FGFR4, CD334 molecule, 534–535

Fibronectin binding:
  CD29/CD49 complexes, 86, 124–127
  CD29/CD51 complex, 131
  CD41/CD61 complex, 104, 144
  CD49e molecule, 127
  CD51/β6 complex, 131
  CD51/CD61 complex, 131, 144
  CD138 molecule, 257–258
  CD280 molecule, 446–447

Fibronectin type II (FNII) domains:
  CD205 molecule, 349
  CD206 molecule, 350–351
  CD280 molecule, 446–447
  structure and function, 8

Fibronectin type III (FNIII) domains:
  CD45 molecule, 115–116
  CD56 molecule, 138–139
  CD114 molecule, 221
  CD116 molecule, 224
  CD118 molecule, 227
  CD119 molecule, 228
  CD122 molecule, 235
  CD124 molecule, 239
  CD125 molecule, 241–242
  CD126 molecule, 243–244
  CD127 molecule, 245–246
  CD129 molecule, 248
  CD130 molecule, 249
  CD131 molecule, 250
  CD132 molecule, 251
  CD142 molecule, 265
  CD148 molecule, 274
  CD202b molecule, 344
  CD210a molecule, 357
  CD212 molecule, 358
  CD213a1/2 molecules, 359
  CD220 molecule, 363–364
  CD221 molecule, 365–366
  CD295 molecule, 474–475
  structure and function, 8

Fimbriae, type 1, CD66a molecule and, 153

Flagellin, CD285 molecule, 456–457

FLG, CD331 molecule, 528–529

FLJ14529, CD323 molecule, 514

flk-1, CD309 molecule, 494–495

flk-2, CD135 molecule, 254

Flow cytometry, antibody applications and, 14–15

FLT1, CD308 molecule, 492–493

FLT2, CD331 molecule, 528–529

FLT3, CD135 molecule, 254

FLT4, CD310 molecule, 496–497

Fluorescence-activated cell sorter, 15

FN14, CD266 molecule, 427

Follicular B-cell non-Hodgkins lymphoma, CD20 molecule, 72

4–1IBB, CD137 molecule, 256

4F2, CD98 molecule, 199, 200

4F9, CD82 molecule, 174, 175

4Ig-B7-H3, CD276 molecule, 441

FPRP, CD315 molecule, 505–506

Frizzled proteins:
  Fz-4, CD344 molecule, 546
  Fz-9, CD349 molecule, 547
  Fz-10, CD350 molecule, 548
FRP-1, CD98 molecule, 199
Fucoganglioside, CD65/CD65s molecules,
  152
Fucoidin, CD204 molecule ligand, 347
Fucose, CD173 molecule, 316
Furin protease, CD167a/b molecules, 303–304
Fusin, CD184 molecule, 329
Fy-glycoprotein, CD234 molecule, 387
FzE4, CD344 molecule, 546
FzE6, CD349 molecule, 547
FzE7, CD350 molecule, 548

GA733-2, CD326 molecule, 519–520
Galactoclycoprotein, CD43 molecule,
  111–112
Galactose, CD301 molecule ligand, 483
Galectin-1 ligand:
  CD7 molecules, 52
  CD45 molecules, 116
  CD66c molecules, 156
  CD107a and b molecules, 213
γ-chain, CD132 molecule, 251
γ-Glutamyl transferase (GGT), CD224
  molecule, 371
γ-Glutamyl transpeptidase, CD224 molecule,
  371
Ganglioside GD3 complex, CD60 molecule,
  143
Gastric tumors, CD44 molecule, 114
GD3, CD60a molecule, 143
γ/δ-T cells, CD8 molecules, 53
Gelatin, CD280 ligand, 446–447
Gene expression, website information sources
  for, 32–33
Gene therapy, CD132 molecule, 251
Genetic information, websites for, 20–22
Genomic sequencing:
  human leukocyte differentiation antigen
    research and, 5–6
  protein domains and, 7–9
  research, diagnosis, and therapy applications,
    13–14
Gerbich (Ge) blood group antigens, CD236
  molecule, 390–391
GGT, CD224 molecule, 371–372
GHI/61, CD163 molecule, 297
Glanzmann's thrombasthenia (GT), CD41
  molecule, 104–105

Gliomas:
  CD15 molecule, 66
  CD71 molecule, 163
Globotriaosylceramide (Gb3), CD77 molecule,
  169
Glucagon-like peptide-1 (GLP-1), CD26
  molecule, 82
γ-Glutamyl cycle, CD224 molecule, 371–372
Glutamine-tryptophan-isoleucine (EWI)
  family:
  CD101 molecule, 205
  CD315 molecule, 505–506
  CD316 molecule, 507
Glutamyl aminopeptidase, CD249 molecule,
  411
Glutathionuria, CD224 molecule and, 372
GlyCAM-1, CD62L molecule binding, 146
Glycation end products, CD204 molecule
  ligands, 347
Glycocalicin, CD42b molecule, 107
Glycophorin A, CD235a molecule, 388–389
Glycophorin B, CD235b molecule, 388–389
Glycophorin C, CD236R molecule, 390–391
Glycophorin C/D, CD236 molecule,
  390–391
Glycophosphoinositol-linked protein
  (GPI):
  CD14 molecule, 64–65, 67–68
  CD16 molecule, 67–68
  CD24 molecule, 79
  CD48 molecule, 121
  CD52 molecule, 132
  CD55 molecule, 136–137
  CD56 molecule, 138–139
  CD58 molecule, 141
  CD59 molecule, 142
  CD66b molecule, 155
  CD66c molecule, 156
  CD66d molecule, 157
  CD66e molecule, 158
  CD73 molecule, 165
  CD87 molecule, 184–185
  CD90 molecule, 188
  CD108 molecule, 215
  CD109 molecule, 216
  CD157 molecule, 289
  CD160 molecule, 293
  CD177 molecule, 320
  CD228 molecule, 378
  CD230 molecule, 381–382
  CD263 molecule, 423
  CD296 molecule, 476

CD297 molecule, 477
CD307 molecule, 490–491
website sources for, 32
Glycosaminoglycans (GAGs):
    CD312 molecule, 500–501
    CD337 molecule, 539–540
    proteoglycans and, 13
    structure, 10
Glycosphingolipid lactosylceramide, CD17
        molecule, 69
Glycosylation:
    carbohydrate structures, 10
    N-linked, 13
    O-linked, 13
    website sources for prediction of, 32
Glypiation, of proteins, 13
GM3 gangliosides, CD17 molecule and, 69
GM-CSF receptor α chain, CD116 molecule,
        224
GNF Symatlas, 32–33
Gov a/b antigens, CD109 molecule and, 216
gp9, CD42a molecule, 106
gp17, CD4 molecule, 47
gp35-37, CD5 molecule, 49
gp37, CD165, 300
gp40, CD7 molecule, 52
gp42, CD47 molecule, 119
gp45, CD38 molecule, 99
gp50-45, CD23 molecule, 77
gp52-40, CD37 molecule, 98
gp55, CD63 molecule, 150
gp67, CD33molecule, 93
gp80, CD39 molecule, 101
gp80-95, CD44 molecule, 113
gp95, CD43 molecule, 111
gp100, CD10 molecule, 55
gp105-120, CD34 molecule, 94
gp110, CD68 molecule, 160
gp130, CD130 molecule, 249
gp140, CD21 molecule, 73
gp150, CD13 molecule, 62
gp180/95, CD11a molecule, 56
GPIa, CD49b molecule, 123
GPIb-α, CD42b molecule, 107
GPIb-β, CD42c molecule, 109
GPIc, CD49f molecule, 128
GPI-gp80, CD108 molecule, 215
GPIIb, CD41 molecule, 104
GPIIIa, CD61 molecule, 144
GPIIIb, CD36 molecule, 97
GPV, CD42d molecule, 110
GPIX, CD42a molecule, 106

gpL115, CD43 molecule, 111
G-protein-coupled receptors (GPCRs):
    CD88 molecule, 186
    CD181 molecule, 326
    CD182 molecule, 327
    CD183 molecule, 328
    CD184 molecule, 329
    CD185 molecule, 330
    CD186 molecule, 331
    CD191 molecule, 332
    CD192 molecule, 333
    CD193 molecule, 334
    CD194 molecule, 335
    CD195 molecule, 336
    CD196 molecule, 337
    CD197 molecule, 338
    CD294 molecule, 473
    CD344 molecule, 546
    CD349 molecule, 547
    CD350 molecule, 548
    CDw198 molecule, 339
    CDw199 molecule, 340
    structure and function, 8
GPV, CD42d molecule, 110
GR6, CD84 molecule, 177
GR11, CD93 molecule, 192
Graft rejection prevention and treatment:
    CD2 molecule, 44
    CD3 molecule, 45
    CD6 molecule, 51
    CD11a molecule, 57
    CD40 molecule, 103
    CD54 molecule, 134
    CD122 molecule, 236
    CD275 molecule, 440
Graft-*versus*-host disease (GVHD):
    CD6 molecule, 51
    CD13 molecule, 62–63
    CD30 molecule, 87
    CD31 molecule, 90
    CD162/162R molecules, 295–296
Granule membrane protein-140 (GMP140),
        CD62P molecule, 148
Granulocyte colony stimulating factor
        (G-CSF) receptor, CD114 molecule,
        221
Granulocyte macrophage colony stimulating
        factor (GM-CSF) receptors:
    CD116 molecule, 224
    CD131 molecule, 250
Granulocyte membrane protein-140, CD62P
        molecule, 148

Granulocytes:
  CD11b molecule, 58–59
  CD15 molecule, 66
  CD62L molecule, 146–147
  CD65/65s molecules, 152
  CD66a/b/c/d molecules, 153–157
  CD88 molecule, 186
  CD89 molecule, 187
  CD97 molecule, 198–199
  CD101 molecule, 205
  CD114 molecule, 221
  CD116 molecule, 224
  CD147 molecule, 273
  CD148 molecule, 274
  CD153 molecule, 281–282
  CD156a molecule, 286
  CD177 molecule, 320
  CD284 molecule, 454–455
  CD302 molecule, 484
Granulophysin, CD63 molecule, 150
Gregory (Gy(a)) antigens, CD297 molecule,
      477
GROα, β, γ, CD182 molecule binding, 327
Group B Streptococci heat labile soluble
      factor (GBS-F), CD286 molecule,
      458–459
GYPC gene, CD236 molecule, 390–391

H2 blood group, CD173, 316
H23 antigen, CD227 molecule, 376
Hairy cell leukemia:
  CD5 molecule, 50
  CD103 molecule, 207
Haptoglobulin, CD22 molecule, 75
HB15, CD83 molecule, 176
H-CAM, CD44 molecule, 113–114
HE5 compound, CD52 molecule, 132
Heat shock proteins (Hsps) ligands:
  CD91 molecule, 190
  CD284 molecule, 444–445
Heat stable antigen receptor (HSAR), CD24
      molecule, 79
Heavy chain of leukocyte function associated
      antigen-1 (LFA-1), CD11a molecule,
      56
HECL, CD303 molecule, 485
hEGP-2, CD326 molecule, 519–520
Helicobacter pylori:
  BabA antigen adhesion and, CD15
      molecule, 66
  CD209 molecule ligand, 355–356
  LeY (CD174) expression, 317

TF (CD176) expression, 319
Helper T cells, CD4 molecule, 47
Hemagglutinin (HA) ligands:
  CD335 molecule, 536–537
  CD336 molecule, 538
Hematopoietic progenitor cells:
  CD135 molecule, 254
  CD173 molecule, 316
  CD235a molecule, 389
  CD318 molecule, 509
Hematopoietic stem cells:
  CD34 molecule, 94
  CD90 molecule, 188
  CD100 molecule, 203–204
  CD114 molecule, 221
  CD117 molecule, 225–226
  CD123 molecule, 238
  CD133 molecule, 252
  CD202b molecule, 344–345
  CD235a molecule, 389
  CDw338 molecule, 541–542
Hematopoietin receptor family:
  CD110 molecule, 217
  CD116 molecule, 224
  CD122 molecule, 235–236
  CD123 molecule, 237–238
  CD124 molecule, 239–240
  CD125 molecule, 241–242
  CD126 molecule, 243–244
  CD127 molecule, 245–246
Hemolytic disease of the newborn,
      396–397
Heparan-sulphate proteoglycans (HSPGs),
      CD335 molecule, 537
Heparin-binding EGF-like growth factors
      (HB-EF), CD9 molecule and, 54
Heparin sulphate binding:
  CD56 molecule, 138–139
  CD62L molecule, 146–148
  CD138 molecule, 257–258
  CD335 molecule, 537
  CD337 molecule, 539
Hepatitis B, CD30 molecule and, 88
Hepatitis C:
  CD81 molecule, 174
  CD209 molecule, 355–356
  CD283 molecule, 452–453
  CD299 molecule, 479–480
HER2/neu, CD340 molecule, 544–545
Hereditary hemorrhagic telangiectasia,
      CD105 molecule, 209
Hermes antigen, CD44 molecule, 113–114

Herpes simplex virus (HSV) receptors:
  CD46 molecule, 117
  CD111 molecule, 218
  CD112 molecule, 219
  CD222 molecule, 367–368
  CD270 molecule, 431–432
Herpes virus entry mediator (HVEM), CD270
    molecule, 431
hFz-4, CD344 molecule, 546
hFz-6, CD349 molecule, 547
hFz-7, CD350 molecule, 548
HG-CSFR, CD114 molecule, 221
hGL50 splice variant, CD275 molecule, 440
hJ1, CD339 molecule, 543
HL9, CD85a molecule, 178
Hly9-b, CD84 molecule, 177
HM1.24, CD317 molecule, 508
HM18, CD85k molecule, 182
HMGL, CD301 molecule, 483
HML, CD301 molecule, 483
HML-1, CD103 molecule, 207
HML-2, CD301 molecule, 483
HMMTOP server, transmembrane helix
    prediction, 31–32
HNA-2a, CD177 molecule, 320
HNK1, CD57 molecule, 140
Hodgkin's lymphoma:
  CD15 molecule expression, 66
  CD30 molecule expression, 87–88
  CD43 molecule expression, 111–112
  CD83 molecule, 176
  CD138 molecule expression, 257–258
  CD273 molecule, 436–437
  CD302/DEC205 fusion molecule, 484
Holley (Hy) antigen, CD297 molecule, 477
hPD-1, CD279 molecule, 444
HPTP-η, CD148 molecule, 274
hRANKL2, CD254 molecule, 415
HTA1, CD1a molecule, 42
Hulym3, CD48 molecule, 121
Human cytomegalovirus (HCMV):
  CD13 molecule, 62
  CD85j molecule, 180–181
  CD155 molecule, 285
  CD209 molecule, 355–356
  CD210 molecule, 357
  CD299 molecule, 479–480
Human immunodeficiency virus (HIV):
  CD4 molecule, 47
  CD16 molecule, 67–68
  CD26 molecule, 81–82
  CD30 molecule, 87–88

  CD38 molecule, 100
  CD59 molecule, 142
  CD91 molecule, 189–190
  CD153 molecule, 281–282
  CD184 molecule, 329
  CD186 molecule, 331
  CD192 molecule, 333
  CD193 molecule, 334
  CD194 molecule, 335
  CD195 molecule, 336
  CD207 molecule, 352–353
  CD209 molecule, 355–356
  CD299 molecule, 479–480
  CDw198 molecule, 339
  CDw199 molecule, 340
Human leukocyte antigen (HLA) molecules:
  CD53 molecule, 133
  CD74 molecule, 167
  CD85d molecule, 179
  CD85j molecule, 180–181
  CD94 molecule, 193–194
  CD158 molecule, 290–291
  CD159 a/c molecules, 292
  CD160 molecule, 293
Human leukocyte cell surface proteins, web
    information sources for:
  conserved protein domains, 27–27, 30
  expression information, 32–33
  functional information, 32, 34
  gene information, 20–23
    orthologues, 20, 23–27
    splice variants and polymorphism, 20
  nomenclature issues, 17–19
  sequence databases, 23–24, 27–28
  sequence similarity comparisons, 27
  structural models, 28, 30
  transmembrane helix prediction, 31–32
Human leukocyte differentiation antigens
    (HLDA):
  current research issues, 5–6
  historical background on, 3
  surface membrane molecules, 4–5
Human Mucosal Lymphocyte (HML) antigen,
    CD103 molecule, 207
Human T-cell leukemia virus (HTLV), CD30
    molecule, 87–88
HUTCH-1, CD44 molecule, 113–114
Hve B, CD112 molecule, 219
Hve C1, CD111, 218
HVEM, CD270 molecule, 431–432
Hyaladhesin family, CD44 molecule,
    113–114

Hyaluronan binding:
  CD44 molecule, 113–114
  CD54 molecule, 134
  CD168 molecule, 305–306
Hyaluronic acid ligands:
  CD38 molecule, 99–100
  CD43 molecule, 111
Hyperandrogenism, CD120b molecule, 231
Hyper-IgM (HIGM) syndrome, CD154 molecule, 283–284

I-309 ligand, CDw198 molecule, 339
IA4, CD82 molecule, 175
iC3b ligands:
  CD 11 molecule, 58, 60
  CD21 molecule, 73
  CD35 molecule, 95–96
iC4, CD35 molecule, 96
ICAM. *See* Intercellular adhesion molecules
ICOS, CD278 molecule, 443
ICOS ligand (ICOS-L), CD275 molecule, 440
IFNγR/IFNγRα, CD119 molecule, 228
IGA, CD79a molecule, 171
Ig-alpha, CD79a molecule, 171
IgA receptor, CD89 molecule, 187
IGB, CD79b molecule, 172
Ig-beta, CD79b molecule, 172
IGF1 receptor (type I), CD221 molecule, 365–366
IGF2R, CD222 molecule, 367–368
Ig-Lambda5, CD179b molecule, 324
Ig-like domain, structure and function, 8
IgSF8, CD316 molecule, 507
IL-2/15Rb, CD122 molecule, 235
ILT/LIR family. *See* Immunoglobulin-like transcript/leukocyte immunoglobulin-like receptor family
Immune adherence receptor, CD35 molecule, 95
Immunoglobulin A (IgA) receptors:
  CD71 molecule, 163
  CD89 molecule, 187
Immunoglobulin E (IgE) receptor, CD23 molecule, 77
Immunoglobulin G (IgG) receptors:
  CD16 molecule, 67–68
  CD32 molecule, 91–92
  CD64 molecule, 151
  CD307 molecule, 490–491

Immunoglobulin iota chain (IGVPB), CD179a molecule, 323
Immunoglobulin Lambda-like polypeptide-1, CD179b molecule, 324
Immunoglobulin-like transcript/leukocyte immunoglobulin-like receptor (ILT/LIR) family:
  CD85a molecule, 178
  CD85d molecule, 179
  CD85j molecule, 180–181
  CD85k molecule, 182
Immunoglobulin M (IgM):
  CD21 molecule, 73–74
  CD79a/79b molecule, 171–172
  CD179a/179b molecule, 324
Immunoglobulin omega chain, CD179b molecule, 324
Immunoglobulin receptor translocation associated (IRTA) gene family, CD307 molecule, 490–491
Immunoglobulin-receptor tyrosine kinase (Ig-RTK) family:
  CD115 molecule, 222–223
  CD140a, 260–261
  CD140b, 262–263
Immunoglobulin superfamily (IgSF), basic properties, 11–13
Immunogolbulin lambda-like polypeptide, CD179b molecule, 324
Immunoreceptor tyrosine-based activation motif (ITAM):
  CD3 molecule, 46
  CD5 molecule, 49
  CD32 molecule, 91–92
  CD79a molecule, 171
  CD79b molecule, 172
  CD247 molecule, 408–409
Immunoreceptor tyrosine-based inhibitory motif (ITIM):
  CD22 molecule, 75–76
  CD31 molecule, 89–90
  CD32 molecule, 91–92
  CD33 molecule, 93
  CD72 molecule, 164
  CD85a molecule, 178
  CD85d molecule, 179
  CD85j molecule, 180–181
  CD85k molecule, 182
  CD92 molecule, 191
  CD94 molecule, 193–194
  CD96 molecule, 196–197
  CD124 molecule, 239–240

CD158 molecule, 290–291
CD159a molecule, 292
CD170 molecule, 309–310
CD172a molecule, 313
CD272 molecule, 435
CD279 molecule, 444–445
CD300 molecule, 481–482
CD305 molecule, 488
CD307 molecule, 490–491
CD327 molecule, 521–522
CD328 molecule, 523–524
CD329 molecule, 525
CD330 molccule, 526–527
Immunoreceptor tyrosine switch motif
    (ITSM):
CD150 molecule, 276–277
CD244 molecule, 403–404
CD279 molecule, 444–445
CD319 molecule, 510
Immunosuppression:
CD3 molecule, 46
CD4 molecule, 48
CD7 molecule, 52
CD11 molecules, 57
CD28 molecule, 85
CD45 molecule, 116
CD52 molecule, 132
CD54 molecule, 134–135
Immunotherapy:
CD89 molecule, 187
CD274 molecule, 438–439
CD278 molecule, 443
CD297 molecule, 477
CD307 molecule, 490–491
CD317 molecule, 508
Imuclone, CD4 molecule, 48
INCAM-110, CD106 molecule, 211–212
Indolcamine 2,3-dioxygenase (IDO), CD152
    molecule, 279–280
Induced by lymphocyte activation (ILA),
    CD137 molecule, 256
Inducible costimulator (ICOS), CD278
    molecule, 443
Inducible costimulator (ICOS) ligand, CD275
    molecule, 440
Infectious disease:
CD1d molecule and, 43
CD66b molecule, 155
CD66c molecule, 156
CD89 molecule, 187
CD209 molecule, 355–356
CD226 molecule, 374–375

Inflammation:
CD49a, b, d molecules, 122–123,
    125–126
CD62L molecule, 146–147
CD62P molecule, 149
CD101 molecule, 205
CD126 molecule, 244
CD134 molecule, 253
CD156a molecule, 286
CD156c molecule, 288
CD191 molecule, 332
CD194 molecule, 335
CD308 molecule, 492–493
Inflammatory myofibroblastic tumor (IMT),
    CD246 fusion molecules, 406–407
Inflammatory response:
CD27 molecule, 84
CD49a molecule, 122
CD49d molecule, 125–126
CD62P molecule, 148–149
CD66b molecule, 155
CD66c molecule, 156
Influenza virus:
CD235a molecule, 388–389
CD335 molecule, 536
CD336 molecule, 538
Insulin-like growth factor (IGF)
    receptors:
CD220 molecule, 363–364
CD221 molecule, 365–366
CD222 molecule, 367
Insulin receptor, CD220 molecule, 363
Insulin secretion:
CD36 molecule, 97
CD220 molecule, 363–364
Integral membrane proteins, attachment and
    orientation, 11
Integrin α-chain family:
α1-chain, CD49a molecule, 122
α2-chain, CD49b molecule, 123
αIIb-chain, CD41 molecule, 104–105
α3-chain, CD49c molecule, 124
α4-chain, CD49d molecule, 125–126
α5-chain, CD49e molecule, 127
α6-chain, CD49f molecule, 128–129
αE-chain, CD103 molecule, 207
αL-chain, CD11a molecule, 56–57
αM-chain, CD11b molecule, 58–59
αV-chain, CD51 molecule, 131
αX-chain, CD11c molecule, 60
Integrin-associated protein (IAP), CD47
    molecule, 119

Integrin β-chain family:
  β1-chain, CD29 molecule, 86
  β2-chain, CD18 molecule, 58, 70
  β3-chain, CD61 molecule, 144
  β4-chain, CD104 molecule, 208
Integrins:
  ligands and associated molecules:
    CD9 molecules, 54
    CD46 molecule, 117–118
    CD47 molecule, 119
    CD50 molecule, 130–131
    CD53 molecule, 133
    CD54 molecule, 134–135
    CD87 molecule, 184–185
    CD98 molecule, 200
    CD147 molecule, 273
    CD171 molecule, 311–312
    CD209 molecule, 355–356
    CD242 molecule, 400
    CD324 molecule, 516
  protein family, 12
Intercellular adhesion molecules (ICAM):
  ICAM-1, CD54 molecule, 134–135, 56, 58, 60
  ICAM-2, CD102 molecule, 56, 58, 206
  ICAM-3, CD50 molecule, 56, 130
  ICAM-4, CD242 molecule, 400
  ICAM-5, 56
Inter-endothelial tight junctions, CD323 molecule, 514
Interferon-γ (IFN-γ):
  CD98 molecule, 200
  CD119 molecule, 228
  CD150 molecule, 276–277
  CD255 molecule, 416–417
  CD273 molecule, 436–437
Interferon-γ (IFN-γ) receptor α chain (IFNγRα), CD119 molecule, 228
Interferon-induced transmembrane protein 1, CD225 molecule, 373
Interleukin-1 (IL-1) receptors:
  Type I IL-1R, CD121a molecule, 233
  TypeII IL-1R, CD121b molecule, 233
Interleukin-2 (IL-2) receptors:
  IL-2R α chain, CD25 molecule, 80
  IL-2R β chain, CD122 molecule, 235–236
  IL-2R γ chain, CD132 molecule, 251
Interleukin-3 (IL-3) receptor α chain (IL-3Rα), CD123 molecule, 237–238
  CD131 molecule, 250
Interleukin-4 (IL-4) receptor α chain (IL-4Rα), CD124 molecule, 239

Interleukin-5 (IL-5) receptor α chain (IL-5Rα), CD125 molecule, 241–242
Interleukin-6 (IL-6) receptor α chain (IL-6Rα), CD126 molecule, 243–244
Interleukin-7 (IL-7) receptor α chain (IL-7Rα), CD127 molecule, 245–246
Interleukin-8 (IL-8), CD234 molecule ligand, 387
Interleukin-8 (IL-8) receptor α chain, CD181 molecule, 326
Interleukin-8 (IL-8) receptor β chain, CD182 molecule, 327
Interleukin-9 (IL-9) receptor α chain, CD129 molecule, 248
Interleukin-10 (IL-10) receptors, CDw210a/b molecules, 357
Interleukin-11 (IL-11) receptor, CD130 molecule, 249
Interleukin-12 (IL-12) receptor β1 chain, CD212 molecule, 358
Interleukin-13 (IL-13) receptors:
  α1 chain, CD213α1 molecule, 359–360
  α2 chain, CD213α2 molecule, 359–360
  CD124 molecule, 239–240
Interleukin-15 (IL-15) receptor:
  CD122 molecule, 235–236
  CD132 molecule, 251
Interleukin-16 (IL-16) receptor, CD4 molecule, 47
Interleukin-17 (IL-17) receptor, CD217 molecule, 361
Interleukin-18 (IL-18) receptor α/β chains, CD218a/b molecules, 362
Interleukin-18 receptor accessory protein (IL-18RAP), CD218b molecule, 362
Interleukin-22 (IL-22) receptor, CDw210b molecule, 357
International Protein Index (IPI) website, protein sequence information on, 23–24, 27–28
Intraepithelial lymphocytes (IELs):
  CD103 molecule, 207
  CD160 molecule, 293
  CD326 molecule, 519–520
Invasin ligands, CD29/CD49d complexes, 86, 126, 128–129
IPO-3, CD150 molecule, 276–277
IRP60, CD300a molecule, 481–482
IRTA2, CD307 molecule, 490
Isoelectric point, determination of, 24
ITGAX molecule, CD11c molecule, 60

Jagged ligands family, CD339 molecule, 543

JAK1 signaling component, CD87 molecule, 184–185

JAK-STAT pathway:
CD114 molecule, 221
CD116 molecule, 224
CD117 molecule, 225–226
CD210 molecule, 357
CD295 molecule, 474–475

Janus-family kinases:
CD122 molecule, 235–236
CD124 molecule, 239–240
CD127 molecule, 245–246

John-Milton-Hagen (JMH) human blood group antigen, CD108 molecule, 215

Joint tissue, CD156c molecule, 288

Joseph (Jo(a)) antigen, CD297 molecule, 477

JTK2, CD334 molecule, 534–535

JTK4, CD333 molecule, 532–533

Junctional adhesion molecules (JAMs):
JAM-1, CD321 molecule, 512
JAM-2, CD322 molecule, 513
JAM-3/JAM-C/JAM-VE, CD323 molecule, 514

Junctional Epidermolysis Bullosa with Pyloric Atresia (JEBPA), CD104 molecule, 208

Juvenile hemangiomas, CD310 molecule, 496–497

Juvenile polyposis syndrome, CD292 molecule, 470–471

K12, CD7 molecule, 52

Kallmann syndrome, CD331 molecule, 529

KDR, CD309 molecule, 494–495

Kell blood group antigen, CD238 molecule, 392

KG-CAM, CD166, 301

KGFR, CD332 molecule, 530–531

Ki-1 antigen, CD30 molecule, 87

KI-24 antigen, CD70 molecule, 162

KIAA0709, CD280 molecule, 446

KIAA1436, CD315 molecule, 505–506

KIEELE motif, CD223 molecule, 369–370

Killer cell lectin-like receptor subfamily B (KLRB), CD161 molecule, 294

Killer cell lectin-like receptor subfamily C (KLRC), CD159 a/c molecules, 292

Killer inhibitory receptor (KIR) family:
CD158 molecules, 290–291

Kininogen, CD87 molecule, 184–185

KIR superfamily, characteristics of, 11–13

Klebsiella pneumoniae, CD209 molecule ligand, 356

Knops blood group antigen, CD35 molecule, 95–96

Ko alloantigen system, CD42b molecule, 107

Kp43, CD94 molecule, 193

KSA, CD326 molecule, 519–520

KSAM-1, CD332 molecule, 530–531

LI, CD171 molecule, 311

Lactobacillus sp. CD209 molecule ligand, 355–356

Lactosamines, CD75/CD75s/CDw76, 168

Lactosylceramide (LacCer), CD17 molecule, 69

LAG-3, CD223 molecule, 369–370

LAIR1, CD305 molecule, 488

LAIR2, CD306 molecule, 489

LAM-1, CD62L molecule, 146

Lambda 5, CD179b molecule, 324

Laminin binding:
CD29/CD49 molecule, 86, 123–124, 128
CD29/CD51 complex, 86, 131
CD51/CD61 complex, 131
CD57 molecule, 140
CD104/CD49f complex, 128, 208
CD171 molecule, 311–312
CD239 molecule, 393–394

LAMP molecules. *See* Lysosomal associated membrane protein (LAMP) family

Landsteiner-Wiener (LW) blood group system, CD242 molecule, 400

Langerhans cells (LCs), CD207 molecule, 352–353

Langerin, CD207 molecule, 352–353

LARC receptor, CD196 molecule, 337

Latency associated peptide (LAP) ligand:
CD222 molecule, 367–368
CD223 molecule, 369–370

LDLR domain, structure and function, 8

Leach phenotype, CD236 molecule, 390–391

LECAM-2, CD62E molecule, 145

LEPR, CD295 molecule, 474

Leptin receptors:
CD295 molecule (LEPR), 474–475
CD327 molecule, 521–522

Leu-1, CD5 molecule, 49

Leu 3a, CD4 molecule, 47

Leu 4, CD3 molecule, 46

Leu 9, CD7 molecule, 52

Leu 13, CD225 molecule, 373

Leu-16, CD20 molecule, 72
Leucine-rich repeat (LRR) family:
    CD42a/b/c/d molecules, 106–110
    CD180 molecule, 325
    CD281 molecule, 448–449
    CD282 molecule, 450–451
    CD283 molecule, 452–453
    CD284 molecule, 454–455
    CD285 molecule, 456–457
    CD286 molecule, 458–459
    CD287 molecule, 460–461
    CD288 molecule, 462–463
    CD289 molecule, 464–465
    CD290 molecule, 466–467
    CD291 molecule, 468–469
Leukemia inhibitory factor (LIF) ligands:
    CD118 molecule, 227
    CD130 molecule, 249
    CD222 molecule, 367–368
Leukemias:
    CD2 molecule, 44
    CD9 molecule, 54
    CD16 molecule, 67–68
    CD38 molecule and, 100
    CD43 molecule, 111–112
    CD73 molecule, 165
    CD74 molecule, 167
Leukocyte adhesion deficiency type I
    (LAD-1):
    CD11 molecules, 58, 60
    CD18 molecule, 70
Leukocyte adhesion deficiency type II
    (LAD-2), CD15 molecule, 66
Leukocyte antigen MIC3, CD9 molecule, 54
Leukocyte-associated Ig-like receptors
    (LAIR):
    CD305 molecule, 488
    CD306 molecule, 489
Leukocyte common antigen (LCA), CD45
    molecule, 115–116
Leukocyte function-associated antigens (LFA):
    LFA-1, CD11a/CD18 complex, 56
    LFA-2, CD2 molecule, 44–45
    LFA-3, CD58 molecule, 44, 141
Leukocyte immunoglobulin-like receptor. *See*
    Immunoglobulin-like transcript/
    leukocyte immunoglobulin-like receptor
    (ILT/LIR) family
Leukocyte inhibitory factor receptor (LIFR),
    CD118 molecule, 227
Leukocyte sialoglycoprotein, CD43 molecule,
    111

Leukocyte surface antigen, CD11c molecule,
    60
Leukocyte tyrosine kinase (LTK), CD246
    molecule, 406–407
Leukosialin, CD43 molecule, 111
Leu T, CD8 molecule, 53
Lewis (a) (Le(a)) antigen, CD328 molecule
    bindeing, 523–524
Lewis X (LeX) antigens, CD15 molecule, 66
Lewis Y (LeY) blood group, CD174 molecule,
    317
LFA molecules. *See* Leukocyte function-
    associated antigens
LICOS, CD275 molecule, 440
LIFR, C118 molecule, 227
LIGHT, CD258 molecule, 420
LIGHT-R, CD270 molecule, 431–432
LILR protein family, 12
LIMP, CD63 molecule, 150
Link domain, structure and function, 8
Lipids, CD1a–e molecules, 43
Lipopolysaccharide (LPS):
    CD11 molecules, 57–58, 60
    CD204 molecule binding, 347
    CD284 molecule, 444–445, 455
Lipopolysaccharide receptor (LPS-R), CD14
    molecule, 64–65
Lipoprotein lipase, CD91 molecule, 189
Lipotechoic acid, CD204 molecule ligand, 347
LIR molecules. *See* Immunoglobulin-like
    transcript/leukocyte immunoglobulin-
    like receptor (ILT/LIR) family
LIT, CD263 molecule, 423
Liver disease, CD224 molecule, 372
Liver sinusoidal endothelial cells (LSECs),
    CD299 molecule, 480
LNGFR, CD271 molecule, 433
Long chain fatty acids, CD36 molecule
    binding, 97
Low-affinity IgE receptor, CD23 molecule, 77
Low density lipoproteins (LDL), ligands:
    CD36 molecule, 97
    CD68 molecule, 160
    CD204 molecule, 347
Low density lipoprotein receptor-related
    protein (LRP), CD91 molecule, 189
LPAP, CD22 molecule, 75
LPS/LPS binding protein complex:
    CD11b molecule, 58
    CD14 molecule and, 64
LPS receptor (LPS-R), CD14 molecule, 64
L-selectin, CD62L molecule, 146

L-SIGN, CD299 molecule, 479
LTa3, CD270 molecule ligand, 431
LTbR, CD258 molecule ligand, 420
Lutheran blood group, CD239 molecules, 393–394
Lutheran glycoprotein, CD239 molecule, 393–394
Lutropin, CD206 molecule ligand, 420
Ly1, CD5 molecule, 49
Ly5, CD45 molecule, 115
Ly-6 superfamily, CD59 molecule, 142
Ly9, CD229 molecule, 379
Ly-19.2, CD72 molecule, 164
Ly32.2, CD72 molecule, 164
LY64, CD180 molecule, 325
Ly94, CD335 molecule, 536–537
Ly95, CD336 molecule, 538
Ly117, CD337 molecule, 539–540
Lyb-2, CD72 molecule, 164
Lyb-2 homologues, CD72 molecule, 164
Lyb8, CD22 molecule, 75
Lymphocyte activation gene 3 (LAG-3), CD223 molecule, 369–370
Lymphocyte antigen 75, CD205 molecule, 349
Lymphocyte phosphatase-associated phosphoprotein (LPAP), CD45 molecule ligand, 115–116
Lymphokines. *See* Interleukins
Lymphoma:
    CD2 molecule, 44
    CD10 molecule, 55
    CD19 molecule, 71
    CD20 molecule, 72
    CD30 molecule, 87–88
    CD43 molecule, 111–112
    CD70 molecule, 162
    CD73 molecule, 165
    CD74 molecule, 167
    CD103 molecule, 207
    CD138 molecule, 257–258
    CD273 molecule, 436–437
    CD274 molecule, 438–439
Lysosomal associated membrane protein (LAMP) family:
    CD68 molecule, 160
    DC-LAMP, CD208 molecule, 354
    LAMP-1/-2, CD107a/b molecules, 213–214
    LAMP-3, CD63 molecule, 150
Lysosomal storage diseases, CD107a/b molecule, 213–214
LyT2, CD8 molecule, 53

M1 peptidase family, CD249 molecule, 411
M4S1, CD326 molecule, 519–520
M6, CD147 molecule, 273
M38, CD81 molecule, 174
M130, CD163 molecule, 297
M241, CD1c molecule, 42
Mac-1 integrin, CD11b/CD18 complex, 58
MACIF, CD59 molecule, 142
α-2-Macroglobulin proteinase complex, CD91 molecule and, 189–190
α-2-Macroglobulin receptor (α2M-R), CD91 molecule, 189–190
Macrophage chemotactic factor proteins (MCP):
    CD193 molecule, 334
    CD195 molecule, 336
Macrophage colony stimulating factor (M-CSF) receptor, CD115 molecule, 222–223
Macrophage inflammatory protein 1α (MIP-1α) receptors:
    CD13 molecule, 62
    CD191 molecule, 332
    CD195 molecule, 336
Macrophage inflammatory protein 1α (MIP-1α), CD195 molecule ligand, 336
Macrophage inflammatory protein 3α (MIP-3α), CD196 molecule ligand, 336
Macrophage inhibitor factor (MIF), CD74 molecule, 167
Macrophage mannose receptor (MMR), CD206 molecule, 350
Macrophage scavenger receptor (MSR), CD204 molecule, 347–348
Macrophage stimulating protein (MSP) receptor, CD136 molecule, 255
Macrosialin, CD68 molecule, 160
MadCAM-1 receptors:
    CD29 molecule, 86
    CD49d molecule, 125–126
    CD62L molecule, 146–147
Major histocompatibility complex (MHC):
    CD3 molecule, 46
    CD4 molecule, 47
    CD8 molecule, 53
    CD13 molecule, 62
    CD20 molecule, 72
    CD37 molecule, 98
    CD43 molecule, 111
    CD53 molecule, 133
    CD82 molecule, 175
    CD85a molecule, 178

CD85d molecule, 179
CD85j molecule, 180–181
CD94 molecule, 193–194
CD158 molecule, 290–291
CD159 a/c molecules, 292
CD160 molecule, 293
CD161 molecule, 294
CD223 molecule, 369–370
MAM domain, CD304 molecule, 486–487
Mannose-6-phosphate receptor, CD222
    molecule, 367–368
Mannose receptors:
    CD206 molecule, 350–351
    CD207 molecule, 352–353
    CD209 molecule, 355–356
    CD222 molecule, 367–368
    CD280 molecule, 446–447
    CD299 molecule, 479–480
Mastocytosis, CD117 molecule, 226
mb-1, CD79a molecule, 171
MCAM, CD146 molecule, 271
McLeod phenotype, CD238 molecule, 392
MDC, CD194 molecule ligand, 335
MDR proteins. *See* Multi-drug resistance
    family
ME 491, CD63 molecule, 150
Measles virus:
    CD46 molecule, 117–118
    CD150 molecule, 276–277
Meconium antigen 100, CD66e molecule,
    158
Mel-14, CD62L molecule, 146
Mel-CAM, CD146 molecule, 271
Melanoma-associated antigen:
    CD63 molecule, 150
    CD307 molecule, 491
Melanoma:
    CD49a molecule, 122
    CD57 molecule, 140
    CD60 molecule expression, 143
    CD63 molecule, 150
    CD87 molecule, 184–185
    CD91 molecule, 189–190
    CD117 molecule, 225–226
    CD146 molecule, 271–272
    CD166 molecule, 301–302
    CD171 molecule, 312
    CD228 molecule, 378
    CD274 molecule, 438–439
    CD310 molecule, 497
    CD338 molecule, 541–542
Melanotransferrin, CD228 molecule, 378

Mel-CAM, CD146 molecule, 271
MEM-133, CD47 molecule, 119
Membrane attack complex (MAC), CD59
    molecule, 142
Membrane cofactor protein (MCP), CD46
    molecule, 117
Membrane-spanning 4A (MS4A) family, CD20
    molecule, 72
Memory B cells:
    CD27 molecule, 83–84
    CD86 molecule binding, 183
Memory T cells:
    CD45 molecule, 115–116
    CD196 molecule, 337
Merosin, CD29/CD49f complex binding, 86,
    128
MGC 24, CD164 molecule, 298
MGSA, CD234 molecule ligand, 387
MGL, CD301 molecule, 483
MHC class I chain-related molecules, CD314
    molecule ligands, 504
MHC class II associated invariant chain (Ii),
    CD74 molecule, 166–167
MHC molecules. *See* Major histocompatibility
    complex (MHC)
MIC2, CD99 molecule, 201–202
MIC18, CD326 molecule, 519–520
MICA/B, CD314 molecule ligands, 504
Microarray expression data, 32
β2-Microglobulin, CD1a–e molecules, 42–43
Microbial lipids, CD1a–e molecules and, 43
Midkine (MK) ligand, CD246 molecule,
    ·   406–407
Migration inhibitory factor (MIF), CD74
    molecule, 167
MIP-1α, CD195 molecule ligand, 336
MIP-3α, CD196 molecule ligand, 337
MIP1b, CD44 molecule binding, 114
MIR7, CD85j molecule, 180
MIR10, CD85d molecule, 179
MIRL, CD59 molecule, 142
MK-1, CD326 molecule, 519–520
MLR3, CD69 molecule, 161
M/N blood group antigens, CD235a molecule,
    388
MN sialoglycoprotein, CD235a molecule,
    388–389
Mo1, CD11b molecule, 58
Mo5, CD157 molecule, 289
Molecular profiles, symbols table, 41
Molt-3 T lymphoblastic leukemia, CD325
    molecule, 517–518

Monocyte chemoattractant protein 1 (MCP-1) receptors:
CD191 molecule, 332
CD192 molecule, 333
CD193 molecule, 334
CD234 molecule, 387
Monosaccharides, structures, 10
Motility-related protein-1 (MRP-1), CD9 molecule, 54
MPIF-1. *See* Myeloid progenitor inhibitory factor 1
MRC OX2, CD200 molecule, 341
MRC OX44, CD53 molecule, 133
MRC2, CD280 molecule, 446
MRX, CD338 molecule, 541–542
MS2, CD156a molecule, 286
MS4A protein family, 12
MSP-R, CD136 molecule, 255
MSR1 gene, CD204 molecule, 348
MUC-1, CD227 molecule, 376–377
MUC-18, CD146 molecule, 271–272
MUC-24, CD164 molecule, 298
Mucin family:
CD34 molecule, 94
CD42b molecule, 107–108
CD43 molecule, 111–112
CD68 molecule, 160
CD99 molecule, 201–202
CD146 molecule, 271
CD164 molecule, 298–299
CD227 molecule, 376–377
Multi-drug resistance protein 1 (MDR1), CD243 molecule, 401–402
Multigene cell-surface receptor, CD3 molecule, 46
Multi-Glycosylated Core protein, 24kDA (MGC-24), CD164 molecule, 298–299
Multiple myeloma:
CD38 molecule and, 100
CD130 molecule, 249
CD138 molecule, 257–258
CD256 molecule, 418
CD267 molecule, 428
CD317 molecule, 508
Multiple sclerosis:
CD134 molecule, 253
CD152 molecule, 279–280
CD154 molecule, 283–284
CD156c molecule, 288
CD192 molecule, 333
Murine heat stable antigen (HSA), CD52 molecule, 132

Murine myeloproliferative leukemia virus (V-mpl), CD110 molecule, 217
MXR/MXR1, CD338 molecule, 541–542
My9, CD33molecule, 93
My10, CD34 molecule, 94
Mycobacterial 19kDa lipoprotein, CD281 molecule ligand, 448
Mycobacterium tuberculosis receptors:
CD209 molecule, 355–356
CD299 molecule, 479–480
Mycoplasmal macrophage-activating lipopeptide-2kDa (MALP-2), CD286 molecule, 458–459
Myelin, CD204 molecule ligand, 347
Myelodysplasia, CD7 marker, 51
Myeloid hematopoiesis:
CD33 molecule, 93
CD115 molecule, 222–223
CD157 molecule, 289
Myelopoiesis, CD114 molecule, 221
Myeloproliferative leukemia virus oncogene (c-mpl), CD110 molecule, 217
Myristoylation, of proteins, 13

N-acetylgalactosamine residues, CD301 molecule ligands, 483
Naive lymphocytes:
CD27 molecule, 83–84
CD45 molecule, 115–116
Na/K ATPase, CD298 molecule, 478
NAP-2, CD182 molecule binding, 327
Natural cytotoxicity receptor (NCR):
CD335 molecule, 536–537
CD336 molecule, 538
CD337 molecule, 539–540
Natural killer (NK) cells:
CD2 molecule, 44
CD16 molecule, 67–68
CD56 molecule, 138–139
CD85a/d/j molecules, 178–181
CD158 molecule, 290–291
CD161 molecule, 294
CD162/162R molecules, 296
CD300a molecule, 481–482
CD314 molecule, 504
CD319 molecule, 510
CD335 molecule, 537
CD337 molecule, 539–540
NB1, CD177 molecule, 320
NCAD, CD325 molecule, 517–518
N-cadherin, CD325 molecule, 517
NCA-50/90, CD66c molecule, 156

NCA-95, CD66b molecule, 155
NCA-160, CD66a molecule, 153
NCBI EntrezGene website:
  Blast, 27
  Blink, 27
  gene expression information on, 32–33
  genetic information on, 20–26
  HomoloGene, 23
  human leukocyte cell surface proteins,
    aliases summarized on, 18
  MapViewer, 20
  protein function information on, 32, 34
  protein sequence similarity comparisons, 27,
    29
  RefSeq database, 23
  SNP:GeneView, 20
NCR1, CD335 molecule, 536
NCR2, CD336 molecule, 538
NCR3, CD337 molecule, 539
Nectin-like 5, CD155 molecule, 285
Nectin-1, CD111 molecule, 218
Nectin-2, CD112 molecule, 219
Nectin-3, CD113 molecule, 220
Neisseria sp. receptors:
  CD46 molecule, 117–118
  CD66a, c, and d molecules, 157
Neprilysin family, CD238 molecule, 392
Nerve growth factor (NGF) receptor. *See*
    Tumor necrosis factor/nerve growth
    factor (TNF/NGF) receptor family
Neural adhesion molecule L1 receptors:
  CD49e molecule, 127
  CD51/CD61 complex, 131
Neural cell adhesion molecules (NCAM):
  CD56 molecule, 138–139
  CD171 molecule, 311–312
Neuroblastomas:
  CD171 molecule, 312
  CD276 molecule, 441
Neurocan, CD171 molecule binding,
    311–312
Neurodegenerative disease, CD156a molecule,
    286
Neuroglandular antigen, CD63 molecule,
    150
Neurolin, CD166, 301
Neuronal adhesion molecule, CD171 molecule,
    311
Neuronal stem cells, CD344 molecule, 546
Neurons, CD15 molecule expression, 66
Neuropilin/Neuropilin-1, CD304 molecule,
    486–487

Neurotrophins, CD271 molecule, 433–434
Neutral endopeptidase (NEP), CD10 molecule,
    55
Neutrophilin, CD47 molecule, 119–120
Neutrophils:
  CD11b molecule, 58
  CD16 molecule, 67–68
  CD17 molecule, 69
  CD23 molecule, 77–78
  CD35 molecule, 95–96
  CD43 molecule, 111
  CD66a molecule, 153–154
  CD66b molecule, 155
  CD92 molecule, 191
  CD97 molecule, 198–199
  CD116 molecule, 224
  CD153 molecule, 281–282
  CD170 molecule, 309–310
  CD177 molecule, 320
  CD181 molecule, 326
  CD182 molecule, 327
  CD281 molecule, 448–449
  CD313 molecule, 502–503
  CD323 molecule, 514
  CD329 molecule, 525
  CD330 molecule, 526–527
NGFR, CD271 molecule, 433–434
19A/19A24, CD319 molecule, 510
Nitric oxides, CD224 molecule, 371–372
NK1, CD160 molecule, 293
NK28, CD160 molecule, 293
N/K ATPase, CD298 molecule, 478
NKG2a/c, CD159a/c molecules, 292
NKG2D, CD314 molecule, 504
NKG2/NKG2C complex:
  CD94 molecule, 193–194
  CD159a/c molecules, 292
NKHI, CD56 molecule, 138
NKp30, CD337 molecule, 539–540
NKp44, CD336 molecule, 538
NKp46, CD335 molecule, 536–537
NKR-P1A, CD161 molecule, 294
Nomenclature issues, human leukocyte and
    stromal cell:
  Multiple gene names,18
  Use of suffixes, 19
Non-glycosylated protein, CD240CE molecule,
    396–397
Non-Hodgkin's lymphoma:
  CD30 molecule, 87–88
  CD43 molecule, 111–112
  CD44 molecule, 114

CD196 molecule, 337
CD273 molecule, 436–437
Nonspecific cross-reacting antigens. *See* NCAs
Norrin, CD344 molecule ligand, 546
Notch proteins, CD339 molecule ligands, 543
NTPDase-1, CD39 molecule, 101
NTR, CD271 molecule, 433
Nucleophosmin (NPM), CD246 molecule, 406–407

OB-BP1, CD327 molecule, 521–522
OBR, CD295 molecule, 474
OB-Rb isoform, CD295 molecule, 474–475
ODFR, CD265 molecule, 425
OFE, CD265 molecule, 425
Oka blood group antigen, CD147 molecule, 273
OKM-5 antigen, CD36 molecule, 97
OKT3 antibody:
    CD3 molecule as, 46
    therapeutic applications, 15
OKT4 antibody, 47–48
OKT8 antibody, CD8 molecule, 53
Oligodendrocyte precursor cells (OPCs), CD162/162R molecules, 296
Oligodendrocytes, CD15 molecule expression, 66
Oncostatin M receptor:
    CD118 molecule, 227
    CD130 molecule, 249
1C7, CD337 molecule, 539–540
Online Mendelian Inheritance in Man (OMIM) website, protein function and disease association information, 32, 34
Opacity-associated (Opa) proteins:
    CD66c molecule, 156
    CD66d molecule, 157
    CD66e molecule, 158
Orthologues, website information sources for, 20, 23, 25–26
Osteoclast activation, CD254 molecule, 415
Osteopontin receptors:
    CD44 molecule, 114
    CD51/CD61 complex, 131
Osteoprotegrin receptors:
    CD253 molecule, 413–414
    CD254 molecule, 415
Outer-surface protein A (OspA) lipoprotein:
    CD281 molecule, 448–449
    CD286 molecule, 458–459
Ovalocytosis, CD233 molecule and, 385
Ovarian carcinoma antigen (OA3), CD47 molecule, 119

OX 2, CD200 molecule, 341
OX 2R, CD200 molecule ligand, 341
OX 40, CD134 molecule, 253
OX 40 ligand (OX40L), CD252 molecule, 412
OX-44, CD53 molecule, 133
OX45, CD48 molecule, 121

P-18, CD59 molecule, 142
p24, CD9 molecule, 54
p67, CD33 molecule, 93
p70, CD92 molecule, 191
p75:
    CD84 molecule, 177
    CD122 molecule, 235
    CD328 molecule, 523–524
p90, CD127 molecule, 245
p90–120, CDw12 molecule, 61
p97, CD228 molecule, 378
p126, CD101 molecule, 205
p150,95 integrin, CD11c molecule and, 60–61
p185^{HER2}, CD340 molecule, 544–545
p220/240, CD245 molecule, 405
Paget's disease of the bone, CD265 molecule, 426
Palmitoylation:
    CD36 molecule, 97
    of proteins, 13
Paroxysmal nocturnal hemoglobinuria (PNH):
    CD48 molecule, 121
    CD52 molecule, 132
    CD55 molecule, 136
    CD58 molecule, 141
    CD59 molecule, 142
    CD160 molecule, 293
    CD177 molecule, 320
PAS-2, CD235a molecule, 388–389
PAS 3, CD235b molecule, 388–389
PASIV compound, CD36 molecule, 97
Pathogen-associated molecular patterns (PAMPs):
    CD281 molecule, 448–449
    CD282 molecule, 450–451
    CD286 molecule, 458–459
PD1, CD279 molecule, 444–445
PD-1β, CD203c molecule, 346
PD1 ligand, CD273 molecule, 436–437
PDB2, CD265 molecule, 425
PDB structural database, 28
PDC1, CD279 molecule, 444
PDCD1L2, CD273 molecule, 436
PDCD1LG1, CD274 molecule, 438

PDCD1LG2, CD273 molecule, 436
PD-L1, CD274 molecule, 438
PD-L2, CD273 molecule, 436
PDNP3, CD203c molecule, 346
Peanut reactive urinary mucin (PUM), CD227
    molecule, 376
Peptide hormones:
  CD10 molecule substrates, 55
  CD13 molecule substrates, 62
Peptidyl dipeptidase A, CD143 molecule, 266
Peripheral neuropathy, CD57 molecule, 140
PETA-3, CD151 molecule, 278
Pfam Protein Families database, 28
P-glycoprotein, CD243 molecule, 401
pgp 170, CD243 molecule, 401
PGRL, CD316 molecule, 507
Phagocyte glycoprotein 1, CD44 molecule,
    113
Phenol-soluble modulin (PSM), CD286
    molecule binding, 458–459
Phosphocan, CD171 molecule binding,
    311–312
Phospholipids, CD36 molecule binding, 97
Phosphotyrosine phosphatase domain,
    structure and function, 9
Pilocytic astrocytomas, CD162/162R molecules,
    296
Pk blood group antigen, CD77 molecule, 169
Placental cells:
  CD327 molecule, 521–522
  CD338 molecule, 541–542
Placental growth factor (PlGF), CD308
    molecule, 492–493
Plasma cells:
  CD28 molecule, 85
  CD38 molecule, 99–100
  CD40 molecule, 102–103
  CD79a molecule, 171
  CD138 molecule, 257–258
  CD269 molecule, 430
  CD317 molecule, 102
Plasmacytoid dendritic cells (PDC):
  CD303 molecule, 485
  CD304 molecule, 487
Plasmacytoid monocyte purification, CD85k
    molecule, 182
Plasminogen activators:
  CD91 molecule, 378
  CD228 molecule, 378
Plasminogen receptors:
  CD222 molecule, 367–368
  CD228 molecule, 378

Plasmodium falciparum infection:
  CD36 molecule, 97
  CD54 molecule, 134
  CD164 molecule, 298–299
  CD233 molecule, 385–386
  CD235a molecule, 388–389
  CD236 molecule, 390–391
Plasmodium knowlesi, Plasmodium vivax
    infection, CD234 molecule, 387
Platelet activation:
  CD63 molecule, 150
  CD69 molecule, 161
  CD109 molecule, 216
  CD110 molecule, 217
Platelet activation-dependent granule-external
    membrane protein (PADGEM), CD62P
    molecule, 148
Platelet activation factor, CD109 molecule,
    216
Platelet-derived growth factor (PDGF)
    receptor:
  CD140a, 260–261
  CD140b, 262–263
Platelet endothelial cell adhesion molecule
    (PECAM-1), CD31 molecule, 89
Platelet endothelial tetra-span antigen, CD151
    molecule, 278
Platelet fibrinogen receptor, CD242 molecule,
    400
Platelet glycoprotein GPIa, CD49b molecule,
    123
Platelet glycoprotein GPIb-α, CD42b
    molecule, 107
Platelet glycoprotein GPIb-β, D42c molecule,
    109
Platelet glycoprotein GPIc, CD49f molecule,
    128
Platelet glycoprotein GPIIa, CD29 molecule,
    86
Platelet glycoprotein GPIIb, CD41 molecule,
    104
Platelet glycoprotein GPIX, CD42a molecule,
    106
Platelet glycoprotein GPV, D42d molecule,
    110
Platelet GPIV, CD36 molecule, 97
Pleiotrophin (PTN) ligand, CD246 molecule,
    406–407
Plexin-B1/Met complex, CD100 molecule,
    203–204
Plexin C1, CD232 molecule, 384
Pltgr40, CD63 molecule, 150

Pluripotential stem cell leukemia:
 CD7 marker, 51
 CD7 molecule expression, 52
 CD166 molecule, 302
Poliovirus receptor-like 3 (PVRL3), CD113
  molecule, 220
Poliovirus receptor (PVR), CD155 molecule,
  285
Poliovirus receptor related 1 proteins (PRR1):
 CD111 molecule, 218
 CD112 molecule, 219
Polycystic ovary syndrome, CD120b molecule,
  231
Polyinosinic acid, CD204 molecule ligand,
  347
Polymorphic epithelial mucin (PEM), CD227
  molecule, 376
Polypeptides, CD3 molecule, 46
Polysaccharides, structure, 10
Poxvirus, CD232 molecule binding, 323–324
preBCR complex, CD179a/b molecule,
  323–324
Pregnancy-specific glycoprotein (PSG), CD66f
  molecule, 159
Prenylation, of proteins, 13
Presenilin 1 (PS1), CD325 molecule, 517–518
Primary congenital lymphoedema (Milroy
  disease), CD310 molecule, 496–497
Primary mediastinal B-cell lymphoma
  (PMBL), CD273 molecule, 436–437
Prion protein, CD230 molecule, 381–382
Profilin, CD291 molecule, 468–469
Proliferin, CD222 molecule ligand, 367–368
Prominin gene family, CD133 molecule, 252
PROML1, CD133 molecule, 252
Prorenin, CD222 molecule, 367–368
Prostaglandin D2 (PGD2), CD292 molecule,
  473
Prostaglandin F2 receptor negative regulator,
  CD315 molecule, 505–506
Prostate cancer:
 CD57 molecule, 140
 CD146 molecule, 271–272
 CD175/175s molecules, 318
 CD204 molecule, 348
 CD304 molecule, 487
 CD310 molecule, 497
 CD331 molecule, 529
Protectin, CD59 molecule, 142
Protein C receptors:
 CD141 molecule, 264
 CD201 molecule, 342–343

Proteins. *See also* Carbohydrates
 domains, 6–9
  website sources for, 27–28, 30
 families, 7, 11–13
 membrane attachment and orientation, 11
 modules, 7
 motifs, 7
 nomenclature issues, 17–18
 phosphorylation, 13
 post-translational modification, 13
 structure and function, 6–13
  functional information sources, 32, 34
  models of, website sources for, 28, 30
 superfamilies, 7
Protein sequences, website sources for, 23–24,
  27–28
 similarity comparisons, 27, 29
Protein tyrosine kinase domain, structure and
  function, 9
Protein tyrosine phosphatase (PTP), structure
  and function, 9
Proteoglycans, defined, 13
Proteomics, human leukocyte differentiation
  antigen research and, 5–6
Pro-UPA, CD228 molecule ligand, 378
PrP(c)/PrP(sc), CD230 molecule, 381–382
PRV1 (polycythemia vera rubra 1), CD177
  molecule, 320
P-selectin, CD62P molecule, 148
P selectin glycoprotein ligand 1 (PSGL-1),
  CD162/162R molecule, 295
Pseudomonas sp., CD91 molecule and,
  190
Pseudorabies virus (PRV) receptors:
 CD112 molecule, 219
 CD111 molecule, 218
PSG, CD66f molecule, 159
PSGL-1, CD162/162R molecules, 295–296
Psoriasis:
 CD4 marker, 47
 CD60 molecule, 143
 CD134 molecule, 253
 CD252 molecule, 412
PTA-1, CD226 molecule, 374
PVRL3, CD113 molecule, 220

R1, CD1b molecule, 42
R2:
 CD1e molecule, 42
 CD82 molecule, 175
R3, CD1d molecule, 42
R4, CD1a molecule, 42

R7, CD1c molecule, 42

Rabson-Mendehall syndrome, CD220 molecule, 363–364

RAE-1-like transcript 1E (RAET1E), CD314 molecule ligand, 504

RANK, CD265 molecule, 425

RANK ligand (RANKL), CD254 molecule, 415

RANTES. *See* Regulated on Activation, Normal T-cell Expressed and Secreted (RANTES) protein

RasGAP binding, CD140b, 262–263

Receptor-associated protein (RAP), CD91 molecule, 189–190

Receptor tyrosine kinase (RTK) family:
   CD117 molecule, 225–226
   CD167a/b molecules, 303–304
   CD202b molecule, 344–345
   CD246 molecule, 406–407
   CD331 molecule, 528–529
   CD332 molecule, 530–531
   CD333 molecule, 532–533
   CD334 molecule, 534–535

Reed-Sternberg cells:
   CD15 molecule, 66
   CD30 molecule, 87–88
   CD138 molecule, 257–258
   CD302 molecule, 302

Regulated on Activation, Normal T-cell Expressed and Secreted (RANTES) protein:
   CD191 molecule, 332
   CD193 molecule, 334
   CD195 molecule, 336
   CD234 molecule, 387

Regulator of complement activation (RCA) gene family:
   CD21 molecule, 73–74
   CD35 molecule, 95–96
   CD46 molecule, 117–118
   CD55 molecule, 136–137

Renal disease:
   CD146 molecule, 271–272
   CD249 molecule, 411

Renin-angiotensin catabolic pathway, CD249 molecule, 411

Reoviruses, CD321 molecule binding, 512

Respiratory syncytial virus (RSV), CD284 molecule, 455

Revised European American Lymphoma (REAL) classification, CD markers and, 15

RGD sequences:
   CD41 molecule binding, 104–105
   CD49e molecule, 127
   CD51 molecule binding, 131
   CD61molecule, 144
   CD97 molecule, 198–199
   CD105 molecule, 209–210
   CD108 molecule, 215
   CD203c molecule, 346
   CD297 molecule, 477
   CD311 molecule, 498–499

RH1, CD240D molecule, 396–397

RHAG gene, CD241 molecule, 399

RHAMM (receptor for hyaluronan involved in migration and motility), CD167 molecule, 305

Rh-associated glycoprotein (RhAG), CD241 molecule, 399

Rh-associated protein, CD47 molecule, 119–120

Rhesus (Rh) blood group antigens:
   Rh30CE, CD240CE molecule, 396
   Rh30D, CD240D molecule, 396–397
   Rh30D/CE/ RhD, CD240DCE molecule, 398
   Rh50/ RhAG, CD241 molecule, 399

Rheumatoid arthritis:
   CD7 molecule expression, 52
   CD60 molecule expression, 143
   CD80 molecule, 173
   CD156b molecule, 287
   CD159 a/c molecules, 292
   CD217 molecule, 361

Rhinoviruses, CD54 molecule, 134

Rh-null phenotype, CD241 molecule, 399

Rhodopsin superfamily:
   basic properties, 12
   CD88 molecule, 186
   CD181 molecule, 326
   CD182 molecule, 327
   CD183 molecule, 328
   CD184 molecule, 329
   CD185 molecule, 330
   CD186 molecule, 331
   CD191 molecule, 332
   CD192 molecule, 333
   CD193 molecule, 334
   CD194 molecule, 335
   CD195 molecule, 336
   CD196 molecule, 337
   CD197 molecule, 338
   CDw198 molecule, 339
   CDw199 molecule, 340

Ribonucleoprotein (RNP), CD288 molecule,
    462–463
RM3/1, CD163 molecule, 297
RON, CD136 molecule, 255
RP105, CD180 molecule, 325

S152, CD27 molecule, 83
Scavenger receptor cysteine-rich (SRCR)
    family:
    CD5 marker, 49–50
    CD6 marker, 51
    CD163 molecule, 297
    CD204 molecule, 347–348
SCF, CD117 molecule, 225–226
Schistoma mansoni, CD209 molecule ligand,
    355–356
Schwartz-Jampel type 2 syndrome, CD118
    molecule, 227
SCR domain, structure and function, 9
SCYA1 ligand, CDw198 molecule, 339
SCYA25 ligand, CDw199 molecule, 340
SDF-1 chemokine, CD184 molecule, 329
Secretin receptor superfamily:
    basic properties, 12
    CD97 molecule, 198–199
Selectins protein family, CD62 molecules,
    145–149
Semaphorins:
    Sema 3A, CD304 molecule ligand, 486–487
    Sema 4D, CD100 molecule, 203–204
    Sema K1/Sema L, CD108 molecule, 215
    structure and function, 9
SEMA protein family, 12
Sendai virus:
    CD335 molecule, 536–537
    CD336 molecule, 538
S-endo, CD146 molecule, 271–272
Sezary syndrome:
    CD24 molecule, 79
    CD158 molecule, 290–291
SH2-containing inositol phosphatase (SHIP),
    CD200 molecule, 341
"Sheddase," CD156b molecule, 287
Sheep red blood cell (SRBC) receptor, CD2
    molecule, 44–45
Shiga-like toxins:
    CD19 molecule, 71
    CD77 molecule, 169
SHPS-1, CD172a molecule, 313
Sialic acid-binding Ig-like lectin (Siglec):
    protein family, 12
    Siglec 1, CD169 molecule, 307–308

Siglec 2, CD22 molecule, 75
Siglec 3, CD33 molecule, 93
Siglec 5, CD170 molecule, 309–310
Siglec 6, CD327 molecule, 521–522
Siglec 7, CD328 molecule, 523–524
Siglec 9, CD329 molecule, 525
Siglec 10, CD330 molecule, 526–527
Sialoadhesin family:
    CD22 molecule, 75–76
    CD33 molecule, 93
    CD169 molecule, 307–308
Sialoglycoproteins:
    CD93 molecule, 192
    CD106 molecule, 211–212
    CD235a/b molecules, 388–389
    CD236 molecule, 390–391
Sialomucin proteins:
    CD34 molecule, 94
    CD164 molecule, 298–299
Sialophorin, CD43 molecule, 111
Sialyllactosamines, CD169 molecule binding,
    307–308
Sialyl-Tn motifs, CD327 molecule ligands, 521
Sickle cell disease:
    CD239 molecules, 393–394
    CD242 molecule, 400
Siglec-like binding protein 2, CD330 molecule,
    526–527
Siglec. *See* Sialic acid-binding Ig-like lectin
Signaling lymphocyte activation molecule
    (SLAM) family:
    SLAMF5, CD84 molecule, 177
    SLAM, CD150 molecule as, 276–277
    CD229 molecule, 379–380
    CD244 molecule, 403–404
    SLAMF7, CD319 molecule, 510
Signal regulatory proteins (SIRPs):
    CD172a molecule, 313
    CD172b molecule, 314
    CD172g molecule, 315
Signal sequence, 13
SIMA135, CD318 molecule, 509
Simian immunodeficiency virus (SIV), CD186
    molecule binding, 331
Single-nucleotide polymorphisms (SNPs):
    CD279 molecule, 444–445
    website information sources for, 20, 23–24
Single-stranded RNA (ssRNA) receptors:
    CD287 molecule, 460–461
    CD288 molecule, 462–463
SIRPα, CD172a molecule, 313
SIRPβ, CD172b molecule, 314

SIRPβ-2/SIRPγ, CD172g molecule, 315
Skeletal disorders:
　CD331 molecule, 528–529
　CD332 molecule, 530–531
　CD333 molecule, 532–533
SLAM. *See* signaling lymphocyte activation
　　molecule family
SLEB2, CD279 molecule, 444
Small lymphocytic leukemias, CD23 molecule
　signaling, 78
SMAP6, CD315 molecule, 505
Smooth muscle cells, CD97 molecule, 199
SN2, CD165 molecule, 300
Snake venom-like protease CSVP, CD156b
　molecule, 287
Snake venom neurotoxins:
　CD59 molecule, 142
Solid tumors, CD57 molecule, 140
Soluble TB factor (STF), CD286 molecule
　ligand, 458–459
Sp-1, CD66f molecule, 159
SP-A/D surfactant proteins, CD172a molecule
　binding, 313
Splice variants in proteins, website information
　sources for, 20, 23–24
SRA, CD204 molecule, 347
S/s blood group antigens, CD235b molecule,
　389
ss-active sialoglycoprotein, CD235a molecule,
　388–389
Stem cell factor, CD117 molecule, 225–226
Stem cells. *See* hematopoietic stem cells
Stem cell transplantation, CD133 molecule,
　252
STK-1, CD135 molecule, 254
Streptococcus pyogenes:
　CD44 molecule, 113–114
　CD46 molecule, 117–118
STRL133, CD186 molecule, 331
Stuve-Wiedemann syndrome, CD118 molecule,
　227
Sulfated carbohydrate, CD2 molecule and, 44
Surface membrane molecules, human
　　leukocyte differentiation antigens and,
　　4–5
Sushi domain, 7, 9
Syndecan-1, CD138 molecule, 257
Systemic lupus erythematosis (SLE):
　CD16 molecule, 68
　CD72 molecule, 164
　CD120b molecule, 231
　CD279 molecule, 444

T1, CD5 molecule, 49
T3, CD3 molecule, 46
T4, CD4 molecule, 47
T6/leu-6, CD1a molecule, 42
T8, CD8 molecule, 53
T10, CD38 molecule, 99
T11, CD2 molecule, 44
T12, CD6 molecule, 51
T14, CD27 molecule, 83
T44, CD28 molecule, 85
T200, CD45 molecule, 115
Tac-antigen, CD25 molecule, 80
TACI, CD267 molecule, 428
TACSTD1, CD326 molecule, 519–520
TACTILE, CD96 molecule, 196
TALLA-1, CD231 molecule, 383
TALL (TNF- and APO-related leukocyte
　　expressed ligand) proteins:
　TALL1, CD257 molecule, 419
　TALL2, CD256 molecule, 418
T-antigen novelle (Tn), CD175/CD175a,
　318
TARC, CD194 molecule binding, 335
Target of an antiproliferative antibody
　　(TAPA-1), CD81 molecule, 174
Tat protein, CD26 molecule, 82
T-BAM, CD154 molecule, 283–284
T-cell activation increased late expression
　　(TACTILE), CD96 molecule, 196
T-cell antigen receptor complex, CD3
　　molecules and, 46
T-cell leukemia antigen, CD7 molecule, 52
T-cell lymphoma, CD274 molecule, 438
T-cell receptors (TCRs):
　α-chain, CD16 molecule, 67–68
　CD3 molecule, 46
　ζ-chain, CD247 molecule, 408–409
T cells:
　CD1a–e molecules, 42–43
　CD2 molecule, 44
　CD3 molecule, 46
　CD4 molecule, 47–48
　CD5 molecule, 49–50
　CD6 molecule, 51
　CD7 molecule, 52
　CD8 molecule, 53
　CD11a molecule, 56–57
　CD27 molecule, 83–84
　CD43 molecule, 111–112
　CD60 molecule, 143
　CD69 molecule, 161
　CD70 molecule, 162

CD96 molecule, 196–197
CD100 molecule, 203
CD134 molecule, 253
CD137 molecule, 256
CD152 molecule, 281–282
CD162 molecules, 295–296
CD172g molecule, 315
CD186 molecule, 331
CD194 molecule, 335
CD197 molecule, 338
CD212 molecule, 358
CD223 molecule, 369–370
CD247 molecule, 408–409
CD278 molecule, 443
TECK ligand, CDw199 molecule, 340
TEK, CD202b molecule, 344
Telencephalin, CD11a binding of, 57
TEM1, CD248 molecule, 410
TEM22, CD280 molecule, 446
Tetralogy of Fallot (TOF), CD339 molecule,
    543
Tetraspanins:
  CD9 molecule, 54
  CD37 molecule, 98
  CD46 molecule binding, 117–118
  CD53 molecule, 133
  CD81 molecule, 173
  CD82 molecule, 175
  CD151 molecule, 278
  CD231 molecule, 383
  CD315 molecule binding, 505–506
  superfamily of, 11–13
Thomsen-Friedenreich (TF) antigen, CD176
    molecule, 319
3A1, CD7 molecule, 52
Threonine peptidase family, CD224 molecule,
    371–372
Thrombin:
  CD42 molecules, 106–111
  CD141 molecule, 264
Thrombomodulin (TM), CD141 molecule,
    264
Thromboplastin, CD142 molecule, 265
Thrombopoietin (TPO) receptor, CD110
    molecule, 217
Thrombosis:
  CD41 molecule, 105
  CD141 molecule, 264
  CD142 molecule, 265
  CD201 molecule, 342–343
Thrombospondin-1 (TS1), CD47 molecule,
    119–120

Thrombospondin receptors:
  CD36 molecule, 97
  CD47 molecule, 119–120
  CD51/CD61 complex, 131
  CD138 molecule, 257–258
Thy-1, CD90 molecule, 188
Thymic stromal lymphopoietin receptor
    (TSLPR), CD127 molecule, 245–246
Thymic T-cell development:
  CD1a molecule, 42
  CD4 molecule, 47
Thymocytes:
  CD1 molecules, 42–43
  CD2 molecule, 44
  CD4 molecues, 47
  CD6 molecule, 51
  CD26 molecule, 81
  CD28 molecule, 85
  CD99 molecule, 201–202
  CD279 molecule, 444–445
TIE2, CD202b molecule, 344
TIL, CD281 molecule, 448–449
TIL3, CD285 molecule, 456–47
TIL4, CD282 molecule, 450–451
TIR domain-containing adaptor protein
    (TRAP), CD284 molecule, 454–455
Tissue factor, CD142 molecule, 265
Tissue factor pathway inhibitor (TFPI), CD142
    molecule and, 265
TK14, CD332 molecule, 530–531
TKF, CD334 molecule, 534–535
TLiSA1, CD226 molecule, 374
TM4SF2, CD231 molecule, 383
TMHMM server, transmembrane helix
    prediction, 31–32
Tn antigen, CD175 molecule, 318
TNF domain, structure and function, 9
TNF-like-2 (TL-2), CD253 molecule, 413
TNF-like weak inducer of apoptosis
    (TWEAK) ligands:
  CD255 molecule, 416–417
  CD266 molecule, 427
TNF/NGF receptor family (TNFRSF). See
    Tumor necrosis family/nerve growth
    receptor family
TNFRI, CD120a molecule, 229–230
TNFRII, CD120b molecule, 231–232
TNF receptor 5, CD40 molecule, 102
TNF receptor associated factors (TRAFs):
  CD27 molecule, 83–84
  CD30 molecule binding, 87
  CD134 molecule, 253

CD265 molecule, 425–426
CD266 molecule, 427
CD269 molecule, 430
TNF-receptor-associated periodic syndrome (TRAPS), CD120a molecule, 229
TNF-receptor (TNFR) domain, structure and function, 9
TNF-related activation protein (TRAP), CD154 molecule, 283
TNF-related apoptosis inducing ligand (TRAIL), CD253 molecule, 413–414
TNF-related weak inducer of apoptosis, CD255 molecule, 416–417
TNFRp55, CD120a molecule, 229–230
TNFRp75, CD120b molecule, 231–232
TNFRSF. *See* Tumor necrosis family/nerve growth receptor family
Tn syndrome, CD175 molecule, 318
Toll-like receptors (TLRs):
    CD180 molecule, 325
    TLR1, CD281 molecule, 448–449
    TLR2, CD282 molecule, 450–451
    TLR3, CD283 molecule, 452–453
    TLR4, CD284 molecule, 454–455
    TLR5, CD285 molecule, 456–457
    TLR6, CD286 molecule, 458–459
    TLR7, CD287 molecule, 460–461
    TLR8, CD288 molecule, 462–463
    TLR9, CD289 molecule, 464–465
    TLR10, CD290 molecule, 466–467
    TLR11, CD291 molecule, 468–469
Tp44, CD28 molecule, 85
Tp50, CD2 molecule, 43–44
Tp55, CD27 molecule, 83–84
Tp67, CD5 molecule, 49
Tp103, CD26 molecule, 81
TRAIL, CD253 molecule, 413–414
TRAIL receptors:
    TRAIL-R1, CD261 molecule, 421
    TRAIL-R2, CD262 molecule, 422
    TRAIL-R3, CD263 molecule, 423
    TRAIL-R4, CD264 molecule, 424
TRANCE, CD254 molecule, 415
TRANCER, CD265 molecule, 425–426
Transferrin, CD71 molecule, 163
Transforming acidic coiled coil (TACC) proteins, CD168 molecule, 305–306
Transforming growth factor-α (TGF-α), CD156b and, 287
Transforming growth factor-β receptor (TGF-β R) family, CD105 molecule, 209–210

Transforming growth factor-β (TGF-β) latency associated peptide (LAP), CD222 molecule ligand, 367–368
Transmembrane 4 superfamily (TM4SF). *See* tetraspanins
Transmembrane helix prediction, website sources for, 31–32
Transmissible spongiform encephalopathies (TSE), CD230 molecule, 381–382
TRID, CD263 molecule, 423
TRIF receptor, CD283 molecule, 452–453
TRIF-related adaptor molecule (TRAM), CD284 molecule, 454–455
TROP1, CD326 molecule, 519–520
TRUNDD, CD264 molecule, 424
TSP-1180, CD104 molecule, 207–208
Tspan-24, CD151 molecule, 278
Tspan-25, CD53 molecule, 133
Tspan-26, CD37 molecule, 98
Tspan-29, CD9 molecule, 54
Tumor-associated carbohydrate antigen (TACA), CD175/175s molecules, 318
Tumor necrosis factor-α (TNFα), CD156c molecule substrate, 288
Tumor necrosis factor-α converting enzyme (TACE), CD156b molecule, 287
Tumor necrosis factor/nerve growth factor (TNF/NGF) receptor family (TNFRSF):
    properties of, 11–13
    TNFRSF1A, CD120a molecule, 229–230
    TNFRSF1B, CD120b molecule, 231–232
    TNFRSF4, CD134 molecule, 253
    TNFRSF5, CD40 molecule, 102–103
    TNFRSF6, CD95 molecule, 195
    TNFRSF7, CD27 molecule, 83–84
    TNFRSF8, CD30 molecule, 87
    TNFRSF9, CD137 molecule, 256
    TNFRSF10A, CD261 molecule, 421
    TNFRSF10B, CD262 molecule, 422
    TNFRSF10C, CD263 molecule, 423
    TNFRSF10D, CD264 molecule, 424
    TNFRSF11A, CD265 molecule, 425–426
    TNFRSF12A, CD266 molecule, 427
    TNFRSF13B, CD 267 molecule, 428
    TNFRSF13C, CD268 molecule, 429
    TNFRSF14, CD270 molecule, 431–432
    TNFRSF16, CD271 molecule, 433–434
    TNFRSF17, CD269 molecule, 430
Tumor necrosis factor (TNF) superfamily (TNFSF):
    superfamily of, 11–13
    TNFSF4, CD252 molecule, 412

TNFSF5, CD154 molecule, 283–284
TNFSF6, CD178 molecule, 321–322
TNFSF7, CD70 molecule, 162
TNFSF8, CD153 molecule, 281–282
TNFSF10, CD253 molecule, 413–414
TNFSF11, CD254 molecule, 415
TNFSF12, CD255 molecule, 416–417
TNFSF13, CD256 molecule, 418
TNFSF13B, CD257 molecule, 419
TNFSF14, CD258 molecule, 420
TWEAK, CD255 molecule, 416–417
TWEAK-R, CD266 molecule, 427
2B4, CD244 molecule, 403
TYMSTR, CD186 molecule, 331
Type 1 diabetes:
    CD36 molecule, 97
    CD38 molecule, 100
    CD141 molecule, 264
    CD279 molecule, 444
Type 2 diabetes:
    CD26 molecule, 82
    CD36 molecule, 97
    CD38 molecule, 100
    CD120a molecule, 230
Type I integral membrane Ig superfamily
    glycoproteins, profile of, 42–43

ULBP-1,-2,-3, CD314 molecule ligands, 504
UniProtKB/Swiss-Prot website:
    human leukocyte cell surface proteins,
        aliases summarized on, 18–19
    protein sequence information on, 23–24,
        27–28
UPARAP, CD280 molecule, 446
Urokinase plasminogen activator-receptor
    (uPA-R), CD87 molecule, 184–185
Uropathogenic Escherichia coli (UPEC),
    CD291 molecule, 468–469
Uvomorulin, CD324 molecule, 515–516

V7, CD101 molecule, 205
Vaccinia virus, CD283 molecule, 452–453
Vascular cell adhesion molecule-1 (VCAM-1),
    CD106 molecule, 211–212
Vascular endothelial growth factor (VEGF)
    receptors:
    VEGFR1, CD308 molecule, 492–493
    VEGFR2, CD309 molecule, 494–495
    VEGFR3, CD310 molecule, 496–497
    VEGFR165R, CD304 molecule, 486–487
VCAM-1, CD106 molecule, 211–212
VEA, CD69 molecule,161

VE-cadherin, CD144 molecule, 268
Verotoxin, CD77 molecule, 169
Very early antigens (VEA), CD69 molecule,
    161
Very late antigen (VLA) protein family:
    CD29 molecule, 86
    CD49a molecule, 122
    CD49b molecule, 123
    CD49c molecule, 124
    CD49e molecule, 127
    CD49f molecule, 128–129
    CD63 molecule, 150
    CD106 molecule, 211–212
VESPR, CD232 molecule, 384
VIM2, CD65s molecule, 154
Vitronectin binding:
    CD51/β5 complex, 131
    CD51/CD29 complex, 131
    CD51/CD61 complex, 131, 144
    CD87 molecule, 184
Vitronectin receptor α chain, CD51 molecule,
    131
von Willebrand factor (vWF):
    CD41 molecule, 104–105
    CD42a molecule, 106
    CD42b molecule, 107–108
    CD42c molecule, 109
    CD42d molecule, 110–111
    CD51/CD29 complex, 131
    CD51/CD61 complex, 131, 144
V pre β, pre lymphocyte gene 1 (VPREB1),
    CD179a molecule, 323

Webb (Wb) antigen, CD236 molecule, 390–391
Websites, table of, 35
Weibel-Palade bodies, CD63 molecule, 150
Wnt protein receptors:
    CD344 molecule, 546
    CD349 molecule, 547
    CD350 molecule, 548
Wound healing, CD140b molecule, 262–263

Xenotransplantation:
    CD55 molecule, 137
    CD59 molecule, 142
X-linked mental retardation, CD231 molecule
    and, 383
X-linked severe combined immune deficiency
    (XSCID), CD132 molecule, 251

YENF endocytosis signaling motif, CD301
    molecule, 483

Yussef (Yus) phenotype, CD236 molecule,
390–391

Zinc metalloproteinases:
CD10 molecule, 55

CD13 molecule, 62
CD143 molecule, 266–267
CD156b molecule, 287
CD156c molecule, 288
CD238 molecule, 392